Pharmacy Practice

Pharmacy Practice

Edited by

Kevin M.G. Taylor

School of Pharmacy,
University of London,
London, UK

and

Geoffrey Harding

Department of General Practice and Primary Care,
St Bartholomew's and the Royal London School of Medicine and Dentistry,
Queen Mary, University of London, London, UK

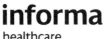

270 Madison Avenue
New York, NY 10016

2 Park Square, Milton Park
Abingdon, Oxon OX14 4RN, UK

www.informahealthcare.com

Published in 2001 by
Taylor & Francis Group
270 Madison Avenue
New York, NY 10016

Published in Great Britain by
Taylor & Francis Group
2 Park Square
Milton Park, Abingdon
Oxon OX14 4RN

International Standard Book Number-10: 0-415-27159-2 (Softcover)
International Standard Book Number-13: 978-0-415-27159-2 (Softcover)

Library of Congress Cataloging-in-Publication Data

Catalog record is available from the Library of Congress

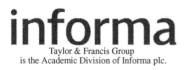

Taylor & Francis Group
is the Academic Division of Informa plc.

**Visit the Taylor & Francis Web site at
http://www.taylorandfrancis.com**

Contents

Foreword   ix

Contributors   xi

Preface   xv

Acknowledgements   xvii

Part One: The development of pharmacy practice

1. **The historical context of pharmacy**   3
   Stuart Anderson

2. **The pharmacy workforce**   31
   Karen Hassell and Sue Symonds

3. **Primary and secondary care pharmacy**   49
   Catherine Duggan

Part Two: International dimensions of pharmacy practice

4. **Community pharmacy in Europe**   61
   Foppe van Mil

5. **Pharmacy in North America**   71
   Joaquima Serradell and Albert Wertheimer

6. **Pharmacy in developing countries**   81
   Felicity Smith

Part Three: Health, illness and medicines use

7. **The social context of health and illness**   105
   Sarah Nettleton

8. **Inequalities in health and health care**   123
   Mark Exworthy

9. **The supply and consumption of over the counter drugs**   139
   Ian Bates

10. **Promoting health**   151
    Alison Blenkinsopp, Claire Anderson and Rhona Panton

11. **Compliance, adherence and concordance**   165
    Robert Horne

Part Four: Professional practice

12. Pharmacy as a profession   187
Geoffrey Harding and Kevin Taylor

13. Professional judgement and ethical dilemmas   203
Richard O'Neill

14. Effective communication   227
Norman Morrow and Owen Hargie

15. Pharmacists and the multidisciplinary health care team   249
Christine Bond

Part Five: Meeting the pharmaceutical care needs of specific populations

16. Ethnic minorities   273
Mohamed Aslam, Farheen Jessa and John Wilson

17. Parents and children   289
Sally Wyke, Sarah Cunningham-Burley and Jo Vallis

18. Pregnancy and breastfeeding mothers   301
Lolkje de Jong-van den Berg and Corinne de Vries

19. The elderly and their carers   313
Ruth Goldstein

20. People with mental health problems   329
Sally-Anne Francis

21. Injecting drug users   345
Janie Sheridan and Trish Shorrock

Part Six: Measuring and regulating medicines use

22. Pharmacovigilance and pharmacoepidemiology   367
Corinne de Vries and Lolkje de Jong-van den Berg

23. Health economics   393
Hakan Brodin

Part Seven: Research methods

24. Measurements of health and illness   411
Sally-Anne Francis

25. Survey methods   433
Jill Jesson and Rob Pocock

26. **Interviews** 457
Madeleine Gantley

27. **Focus groups** 473
Felicity Smith

28. **Analysing qualitative data** 485
Geoffrey Harding, Madeleine Gantley and Kevin Taylor

29. **Statistical tests** 493
Nick Barber

30 **Evaluating community pharmacy services** 509
Felicity Smith

31. **Evaluating hospital pharmacy services** 523
Nick Barber and Keith Ridge

32. **Professional audit and clinical governance** 537
Carl Martin

Foreword

The development of pharmacy practice as an academic discipline has been relatively slow and not without controversy. In the UK it was stimulated in no small part by the 1986 Report of the Nuffield Inquiry into Pharmacy which found a dearth of evidence on what pharmacists really did and, more importantly, how effective they were in achieving their goals — if indeed these goals had been defined. Given progress in the field to date, the appearance of a mature, definitive text is timely and this must be it. Kevin Taylor and Geoffrey Harding have already made their mark with an introductory text on the social aspects of pharmacy and an edited collection of essays on pharmacy practice and now have masterminded the production of this impressive work. There cannot be many topics in pharmacy practice that are not addressed within the eclectic array of chapters by some 40 authors from 33 departments and institutions. Although the authors are drawn predominantly from the UK, we learn much about practice and policy in other countries and it is appropriate that community pharmacy in Europe, pharmacy in North America and in developing countries is addressed by relevant experts.

I have long believed that we have neglected teaching aspects of our heritage. The chapters on the historical context of pharmacy and pharmacy as a profession are valuable backdrops to the sections that deal with issues that are refreshing in their breadth — compliance, adherence and concordance, health promotion, effective communication and also that most crucial of areas, professional judgement. Pharmacists have sometimes hidden behind laws which may paralyse the profession; the application of fine judgement is increasingly important in interactions with ethnic minorities, the elderly, those with mental health problems and with drug misusers. All of these topics are given coverage here.

More and more pharmacists are part of multidisciplinary teams involved in health economics and measures of health and illness, in evaluating care, in advisory rôles, and in audit of practice. The discipline of pharmacy practice has grown to an extent not envisaged all those years ago by the Nuffield Inquiry. Here it all is in one book which, as Dr Taylor and Dr Harding hope, will be placed on library shelves beside the textbooks of pharmacology, pharmaceutics and modern pharmaceutical chemistry which provide the bedrock and uniqueness of the pharmacist. It deserves to be taken down frequently and consulted so that the unique skills of the pharmacist can be put to their optimal use in this new century.

Professor A.T. Florence
The School of Pharmacy
University of London

Contributors

Claire Anderson
The Pharmacy School
University of Nottingham
Nottingham
UK

Stuart Anderson
Department of Public Health and Policy
London School of Hygiene and Tropical
Medicine
London
UK

Mohamed Aslam
Department of Pharmaceutical Sciences
School of Pharmacy
University of Nottingham
Nottingham
UK

Nick Barber
Centre for Practice and Policy
School of Pharmacy
University of London
London
UK

Ian Bates
Centre for Practice and Policy
School of Pharmacy
University of London
London
UK

Alison Blenkinsopp
Department of Medicines Management
Keele University
Keele
Staffordshire
UK

Christine Bond
Department of General Practice and Primary
Care
University of Aberdeen
Aberdeen
UK

Hakan Brodin
TNO Prevention and Health
Sector HTA
Leiden
The Netherlands

Sarah Cunningham-Burley
Department of Community Health Sciences
University of Edinburgh
Edinburgh
UK

Lolkje de Jong-van den Berg
Department of Social Pharmacy and
Pharmacoepidemiology
Groningen University Institute for Drug
Studies
Groningen
The Netherlands

Corinne de Vries
Pharmacoepidemiology and Public Health
Postgraduate Medical School
University of Surrey
Guildford
Surrey
UK

Catherine Duggan
Academic Department of Pharmacy
Barts and the Royal Hospitals NHS Trust
St Bartholomew's Hospital
London
UK

Mark Exworthy
LSE Health
London School of Economics
University of London
London
UK

Sally-Anne Francis
Centre for Practice and Policy
School of Pharmacy
University of London
London
UK

Madeleine Gantley
Department of General Practice and Primary
Care
St Bartholomew's and the Royal London
School of Medicine and Dentistry
Queen Mary
University of London
London
UK

Ruth Goldstein
Medicines Research Unit
School of Health and Community Studies
University of Derby
Derby
UK

Geoffrey Harding
Department of General Practice and Primary
Care
St Bartholomew's and the Royal London
School of Medicine and Dentistry
Queen Mary
University of London
London
UK

Owen Hargie
School of Behavioural and Communication
Sciences
University of Ulster
Jordanstown
Co Antrim
UK

Karen Hassell
School of Pharmacy and Pharmaceutical
Sciences
University of Manchester
Manchester
UK

Robert Horne
Centre for Health Care Research
University of Brighton
Brighton
East Sussex
UK

Farheen Jessa
Department of General Practice
University Hospital
Queens' Medical Centre
Nottingham
UK

Jill Jesson
Pharmacy Practice Research Group
Aston University
Aston Triangle
Birmingham
UK

Carl Martin
Centre for Practice and Policy
School of Pharmacy
University of London
London
UK

Norman Morrow
Pharmaceutical Branch
Department of Health, Social Services and
Public Safety
Stormont
Belfast
UK

Sarah Nettleton
Department of Social Policy and Social Work.
University of York
York
UK

Richard O'Neill
Centre for Practice and Policy
School of Pharmacy
University of London
London
UK

Rhona Panton
Worcester NHS Community Trust
Worcester
UK

Rob Pocock
M.E.L. Research Limited
Aston Science Park
Birmingham
UK

Keith Ridge
NHS Executive
Department of Health
London
UK

Joaquima Serradell
Serradell and Associates
Blue Bell
Pennsylvania
USA

Janie Sheridan
National Addiction Centre
Institute of Psychiatry
London
UK

Trish Shorrock
Leicester Community Drug Team
Leicester
UK

Felicity Smith
Centre for Practice and Policy
School of Pharmacy
University of London
London
UK

Sue Symonds
Formerly of School of Sociology and Social
Policy
University of Nottingham
Nottingham
UK

Kevin Taylor
Centre for Practice and Policy
School of Pharmacy
University of London
London
UK

Jo Vallis
Department of Geriatrics
University of Edinburgh
Edinburgh
UK

Foppe van Mil
Quality Institute for Pharmaceutical Care
Margrietlaan
Zuidlaren
The Netherlands

Albert Wertheimer
MERCK and Co
West Point
Philadelphia
USA

John Wilson
Nottingham Health Authority
Nottingham
UK

Sally Wyke
Department of Community Health Sciences
University of Edinburgh
Edinburgh
UK

Preface

Pharmaceutical services are increasingly patient-centred rather than drug-centred, as exemplified by the concept of pharmaceutical care. Pharmacists need to both understand and meet patients' specific pharmaceutical requirements. To do this requires a blend of clinical, scientific and social skills. This shift to patient-centred care comes as health care is increasingly delivered by an integrated team of health workers. Effective pharmacy practice requires an understanding of the social context within which pharmacy is practised, recognising the particular needs and circumstances of the users of pharmaceutical services, and of pharmacy's place within health service provision.

With these issues in mind we have aimed to provide pharmacy students with a background in some of the pertinent issues for effective contemporary pharmacy practice. We have purposefully avoided clinical pharmacy and therapeutics *per se*, along with specific aspects of pharmacy law, because these are already comprehensively covered in existing texts. Our focus here is the practice of pharmacy *in its social and behavioural context*. For instance, how do an individual's beliefs or social circumstances influence their decision to use a pharmacy, and how might pharmaceutical services best be delivered to meet that individual's specific health needs?

Effective pharmacy practice is based on research evidence and best practice, and original research is referred to, where appropriate, throughout the text. As practice becomes more evidence-based, pharmacists increasingly need to evaluate and implement research findings, and undertake their own research and professional audits. To this end, we have included sections detailing how medicines use is surveyed and costed, together with practical guidance on doing pharmacy practice research and evaluating pharmaceutical services.

Undergraduate pharmacy courses remain rooted in the pharmaceutical sciences. Within libraries, social and behavioural science texts are segregated from pharmacy texts, and often found at separate sites. Furthermore, interdisciplinary teaching within pharmacy schools remains the exception rather than the rule. Consequently, many of the disciplines and concepts included here will be unfamiliar, perhaps even alien to readers. The backgrounds of the contributors to this textbook are diverse, including pharmacy, sociology, psychology, anthropology, history, health economics and communication. However, they share a common appreciation of how selected aspects of their specialty inform pharmacy practice. It is hoped that by bringing together disciplines whose knowledge base can, and should, underpin pharmacists' activities, this comprehensive book will equip readers to be effective health care practitioners.

Acknowledgements

We are indebted to all the authors who have contributed to this textbook, for their diligence, attention to detail and adherence to deadlines. We additionally thank Henry Chrystyn (University of Bradford), Dai John (University of Wales, Cardiff), Judith Rees (University of Manchester) and John Varnish (Aston University, Birmingham) for the assistance and information they provided when this book was in the planning stage. The secretarial support provided by Marlene Fielder (School of Pharmacy, London) is also gratefully acknowledged. Our thanks are also due to the editorial staff of Harwood Academic Press, for their guidance, in particular Matthew Honan who commissioned the project, and latterly Julia Carrick and Tracy Breakell.

On a personal note, we would like to acknowledge the contribution of Harts the Grocer, Russell Square, whose cinnamon honey rolls and blueberry muffins provided relief and sustenance during the long days of planning, writing and editing.

Finally, we acknowledge the forbearance and support of our wives, Pauline and Sally, throughout the long duration of this project, particularly as we had stated 'never again' after our previous book.

PART ONE

The Development of
Pharmacy Practice

1 The Historical Context of Pharmacy

Stuart Anderson

INTRODUCTION   4
THE ORIGINS OF PHARMACY UP TO 1841   4
  The dawn of pharmacy, Antiquity to 50 BC   4
  The emergence of pharmacy, 50BC to 1231AD   4
  The separation of pharmacy from medicine: the edict of Palermo 1231   5
  The medicalisation of the apothecary   7
  The organisation of pharmacy   8
THE PROFESSIONALISATION OF PHARMACY, 1841 to 1911   9
  The foundation of the Pharmaceutical Society of Great Britain, 1841   9
  Pharmacists' education and qualifications   10
  The origins of the multiples in community pharmacy   11
  The practice of pharmacy   12
NATIONAL INSURANCE TO NATIONAL HEALTH, 1911 to 1948   13
  The separation of dispensing from prescribing   13
  The limitation of the Pharmaceutical Society's functions   15
  The triumph of professional regulation   16
  Preparing pharmaceutical products: from bespoke to off-the-peg   17
PHARMACY IN THE NATIONAL HEALTH SERVICE   18
  The impact of the National Health Service   18
  The 'disappearing' pharmacist   19
  Professionalism versus commercialism   20
THE EMERGENCE OF 'THE NEW PHARMACY', 1986 TO PRESENT   21
  The Nuffield Report, 1986   21
  The extended role   22
  Is pharmacy returning to its roots?   23
A BRIEF HISTORY OF HOSPITAL PHARMACY   23
  The origins of hospital pharmacy to 1897   23
  The emergence of professional identity, 1897 to 1923   24
  Unification and standardisation, 1923 to 1948   25
  Consolidation and survival, 1948 to 1970   25
  Expansion and development, 1970 to the present   26
CONCLUSION   26
FURTHER READING   27
REFERENCES   28
SELF-ASSESSMENT QUESTIONS   28
KEY POINTS FOR ANSWERS   29

INTRODUCTION

Why is pharmacy practised in the way it is today? Has the dispensing of prescriptions always been the main activity in community pharmacy? How did multiples come to dominate community pharmacy in Britain, but not in other countries? Could pharmacy practice just as easily have developed very differently? The answers to these questions are to be found in pharmacy's history, from its origins in the mists of time to the diversity of practice that is pharmacy today.

This chapter has three objectives: to define the main *'time frames'* (periods bounded by key events) within the history of pharmacy; to describe the key *'watersheds'* (the defining events) in that history; and to examine the impact which these events have had on the practice of pharmacy. Following a general account of the evolution of pharmacy, the chapter focuses on developments in Britain, illustrating the balance of social, political, economic and technological factors that determine the nature of pharmacy practice in all countries.

THE ORIGINS OF PHARMACY UP TO 1841

The dawn of pharmacy, Antiquity to 50 BC

The nature of the earliest medicines is lost in the remoteness of history. Cavemen almost certainly rolled the first crude pills in their hands. Pharmacy, as an occupation in which individuals made a living from the sale and supply of medicines, is amongst the oldest of professions. The earliest known prescriptions date back to at least 2700 BC and were written by the Sumerians, who lived in the land between the Euphrates and Tigris rivers. The practitioners of healing at this time combined the roles of priest, pharmacist and physician.

Chinese pharmacy traces its origins to the emperor Shen Nung in about 2000 BC. He investigated the medicinal value of several hundred herbs, and wrote the first *Pen T'sao*, or native herbal, containing 365 drugs. Egyptian medicine dates from around 2900 BC, but the most important Egyptian pharmaceutical record, the *Papyrus Ebers*, was written much later, in about 1500 BC. This is a collection of around 800 prescriptions, in which some 700 different drugs are mentioned. Like the Sumerians, Egyptian pharmacists were also priests, and they learnt and practised their art in the temples.

The emergence of pharmacy, 50 BC to 1231 AD

It was more than another thousand years before the early Greek philosophers began to influence medicine and pharmacy. They not only observed nature, but sought to explain what they saw, gradually transforming medicine into a science. The traditions of Greek medicine continued with the rise of the Roman Empire. Indeed, the greatest physicians in Rome were nearly all Greek. The transition of pharmacy into a science received a major boost with the work of Dioscorides in the first century AD. In his *Materia Medica* he describes nearly 500 plants and remedies prepared from animals and metals, and gives precise instructions for preparing them. His texts were considered basic science up to the sixteenth century.

Perhaps the greatest influence on pharmacy was Galen (130 to 201 AD), who was born in Pergamos and started his career as physician to the gladiators in his home town. He moved to Rome in 164 AD, eventually being appointed as physician to the imperial family. Galen practised and taught both pharmacy and medicine. He introduced many previously unknown drugs, and was the first to define a drug as anything that acts on the body to bring about a change. His principles for preparing and compounding medicines remained dominant in the Western world for 1,500 years, and he gave his name to pharmaceuticals prepared by mechanical means (galenicals).

The first privately owned drug stores were established by the Arabs in Baghdad in the eighth century. They built on knowledge acquired from both Greece and Rome, developing a wide range of novel preparations, including syrups and alcoholic extracts. One of the greatest of Arab physicians was Rhazes (865-925 AD) who was a Persian born near Tehran. His principal work, *Liber Continens,* was to play an important part in Western medicine. He wrote *'if you can help with foods, then do not prescribe medicaments; if simples are effective, then do not prescribe compounded remedies'.*

These new ideas became assimilated into the practice of pharmacy across western Europe following the Moslem advance across Africa, Spain and southern France. Perhaps the greatest figure in the science of medicine and pharmacy during this period was the Persian, Ali ibn Sina (980 to 1037 AD), who was known by the western world as Avicenna. He was the author of books on philosophy, natural history and medicine. His *Canon Medicinae* is a synopsis of Greek and Roman medicine. His teachings were treated as authoritative in the West well into the seventeenth century and they remain dominant influences in some eastern countries to this day. The figures of Avicenna and Galen appear in the Coat of Arms of the Royal Pharmaceutical Society of Great Britain (Figure 1.1).

The separation of pharmacy from medicine: the edict of Palermo 1231

In European countries exposed to Arab influence, pharmacy shops began to appear around the eleventh century. Frederick II of Hohenstaufen, who was Emperor of Germany and King of Sicily, provided a key link between east and west, and it was in Sicily and southern Italy that pharmacy first became legally separated from medicine in 1231 AD. At his palace in Palermo, Frederick presented the first

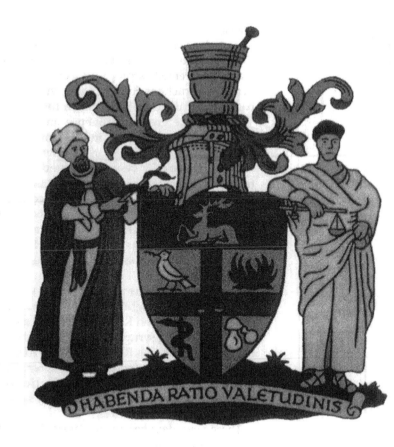

Figure 1.1 The coat of arms and motto of the Royal Pharmaceutical Society of Great Britain. Note the figures of Avicenna (left) and Galen (right). The motto is commonly but incorrectly translated as *'We must pay attention to our health'*. Reproduced with permission of the Royal Pharmaceutical Society of Great Britain.

European edict creating a clear distinction between the responsibilities of physicians and those of apothecaries, and he laid down regulations for their professional practice.

Frederick's decree provided the basis of similar legislation elsewhere. The Basle Apothecaries Oath, for example, drawn up in 1271, spelled out the relationship between physicians and apothecaries. It stated that *'no physician who cares for or has cared for the sick shall ever own an apothecary's business in Basle, nor shall he ever become an apothecary'*. In other European countries, pharmacy emerged as a separate occupation over the centuries which followed. German pharmacists, for example, formed themselves into a society in 1632.

The first official pharmacopoeia, to be followed by all apothecaries, originated in Florence. The *Nuovo Receptario*, published in 1498, was the result of collaboration between the Guild of Apothecaries and the Medical Society, one of the earliest examples of the two professions working constructively together.

The medicalisation of the apothecary

In most European countries, the apothecary or pharmacist developed from pepperers or spicers. The evolution of the English apothecary and pharmacist from the twelfth to the nineteenth centuries is illustrated in Figure 1.2. Traders in spicery, which included crude drugs and prepared medicines, evolved into either grocers or apothecaries. By the thirteenth century, apothecaries formed a distinct occupational group in many countries, including England and France.

During the Middle Ages the evolution of French and British pharmacy was almost identical. In due course, the French *apothicaire* developed into the *pharmacien*, whilst the English apothecary became a general medical practitioner. In Britain, trade in drugs and spices was monopolised by the Guild of Grocers, who had jurisdiction over the apothecaries. However, the apothecaries formed an alliance with court

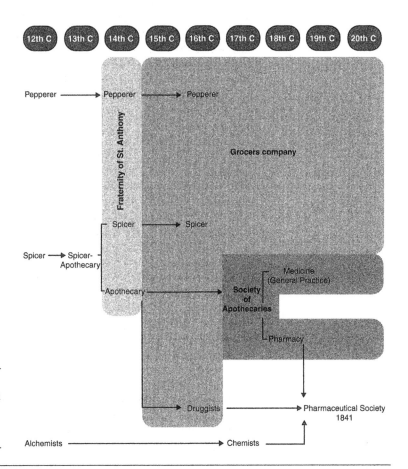

Figure 1.2 The evolution of pharmacy in Great Britain, twelfth century to 1841. Source: Trease (1964).

physicians, and they succeeded in persuading James I to grant a Charter in 1617 to form a separate company, the Society of Apothecaries. This was the first organisation of pharmacists in the Anglo-Saxon world.

The apothecaries were both physicians (but not surgeons) and pharmacists, diagnosing and dispensing the medicines which they themselves prescribed. There were, however, other groups involved in the sale and supply of medicines, the chemists and druggists. The Apothecaries Act of 1815 confirmed apothecaries as physicians, and laid down the training required to practise as such. Most apothecaries subsequently opted to practise exclusively as general medical practitioners, and an opportunity was presented to the other groups whose business was the sale and supply of medicines.

The organisation of pharmacy

In France, the *pharmacien* received official recognition with the establishment of the College de Pharmacie in 1777, which ushered in modern French pharmacy. During the 17th and 18th centuries many people in continental Europe passed the examinations for both pharmacy and medicine, and practised both. In some countries, developments took place on a regional basis. In Italy, for example, Austrian regulations for the Lombardy district in 1778 provided the stimulus for changes in pharmacy practice in the north of the country. But it was only after the establishment of the new Italian Kingdom in 1870 that uniform arrangements were established across Italy.

In Germany, pharmacists in Nuremberg formed themselves into a society as early as 1632. A regional organisation for north Germany was formed in 1820, and for southern Germany in 1848. After the federation of German states, these two societies amalgamated to form a national German pharmacists' society, the *Deutscher Apothekerverein*, in 1872. A few years later, in 1890, the *Deutsche Pharamzeutische Gesellschaft* was established to promote pharmaceutical science and research. Early American pharmacy was heavily influenced by immigrants from Europe. An Irish apothecary, Christopher Marshall, established the first such shop in Philadelphia in 1729. The American Pharmaceutical Association, open to '*all pharmaceutists and druggists of good character*', was established some time later, in 1852.

International cooperation between pharmacists has a long history. It had long been a dream of many pharmacists to establish an international pharmacopoeia. German pharmacists took the initiative to convene the first International Congress of Pharmacy, which took place in Braunschweig, Germany in 1865. International congresses continued to be held every few years in different countries, but there was no formal mechanism for international contact. It was the Dutch Pharmaceutical Association that proposed at the tenth congress in 1910 that a permanent association be formed. The International

Pharmaceutical Federation (FIP), with headquarters and secretariat at The Hague, was founded in 1911, when the first meeting of delegates from around the world took place.

THE PROFESSIONALISATION OF PHARMACY, 1841 TO 1911

It is with the foundation of the Pharmaceutical Society of Great Britain in 1841 that the modern history of British pharmacy begins. The seventy years leading up to the beginnings of the welfare state in 1911 were a time of rapid social change which saw the increasing professionalisation of many occupations, including pharmacy. This section focusses on four developments: the foundation of the Pharmaceutical Society of Great Britain; pharmacists' education and qualifications; the origins of the multiples in pharmacy; and the nature of practice during this period.

The foundation of the Pharmaceutical Society of Great Britain, 1841

Early in 1841, a Mr Hawes introduced a Bill to Parliament that would have made it compulsory for chemists and druggists to pass an examination before being able to carry on their business. If they bandaged a finger or recommended a remedy they would be deemed to be practising medicine, and hence would need to be medically qualified. The leaders of the chemists and druggists took action, and on April 15, 1841 a small group met at the Crown and Anchor Tavern in the Strand in London. They included William Allen FRS, John Savory, Thomas Morson, and Jacob Bell, the son of a well-known Quaker chemist and druggist, John Bell.

William Allen moved a resolution that *'an Association be now formed under the title of The Pharmaceutical Society of Great Britain'*. It was seconded by John Bell and carried by the meeting. The Society was to have three objectives:

'To benefit the public, and elevate the profession of pharmacy, by furnishing the means of proper instruction; to protect the collective and individual interests and privileges of all its members, in the event of any hostile attack in Parliament or otherwise; and to establish a club for the relief of decayed or distressed members'.

At its foundation, the Society was to consist of both members and associates. Full membership was restricted to chemists and druggists who owned their own businesses. Pharmacy managers, or assistants, even those who had passed the major examination, could only become associates. Nevertheless, by the end of 1841 the new society had around 800 members, and by May of 1842 membership had risen to nearly 2,000. In December 1841 it acquired 17 Bloomsbury Square,

London, as its headquarters. It was to remain there until September 1976. Jacob Bell began a series of monthly scientific meetings at his own home, and in July 1841 he published *The Transactions of the Pharmaceutical Meetings*, later to be re-titled the *Pharmaceutical Journal*. The Society gained legal recognition with its incorporation by Royal Charter in 1843.

Pharmacists' education and qualifications

From its foundation, one of the main priorities of the Pharmaceutical Society was the setting up of an examination system and a school of pharmacy. The examination system consisted of an entrance requirement, followed by the Minor examination, which was taken at the end of a four or five year apprenticeship. To become a full member the associate was required to take the more advanced Major examination. Apprentices and assistants were advised to attend appropriate lectures, but the opportunities to do so were few. The Society set up its own School of Pharmacy within its Bloomsbury Square headquarters in 1842, but this was only available to those with ready access to London.

Branch schools were opened in Manchester, Norwich, Bath and Bristol in 1844, and in Edinburgh soon afterwards. After 1868, privately owned schools of pharmacy began to appear. In 1870 there were seven, only two of which were outside London. But by 1900 the number of schools offering courses in pharmacy had reached forty-five. The number of schools of pharmacy in Britain between 1880 and 1963 is illustrated in Figure 1.3. The last privately-owned school, in Liverpool, closed in 1949.

The first Register of Pharmaceutical Chemists was established under the Pharmacy Act of 1852. However, there was no requirement at that stage for pharmaceutical chemists (i.e. those whose names appeared on the Register) to become members of the Pharmaceutical Society. The Society was a voluntary association, and those who passed the Major examinations were free to choose whether or not to become members. Only with passage of the Pharmacy and Poisons Act of 1933 was it made compulsory to be a member of the Pharmaceutical Society in order to practice.

The 1868 Pharmacy Act created a second legal category of pharmacist – the chemists and druggists, whose names appeared on a separate register. The original members of this group came from a wide range of backgrounds. Some had been in business before the Act, some were associate members of the Society, some were assistants who had passed a new modified examination, and some had passed the Pharmaceutical Society's Minor examination, which became the sole means of entry. The difference between the pharmaceutical chemist and the chemist and druggist was simply one of educational attainment. This two-tier structure to the pharmaceutical profession in Britain continued until 1954, when pharmaceutical chemists became fellows of the Society and the two registers merged.

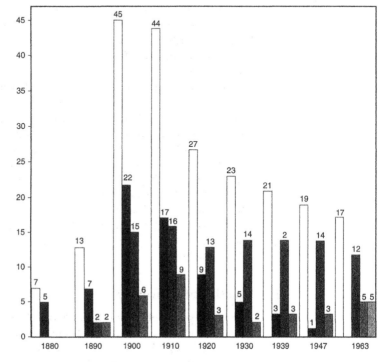

	1880	1890	1900	1910	1920	1930	1939	1947	1963
School of Pharmacy, London	1	1	1	1	1	1	1	1	–
Royal Dispensary, Edinburgh	1	1	1	1	1	1	–	–	–
Technical Colleges	–	2	15	16	13	14	14	14	12
University Schools	–	2	6	9	3	2	3	3	5
Proprietary Schools	5	7	22	17	9	5	3	1	–
CATs	–	–	–	–	–	–	–	–	5
Total	7	13	45	44	27	23	21	19	17

Figure 1.3 Schools of Pharmacy in Great Britain, 1880 to 1963. Source: Earles (1965).

The origins of the multiples in community pharmacy

In securing the 1868 Pharmacy Act, The Pharmaceutical Society was satisfied that it had achieved privileges, including the use of titles, on behalf of proprietor pharmacists. The Society's view was that the professional practice of pharmacy required that qualified pharmacists must retain ownership and control. It maintained that since a corporate body could not sit examinations or be registered as a pharmaceutical chemist, it had no right to operate a chemist's business.

But in the 1870s a number of limited companies, including Cooperative societies and Harrods, began to sell medicines, using the term '*chemist*' to describe that part of the shop where this took place. In 1880 the issue of whether companies could own pharmacies was tested in an important legal case, *The Pharmaceutical Society v. The London and Provincial Supply Association*, under the 1868 Pharmacy Act. The Association had been deliberately registered as a company with the intention of enabling an unqualified person to keep open shop for the sale of poisons. The legal argument was about whether the word *'person'* could include a company. If it could not, then companies would not be able to own pharmacies. The Pharmacy Act applied only to persons; a company could not be held guilty of an offence under the Act. The Society lost the case in the County Court, but appealed against the decision to a higher Court, where it won. However, the defendants appealed to the Court of Appeal. This court overturned the decision of the previous court, so the Pharmaceutical Society appealed again, this time to the House of Lords. At the hearing on 20 July 1880, the Law Lords confirmed the decision of the Court of Appeal, deciding that the carrying on of a pharmacy business by a limited company was indeed legal.

The decision meant that titles restricted to chemists and druggists by the 1868 Act could now legally be used by companies, provided that a qualified person was employed to carry out the sale of poisons. The decision meant that businesses consisting of large numbers of branches were now possible. The impact was immense; over the next fifteen years more than two hundred companies were registered for retail trade in drugs and dispensing. The first limited company was that set up by an unqualified druggist, Jesse Boot, in Nottingham. Boot called himself a cash chemist, and began opening branches. His first was in Nottingham. By 1883 he had ten, and by 1900 he already had by far the largest retail chemist chain, with more than 250 branches.

The practice of pharmacy

The emergence of the multiples was not the only threat facing proprietor pharmacists. The nature of retailing was changing, with the emergence of department stores and the growth of the cooperative movement. Sales of proprietary medicines expanded rapidly during this period, but so did the number of outlets from which they were available, and proprietor pharmacists needed to diversify to make a living. Many built up a substantial photographic business, as well as developing their trade in toiletries and cosmetics, and often tobacco products, wines and spirits. Figure 1.4 indicates the principal sources of income for independent community pharmacists during the course of the twentieth century.

In late Victorian Britain, many pharmacists also practised as dentists. Indeed, when the first dental register appeared in1879, following passage of the first Dentists Act in 1878, two thirds of those appearing on it combined the practice of dentistry with that of pharmacy. For thousands of pharmacies the extraction of teeth, making fillings and crowns, and supplying false teeth were one of the most profitable parts of the business. Although the Dental Act of 1921 restricted entry to the register to those who had undertaken approved courses of study, it admitted those who had been practising for at least seven years, and

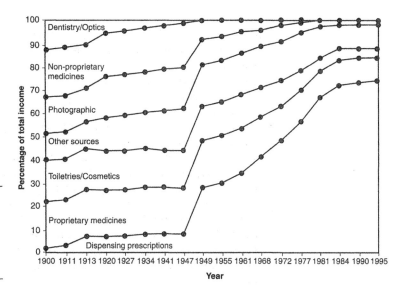

for whom dentistry represented a substantial part of their business. As a result many pharmacists were able to register as dentists and to carry on as before. The Chemists Dental Association, which represented the interests of the chemist-dentists, was finally disbanded in 1949, by which time it had five members.

NATIONAL INSURANCE TO NATIONAL HEALTH, 1911 TO 1948

The period between 1911 and 1948 is one that was dominated by two world wars. For the country and for pharmacy, many things had to be put on hold. But the introduction of the National Insurance Scheme in 1911 represents a major watershed in the development of pharmacy practice. Post war plans for the reform of industrial relations were another, leading to another important legal case, which resulted in a change of direction for the Pharmaceutical Society. It is also a period during which the nature of pharmaceutical products changed.

The separation of dispensing from prescribing

The provision of health insurance was to have a major impact on the fortunes of community pharmacists in Britain. An early form of such insurance was provided by the Friendly Societies, which had largely emerged in the eighteenth century. It has been estimated that by 1815, nearly nine per cent of the population belonged to one. During the nineteenth century membership continued to grow, such that by 1900 about half the adult male population were covered by either a Friendly Society or a trade union. Community pharmacists began seeing more prescriptions, although most of the dispensing continued to be done be the doctors themselves. The way in which the proportion of written prescriptions dispensed by doctors and pharmacists changed during the course of the twentieth century is illustrated in Figure 1.5.

The first major step in the state provision of health care came with the National Health Insurance Act of 1911. The minister responsible for its introduction was David Lloyd George. The Act created a national scheme of insurance against sickness and disability, and applied to all workers over the age of 16 earning no more than £160 per year, amounting to some 14 million men and women. It did not apply to their dependents, although payments were made for the support of the family while the breadwinner was ill. The insurance covered the cost of visiting the doctor and the supply of medicines. However, before the introduction of the welfare state the pharmacist was effectively the poor man's doctor. Many acted as father confessors, with patients often telling the pharmacist things they felt unable to tell the doctor.

It was in the National Health Insurance Act that the first legal distinction was made between the prescribing and dispensing of medicines. Lloyd George was keen to '*separate the drugs from the doctors*'. He was of the opinion that paying doctors to supply medicines encouraged excessive prescribing. When the National Insurance Scheme was introduced, doctors were given financial incentives to prescribe economically. The total sum for medical care was to be nine shillings per person, of which one shilling and sixpence was available for the supply of drugs. However a further sixpence (the so-called '*floating sixpence*') was to be available for paying chemists if the drug bill exceeded this limit. If it

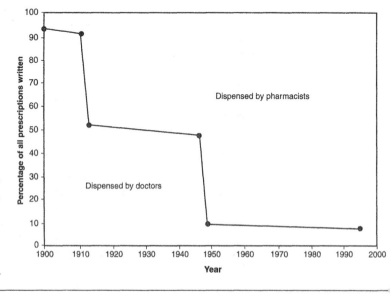

Figure 1.5 Proportion of all written prescriptions dispensed by doctors and pharmacists, 1900 to 1995. Source: Anderson and Berridge (1999).

Chapter One

wasn't needed, it was credited to the doctor, thus giving the doctor an incentive to deny patients the use of expensive drugs. This arrangement was to have clear parallels 80 years later with the advent of general medical practitioner (GP) fund-holding practices.

For community pharmacists, the National Health Insurance Act was a watershed. Whilst the immediate impact was a threefold increase in the number of prescriptions presented, decisions made at this time were largely to determine the shape of community pharmacy in Britain for the rest of the century. A separate salaried service for the dispensing of National Insurance prescriptions was resisted: companies as well as proprietor pharmacists were to be allowed to contract for pharmaceutical services, and special arrangements were agreed to allow doctors to dispense in rural areas where no chemist was available.

The limitation of the Pharmaceutical Society's functions

One of the major factors in determining the nature of pharmacy practice in Britain has been the powers of the Pharmaceutical Society, and the way in which these have been exercised. These powers have regularly been tested in the courts, and many of the cases represent watersheds in the evolution of pharmacy practice. One such was the Jenkin case of 1920.

In the aftermath of the first world war, the government was keen to reform industrial relations in Britain, by setting up a number of schemes for negotiating wage rates and other working conditions. The Pharmaceutical Society promoted the instigation of a Joint Industrial Council for this purpose, for the whole of the pharmaceutical industry, including manufacturing, wholesaling and retailing. The Society's membership included both employers and employees, and it was well placed to preside over negotiations between them.

The Society's plans came up against some powerful opponents, notably Jesse Boot and pharmacists in Scotland. The latter obtained legal opinion on whether the Society had the powers under its Charter, to become involved in negotiations about pay and conditions. The Society decided to test its powers in the courts. Arthur Henry Jenkin was a hospital pharmacist, and a member of the Society's Council. He took out an injunction to restrain the Council of the Society from undertaking a range of activities, including the regulation of pay and conditions of service, to function as an employers' association, and to provide legal and insurance services to members.

The injunction was granted. At a hearing on 19 October 1920, the Court decided that the Society did not have powers to regulate wages, hours of business, and the prices at which goods were sold, or to provide insurance or legal services. As a result of this decision, and just two months later, a separate body, the Retail Pharmacists Union, was set up as a *union of retail employer chemists for the protection of trade interests*. It was renamed the National Pharmaceutical Union in 1932, and the National Pharmaceutical Association (NPA) in 1977. At the same time Jesse Boot established a Managers' Representative Council to represent pharmacist-managers in his branches.

The triumph of professional regulation

After the Jenkin case the Society set about redefining its purpose, and changed direction. Indeed, it has been argued that the NPA is the true successor to the aims of the founding fathers of the Pharmaceutical Society. A new Pharmacy and Poisons Act in 1933 clarified the relationship between the Society's Council, the Privy Council and its members. For the first time every person registered as a pharmacist automatically became a member of the Pharmaceutical Society: the distinction between registration under the Pharmacy Acts and membership of the Society, which until that time had been voluntary, was ended. Membership jumped from 13,800 in 1932 to 20,900 in 1933.

The 1933 Act added substantially to the Pharmaceutical Society's statutory duties. The Society was required to enforce the Act, and had to appoint inspectors, who must be pharmacists themselves, for the purpose. The inspectors had to inspect the conditions under which poisons were stored, the registers of sales, and the premises of registered '*authorised sellers of poisons*', which included individual proprietor pharmacists and corporate bodies having a superintendent pharmacist.

Furthermore, a disciplinary committee, the Statutory Committee, was to be established with authority not only over pharmacists, but also over companies carrying on businesses under the Pharmacy Acts. The Committee was given the duty of inquiring into any case where a pharmacist (or other authorised seller of poisons) had been convicted of a criminal offence. The first Statutory Committee met in July 1934, and the first name was removed from the Register shortly after. A code of ethics for the profession followed within a few years. The first '*Statement upon Matters of Professional Conduct*' was eventually published in the *Pharmaceutical Journal* of June 17, 1944. It was revised and extended in 1953, a process which has continued ever since.

It has been said that with the 1933 Act '*professional regulation triumphed over protection and trade unionism*'. The Jenkin case had removed any prospect of the Society being involved in negotiating terms of service for its members. The 1933 Act ended any hope of the Society amalgamating with the Retail Pharmacists' Union and the Chemists' Defence Association into a '*British Medical Association for Pharmacy*'. The objectives of the Society were formally changed through a Supplemental Charter in 1953. The words '*the protection of those who carry on the business of chemists and druggists*' were replaced by '*to maintain the honour and safeguard and promote the interests of the members in the exercise of the profession of pharmacy*'.

Preparing pharmaceutical products: from bespoke to off-the-peg

During the course of the twentieth century the nature of pharmaceutical products, and their mode of preparation, changed beyond all recognition. At the turn of the century, many poor people still bought small quantities of ingredients to make their own home remedies. An important role of pharmacists was to counter prescribe, to suggest a remedy for a cold or a pain. They would usually make their own nostrums, such as cough and indigestion medicines, to their own formulae, and using their own labels. There were relatively few proprietary medicines available, and the vast majority of drugs in use were galenicals (liquid medicines extracted mainly from plants), and minerals such as potassium citrate and sodium bicarbonate. However, the '*therapeutic revolution*' of the 1950s and 1960s led to the marketing by pharmaceutical companies of increasing numbers of new chemical entities under brand names, and branded products came to dominate the prescribing habits of many doctors. This trend was only reversed in the 1990s. Changes in the proportion of branded and generic drugs prescribed by doctors during this period are illustrated in Figure 1.6.

Figure 1.7 shows changes in the nature of the principal dosage forms in use during the twentieth century. It shows the frequency with which particular dosage forms appeared in the prescription books of a single pharmacy in south London. At the beginning of the century over 60% of all medicines supplied were oral liquids, mainly mixtures and draughts (single dose liquid medicines). Only a very small proportion were solid dosage forms, and these were mainly pills and cachets; less

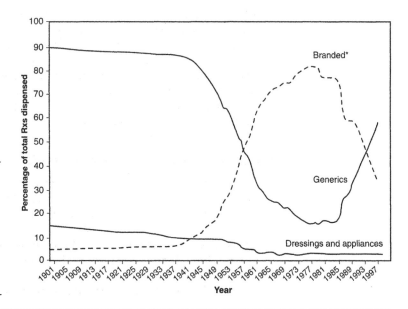

Figure 1.6 Proportion of generic and branded medicines prescribed, 1900 to 1997. Note ★ includes prescriptions written in generic names. Sources: Office of Health Economics, Department of Health, UK (1999).

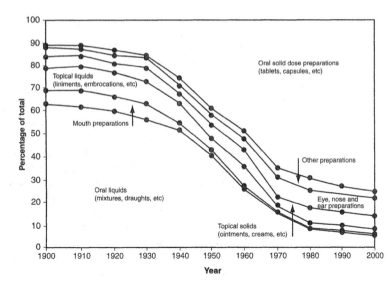

Figure 1.7 Principal dosage forms appearing in prescription books, 1900 to 2000.
Source: Anderson and Homan (1999).

than 2 per cent were tablets. By 1980 over 70 per cent of all medicines were supplied in oral solid dosage form, mainly tablets and capsules; less than 8 per cent were supplied as liquids. The period between 1930 and 1970 was one of great change in the practice of community pharmacy, as the need for extemporaneous dispensing diminished and preparation shifted from the dispensary to the factory.

PHARMACY IN THE NATIONAL HEALTH SERVICE

With the end of the Second World War the new Labour government set about implementing a programme of reform, including a comprehensive National Health Service (NHS). For pharmacy, its consequences were to be far-reaching. The NHS was to be a major factor in determining the nature of community pharmacy practice for the rest of the century. But it was not the only one. The basic tensions between trade and profession within pharmacy were to surface as the powers of the Society were tested yet again.

The impact of the National Health Service

By 1946 around 24 million workers, representing about half the total population, were covered by the National Insurance Scheme, as the income limit was gradually increased. The NHS, introduced on 5 July 1948, made the service available to everyone. Its introduction had a major impact on the practice of community pharmacy in Britain. Before 1948, dispensing prescriptions still accounted for less than 10 per cent of the income of most chemists. After 1948, 94 per cent of the population obtained their medicines from registered pharmacies, and dispensing prescriptions quickly came to form the major part of pharmacists' income (see Figure 1.4).

Figure 1.8 illustrates the increase in prescription numbers dispensed during the twentieth century. Within a year the number of prescriptions presented at chemists almost quadrupled, from seventy million in 1947 to nearly two hundred and fifty million in 1949. Just as prescription numbers increased, so other parts of pharmacists' traditional business began to decline. The number of private prescriptions presented dropped markedly, as did both requests for counter prescribing, and the sale of proprietary medicines, since all medicines prescribed by the doctor were now available free of charge.

Not surprisingly, most people preferred to go to the doctor for a prescription, even for the most minor of complaints, rather than pay for something from the chemist. The drop in the sale of proprietary medicines was to be short lived, however, as manufacturers increased their advertising on television and in magazines from the early 1950s. The sale of traditional chemists' items, such as toiletries and cosmetics, and photographic requisites, was threatened as other retailers entered these markets and specialist shops opened. Dependence on income from secondary occupations, particularly dentistry and optics, which had been common earlier in the century, had virtually ended, and many proprietor pharmacists were persuaded to sell their businesses to the multiples.

The 'disappearing' pharmacist

The consequences of the increase in prescription numbers were far-reaching. Almost overnight, many pharmacists effectively migrated from the front of the shop to the back, as they spent much of the

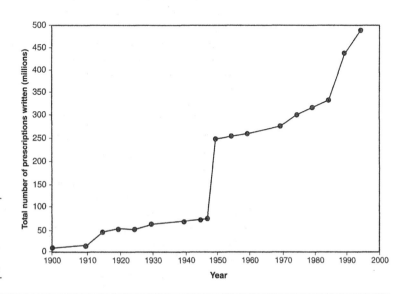

Figure 1.8 Number of prescriptions written by doctors in Great Britain, 1900 to 1995.
Source: Anderson (2000).

working day dispensing prescriptions in the dispensary. At the inception of the NHS, a majority of prescriptions still required the medicines to be compounded. Only a small proportion was available commercially as tablets or capsules. Many pharmacists took the opportunity to enlarge their dispensaries to meet the demand. Most felt that dispensing was what they had been trained to do, and only a few took the opportunity to train assistants to help with the dispensing. Most were happy with the increase in prescription numbers as it brought a substantial increase in their income.

During the 1950s and 1960s, the numbers of prescriptions continued to increase, although the nature of dispensing changed significantly. With new drugs being constantly marketed, more and more of the drugs prescribed were available as tablets and capsules, and the need for the individual making-up of medicines diminished greatly. By this time the dispensing of prescriptions accounted for more than half the income of most pharmacists, and the expectation of most new entrants to community pharmacy was to dispense prescriptions at the back of the shop. Pharmacists slowly began to disappear from the public's view as access to them diminished.

Professionalism versus commercialism

The conflict between trade and profession has been a central issue throughout pharmacy's history (see also Chapter 12). Pharmacists have always been paid for the products they sell, not the advice they give, and almost all engage in retail trade stretching beyond the strict confines of pharmacy. As we have seen, the trade issue became accentuated after 1880 when it was established that companies had the right to establish pharmacy businesses. Throughout its history, the Pharmaceutical Society has resisted commercial developments which it perceived as having an adverse effect on the professional standing of pharmacy.

By 1955, there was sufficient concern about the state of community pharmacy for the Council of the Society to appoint a committee to report on the general practice of pharmacy, with particular reference to the maintenance of professional standards. The Committee submitted its report in 1961, and it was eventually published in the *Pharmaceutical Journal* on April 20, 1963. The report suggested that it was undesirable for nonprofessional business to predominate in a pharmacy, and that the extension of this kind of business in pharmacies should be controlled.

An attempt to incorporate this principle into the Statement Upon Matters of Professional Conduct was challenged and led to the Dickson case. A motion was put to the Annual General Meeting of the Society in 1965, but owing to the large attendance no vote could be taken, and a special meeting to consider the recommendation was held at the Royal Albert Hall on July 25, 1965. Mr RCM Dickson, who was a director of the Boots Pure Drug Company, sought an injunction to prevent the holding of the meeting, claiming that the motion was outside the scope of the Society's powers, and that if implemented, would be a restraint on trade.

The Society was unable to satisfy the courts that the professional side of a pharmacy business was adversely affected by other activities. The Society appealed to the House of Lords, who upheld the decision of the lower court. The Society was judged to have no powers to restrict the sale of certain goods from pharmacies. It could make rules affecting the nonprofessional activities of pharmacists, but only if the rules could be shown to be in the interest of the public and the profession. The Society had attempted to control the commercial aspects of pharmacy. The Dickson case demonstrated that it did not have the power to do so.

THE EMERGENCE OF 'THE NEW PHARMACY': 1986 TO PRESENT

By the early 1980s there was widespread uncertainty about the future of pharmacy, particularly community pharmacy. The Minister for Health, Dr Gerard Vaughan, announced at the British Pharmaceutical Conference that *'one knew there was a future for hospital pharmacists, one knew there was a future for industrial pharmacists, but one was not sure that one knew the future for the general practice pharmacist'*. Pharmacy needed to re-invent itself. Some important initiatives were taken. In 1982, for example, the National Pharmaceutical Association began its *'Ask Your Pharmacist'* campaign, in which it promoted the use by the public of their local pharmacy. But what was really needed was an independent and far-ranging inquiry into the profession. The result was the *'Nuffield Report'*.

The Nuffield Report 1986

In October 1983 the Trustees of the Nuffield Foundation commissioned an inquiry into pharmacy (Nuffield Committee of Inquiry into Pharmacy 1986). Its terms of reference were *'to consider the present and future structure of the practice of pharmacy in its several branches and its potential contribution to health care and to review the education and training of pharmacists accordingly'*. The Committee of Inquiry was chaired by Sir Kenneth Clucas, a former Permanent Secretary at the Department of Trade, and had twelve members, only half of whom were pharmacists. It made a total of 96 recommendations, 26 of which related to community pharmacy.

The tone of the Nuffield report was very positive: *'we believe that the pharmacy profession has a distinctive and indispensable contribution to make to health care that is capable of still further development'*. The years which followed its publication were dominated by the action necessary to implement the recommendations. Two aspects came to dominate the discussion: whether a pharmacist needed to be on the premises in order to supervise activities, and the extended role.

In order to have time to carry out the extended role, the pharmacist would need to be able to leave the pharmacy at times, so that supervision could be exercised in other ways. Eventually the pharmacy profession rejected this radical suggestion, and in 1989 the Council of the Royal Pharmaceutical Society of Great Britain issued a statement to the effect that *'every prescription for a medicine must be seen by a pharmacist, and a judgement made by him as to what action is necessary'*. Pharmacists had not only disappeared from view, but were now shackled to the dispensary bench.

The extended role

The task of considering in what ways the role of community pharmacists might be extended was delegated to a Joint Working Party of the Department of Health and the pharmaceutical profession. This was set up in November 1990 with the following terms of reference; *'to consider ways in which the National Health Service community pharmaceutical services might be developed to increase their contribution to health care; and to make recommendations'*.

Its report *'Pharmaceutical Care: the Future for Community Pharmacy'* (Department of Health and Royal Pharmaceutical Society of Great Britain 1992) was published in March 1992, and it made a total of 30 recommendations. These included increasing the range of medicines available for sale by pharmacists, the maintenance of patient medication records by pharmacists, the extension of needle and syringe exchange schemes, participation in health promotion campaigns, and having separate areas for providing advice and counselling. The recommendations formed the basis for negotiations about the scope of community pharmacy over the years that followed.

By the mid-1990s it was clear that most of the recommendations of the Nuffield Report which could be implemented had been. Nuffield was a catalyst for change, but in order to maintain the momentum it was necessary to involve the membership as a whole. The Society's response was to launch the *Pharmacy in a New Age* (PIANA) initiative in October 1995. This was an attempt to involve as many members of the profession as possible in the process of developing a strategy for the future of pharmacy. To assist this process, six papers on factors affecting the future of pharmacy were published in February 1996 as *'The Shape of Things to Come'*.

Over 5,000 pharmacists took part in the consultation process. The Council's response was a further document published in September 1996, *The New Horizon* (Royal Pharmaceutical Society of Great Britain 1996). Four key areas for pharmacy involvement were identified: the management of prescribed medicines; the management of chronic conditions; the management of common ailments; and the promotion and support of healthy lifestyles. The outcome of this process was the publication in September 1997 of a strategy for a twenty-first century pharmaceutical service under the title *Building the Future* (Royal Pharmaceutical Society of Great Britain 1997), which set specific aims and targets for each of the four areas.

Is pharmacy returning to its roots?

The '*Ask Your Pharmacist*' campaign, the *extended role*, and the *Pharmacy In A New Age* initiative can be seen collectively as an attempt to draw pharmacists out of the dispensary (which was usually at the back of the shop), to the front of the shop where they would be more accessible to the public. Here they would be the '*first port of call*' for the public seeking medical attention; they would be a source of advice and information about medicines to the public; and they would prescribe from an increasingly long list of recently deregulated medicines. At the same time as pharmacists were becoming more accessible, doctors were becoming less accessible, as group practice became the norm, appointment schemes were introduced, and prescription charges continued to increase.

The idea of the extended role for community pharmacists has been taken up enthusiastically by many countries, and seems set to develop further. The changes in pharmacy practice in the last quarter of the twentieth century represented a shift away from a product-oriented approach to medicines towards a patient-focused one. In many ways, developments in the practice of community pharmacy since 1986 can be seen as a return to the traditional role of the community pharmacist, which had been eroded following introduction of the NHS in 1948: whilst the increasing prescribing role of the community pharmacist has clear parallels with the role of the apothecary in earlier centuries.

A BRIEF HISTORY OF HOSPITAL PHARMACY

The history of pharmacy prior to the start of the twentieth century is largely the history of shop-based pharmacy. Yet pharmacy practice in hospitals can be traced back over many centuries, and the history of hospital pharmacy is closely allied to the history of hospitals. The history of hospital pharmacy can be considered within three time frames: an emergent period up to 1897; a period of standardisation up to 1948; and a period of expansion and consolidation since then.

The origins of hospital pharmacy to 1897

The first hospitals in Britain in which it is known pharmacy was practised were the Roman military hospitals known as *valetudinaria*. As Britain converted to Christianity, so the Church began to care for the sick and needy. Between 794 and 1547 nearly 800 hospitals were established, of which around 200 were for the care of lepers. However, in medieval times hospitals were ecclesiastical rather than medical institutions, being essentially for the refreshment of the soul rather than the relief of the body. In addition to these hospitals, there were infirmaries attached to many monasteries throughout Europe.

Further hospitals were established by religious and craft guilds in the fourteenth and fifteenth centuries, and a number of pest houses opened in the sixteenth and seventeenth centuries to care for the victims of the plague. Many employed an apothecary and contained a dispensary. The apothecary usually combined the roles of resident medical officer and dispenser of medicines. Larger hospitals, such as St. Bartholomew's and St. Thomas's in London, often also employed an apothecary's assistant or apprentice, and would undertake the preparation of most of their own medicines. Smaller hospitals often employed the services of a visiting apothecary.

Passage of the Apothecaries Act in 1815 put a stop to the early development of hospital pharmacy in Britain, since most hospital apothecaries devoted most of their time to medical matters, and neglected the dispensing side. As the Linstead Report on the hospital pharmaceutical service in 1955 was to note '*the original development of the pharmaceutical service in hospitals was checked when the apothecary obtained recognition as a general practitioner of medicine, and explains why hospital pharmacy had to make a fresh start in the middle of the last century*'. During the second half of the nineteenth century, at least in the larger hospitals, the remaining apothecaries were slowly replaced by qualified pharmacists, and some hospitals now began to insist that those appointed be members of the Pharmaceutical Society.

The emergence of professional identity, 1897 to 1923

There was, however, no legal requirement that only registered pharmacists must be employed in hospitals, and many institutions continued to employ unqualified people with a wide range of backgrounds. Changes in the practice of pharmacy in hospitals in the late nineteenth century led to the creation of a number of separate professional associations. The Poor Law Dispensers Association was formed in 1897, and in the following year The Public Dispensers Association came into being. The Association consisted of London County Council asylum dispensers, prison and charity dispensers, and a few hospital dispensers.

These two associations amalgamated in 1900, becoming the Public and Poor Law Dispensers Association. By 1909 the title had became The Public Pharmacists and Dispensers Association. At this time many of the pharmacists employed in the public service were women. By 1908 over sixty per cent of practising women pharmacists were working in hospitals and institutions. In 1916 the organisation decided that in future only individuals whose names appeared on the register of chemists and druggists should be elected as members. In 1917 it became the Public Pharmacists Association.

Unification and standardisation, 1923 to 1948

Pharmacists in voluntary hospitals regarded themselves as rather different from their colleagues in other institutions. They formed a separate organisation, as a pharmacy section of the Hospital Officers Association. However, in due course the two organisations agreed to merge. The inaugural meeting of the Guild of Public Pharmacists was held on 23 January 1923. There was now a single body to represent pharmacists working in voluntary hospitals, Poor Law institutions, prisons, and other branches of the public service. With the creation of the Guild, public service pharmacy had come of age. The first quarter of the twentieth century represented a period during which the salaries, status, and prospects of such pharmacists had improved substantially.

The period from 1923 to 1948 represented a period of standardisation for the service. But differences still remained between pharmacy in voluntary rather than municipal hospitals, since there was no legal requirement to employ a pharmacist in hospitals, and in many the supply of medicines was undertaken by medical staff, nurses, or under-qualified dispensers. In 1939 the Pharmaceutical Society carried out the first survey of hospital pharmacy. It found that over two-thirds of the 397 hospitals having one hundred or more beds employed a full-time pharmacist, and a further 13 hospitals used the services of a local community pharmacist. Although only 15 per cent of the 543 hospital with less than 100 beds employed a pharmacist, nearly half used a pharmacist outside to supervise the dispensing.

Consolidation and survival, 1948 to 1970

The introduction of the NHS in 1948 provided the opportunity for further development and enhancement of professional aspirations. The Pharmaceutical Whitley Council, at which salaries and conditions of service were negotiated, was the first to be convened. However, initial optimism was soon dashed. Although national pay scales were agreed, poor pay and prospects were to overshadow the practice of hospital pharmacy in Britain throughout the 1950s and 1960s.

Despite these difficulties a number of important innovations were possible at several centres, mainly in teaching hospitals where recruitment difficulties were less severe, where locums could usually be recruited, and which tended to have larger establishments. From 1965 onwards, at the Westminster and London Hospitals in London, and at Aberdeen Royal Infirmary, developments were under way which required hospital pharmacists to inspect prescription sheets on the ward rather than in the pharmacy.

Quality control for manufacturing was becoming more vigorous, and drug information services were beginning to be developed, initially to support ward pharmacists. But for most hospitals the capacity to introduce such innovations was severely limited by small establishments, poor recruitment and no obligation on hospital managers to do much to improve matters.

Expansion and development, 1970 to the present

Concern about the state of the hospital pharmaceutical service eventually persuaded the government to set up a Committee of Enquiry. The Noel Hall Report was published in 1970 (Report of the Working Party on the Hospital Pharmaceutical Service 1970). At the core of the recommendations was the belief that hospital pharmacy needed to be organised on a larger scale, with several pooling their resources in Noel Hall areas, and that these should be co-ordinated on a regional basis.

Other reports and health circulars promoted and legitimised many of the innovations which had been developed in a small number of centres. Substantial pay increases were awarded, a proper career structure was established, and the early 1970s saw a period of rapid expansion and specialisation. By the end of the 1970s, ward pharmacy was practised in most hospitals, a drug information network had been established, and other specialities such as purchasing and radiopharmacy had emerged.

By the 1980s, financial restraint was being applied to the health service. Hospital pharmacy was not immune. It was nevertheless able to establish new activities which contributed to cost control, such as formulary development, and many pharmacists began to specialise in a particular area of clinical pharmacy, such as paediatrics or cardiology.

The 1990s were to see some contraction of the service, as the more senior posts, at district and region levels, disappeared following health service changes. Since then, the service has had to contend with further rounds of health service reform, and finds itself with a chronic recruitment crisis, mirroring experience in the 1950s and 60s.

CONCLUSION

Since the formation of the Pharmaceutical Society in 1841, pharmaceutical politicians and commentators have at regular intervals referred to pharmacy being '*at the crossroads*'. This has led to a belief that pharmacy progresses from one crisis to another. In fact, examination of these so-called crossroads indicates that each is different: pharmacy has moved on from one crossroads to the next. Indeed, the metaphor of '*being at the crossroads*' is one to be found in all occupations and indeed in many walks of life. It indicates the need to make often difficult choices at regular intervals, and it is one of the strengths of pharmacy that it has had many choices to make.

The metaphor of the crossroads is less helpful in suggesting that progress is made by choosing the *'right'* route and rejecting the others. In fact, successful professions are those that proceed along several routes from the crossroads simultaneously. With hindsight, it can be seen that pharmacy suffered during the 1950s and 1960s by proceeding down a single *'structural'* route. It was assumed that status, respect and prosperity would automatically follow from increased educational achievement, by making the profession degree entry only. At the same time there was neglect of issues concerned with *'output'* and *'outcome'*; what were pharmacists, particularly those in the community, actually doing? And how did this contribute to the well-being of the public? The lessons of recent history for pharmacy are that survival and prosperity depend on its capacity to respond to the wide range of technological, political, social and economic factors which form the world in which it operates, and to keep it eyes firmly on the *'added value'* it provides.

FURTHER READING

Anderson, S.C. (2000) Community Pharmacy in Great Britain: Mediation at the Boundary Between Professional and Lay Care 1920 to 1995. In: T. Tansey and M. Gijswijt-Hofstra (Eds.) *Biographies of Remedies: Drugs, Medicines and Contraceptives in Dutch and Anglo-American Healing Cultures*, Amsterdam.

Anderson, S.C. and Berridge, V.S. (2000) The Role of the Community Pharmacist in Health and Welfare 1911 to 1986. In: J. Bornat, R.B. Perks, P. Thompson and J. Walmsley (Eds.) *Oral History, Health and Welfare*, Routledge, London.

Grier, J. (1937) *A History of Pharmacy*, The Pharmaceutical Press, London.

Holloway, S.W.F. (1991) *Royal Pharmaceutical Society of Great Britain 1841–1991. A Political and Social History*, The Pharmaceutical Press, London.

Kremer and Urdang, (1976) *History of Pharmacy*, Blackwell Scientific Publications, Oxford.

Matthews, L.G. (1965) *History of Pharmacy in Britain*, Livingstone, London and Edinburgh.

Poynter, F.N.L. (1965) *The Evolution of Pharmacy in Britain*, Pitman Medical Publishing, London.

Trease, G.E. (1964) *Pharmacy in History*, Bailliere, Tindall and Cox, London.

REFERENCES

Anderson, S.C. (2000) Community Pharmacy in Great Britain: Mediation at the Boundary Between Professional and Lay Care 1920 to 1995. In: T. Tansey and M. Gijswijt-Hofstra (Eds.) *Biographies of Remedies: Drugs, Medicines and Contraceptives in Dutch and Anglo-American Healing Cultures*, Rodopi, Amsterdam.

Anderson, S.C. and Berridge, V.S. (1999) L'Heritage perdu du pharmacien: professionnalisation, specialisation et accroissement de la protection sociale. In: O. Foure and A. Opinel (Eds.) *Les Therapeutiques: Savoirs et Usages*, Collection Fondation Marcel Merieux, Saint Julien en Beaujolais.

Anderson, S.C. and Berridge, V.S. (2000) The Role of the Community Pharmacist in Health and Welfare 1911 to 1986. In: J. Bornat, R.B. Perks, P. Thompson and J. Walmsley (Eds.) *Oral History, Health and Welfare*, Routledge, London.

Anderson, S.C. and Homan, C. (1999) Prescription books as historical sources. *Pharmaceutical Historian*, **29**, 51–54.

Compendium of Health Statistics (1999) Office of Health Economics, London.

Department of Health and Royal Pharmaceutical Society of Great Britain (1992) *Pharmaceutical Care: the Future for Community Pharmacy*. Royal Pharmaceutical Society of Great Britain, London.

Earles, M.P. (1965) The pharmacy schools of the nineteenth century. In: F.N.L. Poynter (Ed.) *The Evolution of Pharmacy in Britain*, Pitman Medical Publishing, London.

Nuffield Committee of Inquiry into Pharmacy (1986) *Pharmacy: a Report to the Nuffield Foundation*, Nuffield Foundation, London.

Prescriptions Dispensed in the Community: Statistics for 1988 to 1998: England (1999) Department of Health, London.

Report of the Working Party on the Hospital Pharmaceutical Service (Noel Hall Report) (1970) HMSO, London.

Royal Pharmaceutical Society of Great Britain (1996) *Pharmacy in a New Age: the New Horizon*, The Royal Pharmaceutical Society of Great Britain, London.

Royal Pharmaceutical Society of Great Britain (1997) *Pharmacy in a New Age: Building the Future*, The Royal Pharmaceutical Society of Great Britain, London.

Trease, G.E. (1964) *Pharmacy in History*, Bailliere, Tindall and Cox, London.

Question 1: In what ways can the passage of the National Health Insurance Act in 1911 be said to represent a watershed in the development of pharmacy practice in Britain?

Question 2: To what extent did the introduction of the National Health Service in 1948 influence the nature of community pharmacy practice in Britain?

Question 3: In what ways could the pharmacist be said to have '*disappeared*' in the decades following the introduction of the National Health Service?

KEY POINTS FOR ANSWERS

Question 1:

- The Act made a clear distinction between prescribing and dispensing for the first time
- The idea of a salaried service for the dispensing of National Insurance prescriptions was rejected
- Companies as well as proprietor pharmacists were to be allowed to contract to provide dispensing services
- Within a year the numbers of prescriptions presented at pharmacies almost tripled

Question 2:

- Prescription numbers increased by over three times, from 70 million to 241 million
- Many pharmacists used existing shop floor space to enlarge their dispensaries
- With an on-cost payment of over 30 per cent, many pharmacists now saw the dispensing of prescriptions as their main business and their principal source of income
- Most pharmacists saw dispensing as the activity for which they had been trained, and continued to undertake this work themselves, rather than employ and train support staff to do so

Question 3:

- Since 1948, the majority of pharmacists had spent most of their working day at the back of the shop in the dispensary. They only emerged when asked to do so. In the public's mind the pharmacist had effectively '*disappeared*' as a front-line health professional

- New entrants to the profession came to see the role of the pharmacist as someone who dispenses prescriptions out of sight of the public. Few made a positive effort to make themselves readily available to the public
- The nature of dispensing itself was changing dramatically during this period as the need for extemporaneously prepared medicines diminished

2 The Pharmacy Workforce

Karen Hassell and Sue Symonds

INTRODUCTION	32
WORKFORCE PROFILE IN THE UK AND OTHER COUNTRIES	32
FACTORS AFFECTING SUPPLY AND DEMAND IN THE PHARMACY	
WORKFORCE	35
Demand factors	35
Supply factors	36
Women's entry into pharmacy and their impact on workforce issues	36
The increasing participation of ethnic minority groups in pharmacy	38
Age and retirement	40
The significance of part-time work in workforce issues	41
Other factors affecting supply	43
CONCLUSION	43
FURTHER READING	44
REFERENCES	44
SELF-ASSESSMENT QUESTIONS	45
KEY POINTS FOR ANSWERS	46

INTRODUCTION

The contribution of pharmacists to health care and health gain has been the subject of considerable debate. However, the impact of changing employment patterns in pharmacy on the supply and demand for pharmacists has been largely neglected even though this affects the way pharmacy is practised. The aim of this chapter is to describe the features which characterise the current pharmacy workforce, to explore what changes have taken place over time, and to discuss the likely impact of the changes on the supply of, and demand for, pharmacy labour.

While the focus of this chapter is on UK pharmacists, many of the key workforce issues discussed are more generally applicable. Direct comparisons of international workforce data are not always possible, partly because of differences in terminology and non comparable health care systems, but also because it is difficult to obtain data matched by year. Some of the available international data on the workforce are presented in Table 2.1.

WORKFORCE PROFILE IN THE UK AND OTHER COUNTRIES

In UK pharmacies, the workforce is divided into registered pharmacists and support workers. Within community pharmacies, support workers include dispensers and counter assistants, while in hospital pharmacies, dispensing technicians provide technical support. At present there is no central register of support workers, so there is little information on what proportion of the total pharmacy workforce they comprise. Any questions, therefore, about skill mix, (the balance between work undertaken by professionally qualified staff and by support workers), are difficult to address.

Pharmacists are, in most countries, obliged to register with a governing body – in the UK this is the Royal Pharmaceutical Society of Great Britain (RPSGB). In 1997, 41,700 pharmacists were registered with the RPSGB. The number of pharmacists registered but not practising is relatively constant, while in recent years around 500 pharmacists have been added to the register in successive years, suggesting a growth in labour resources. The majority (61%) in pharmacy employment are based in community pharmacy, while approximately 16% are thought to work in the hospital sector (Royal Pharmaceutical Society of Great Britain 1996a).

Workforce surveys conducted by the RPSGB do not distinguish between community pharmacists who work as independent contractors, or owner/proprietors and those employed in multiple pharmacy companies. However, recent research has estimated the proportion of employee pharmacists to be more than 60% (Magirr and Ottewill 1995).

Given the marked shift within community pharmacy over the last twenty years or so, from independent contractor to small or large multiple pharmacies, the increase in the number of pharmacists who are employees is unsurprising. The dynamics of the business sector are such that rapid changes in ownership, particularly from the small groups to the large multiples, are common. Lloyds Chemist plc, for example, began in 1973 as one chemist shop, and by 1986 when the company was floated on the stock market, it comprised 100 shops. By the early 1990s, after an intense period of take-over activity, Lloyds pharmacy became the second largest owner of pharmacy outlets in the UK.

Data from the Department of Health in the UK confirm the growing trend towards 'corporatisation'. The proportion of community pharmacies in England belonging to large multiples (defined as those with over five stores) has grown from 17% in 1969 to 34% in 1995. This corporatisation process can be seen in some, but not all, of the countries listed in Table 2.1. In Canada, the growth in the number of multiples is similar to trends witnessed in the UK. In New Zealand, on the other hand, the majority of the 1100 retail pharmacies, because of legal restrictions on ownership, remain small independently owned outlets (Norris 1997).

Since 1972, the RPSGB workforce surveys have provided estimates of the extent of employment (whether full-time, part-time, or not in employment at all) of pharmacists in different categories of occupation. Between 1972 and 1994 the number of pharmacists working part-time increased from 17% to 30%. Whilst the majority of women pharmacists on the register (60%) in paid employment work full-time, most part-timers (72%) are women. There is a demonstrable relationship between part-time work, gender and age: the majority of women who work part-time are aged between 30 and 39 years, while the majority of men part-timers are aged 55 and over. Similar trends to these have been observed in Australia (Anderson 1990), New Zealand (Norris 1997) and the USA (Knapp 1994).

The increasing proportion of women on the UK Pharmacy register indicates that they will be in the majority by the year 2000. In fact, in a number of countries where data are available, (e.g. Canada, New Zealand, UK) women are already in the majority in the younger age groups. The impact that an increasingly female membership might have on the pharmacy workforce is discussed below.

Whereas the exact composition of the pharmacy workforce varies across different countries, there are also several notable similarities. Women now comprise nearly half, or over half, of the pharmacy workforce in all the countries listed in Table 2.1, with the exception of the USA. Most pharmacists work in community pharmacy and the percentage in active employment is relatively high in those countries for which data are available. Although the proportion of women pharmacists in the USA is smaller than in the UK, the tendency for women with young families to work part-time is similar in the two countries. In view of the continuing increase in the number of women entering

	Number of pharmacists	% female	% in active practice	% in community	% in hospital	% part-time	Number of pharmacies	Data
Belgium	13,000	52%		61%	4%			1996
Germany	50,372	59%		87%	4%			1996
France	55,106	61%						1993
Italy	55,000	52%						1993
Portugal	7,159	79%		50%	6%			1996
Sweden	7,425	45%	97%	81%	7%			1996
UK	41,743	47%	87%	61%	16%	24%	12,300	1997
Canada	18,000	51%			25%			1991
USA	194,570	29%	88%	66%	24%			1992
New Zealand	2,500	45%			12%		1,100	1991

Table 2.1 Pharmacy workforce data in 10 countries

the pharmacy profession, and the younger age profile of women pharmacists compared with men, the proportion of pharmacists working part-time is predicted to increase (Knapp 1994). Similar trends have been noted in New Zealand by Norris (1997) and by Muzzin *et al.* (1994) in Canada.

FACTORS AFFECTING SUPPLY AND DEMAND IN THE PHARMACY WORKFORCE

Demand factors

A number of factors influence the supply of, and demand for, pharmacists (Table 2.2).

The increasing emphasis on primary care within the UK is likely to result in changes to the nature of pharmacists' employment, and will influence the demand for pharmacists. An increasing number of pharmacists are being employed within general practitioners' practices and similarly more are being appointed to managerial positions within the health service. In addition, the drive towards enhancing efficiency within health care, has resulted in the recognition of pharmacists as supplementary providers of health care alongside general practitioners and other health care workers (Hassell *et al.* 1997). In particular, recent UK health policy has called for community pharmacists to be used as the '*first port of call*' in the management of minor ailments.

While professional development factors such as these may have a positive impact on the growth in workforce demand, developments within the general population may also influence demand. Discussing pharmacy workforce issues in Australian pharmacy, Anderson (1990) has argued, for example, that an increase in the prescription volume due to the ageing population will also increase the demand for more pharmacists.

Commercial developments taking place within the retail sector are also likely to have an impact on pharmacy workforce demand. A growing number and proportion of pharmacies are owned by supermarkets and larger multiples. These pharmacies tend to have longer opening hours, and provide a greater number of pharmaceutical services, which require pharmacists to leave the premises. Under these circumstances additional pharmacists are required to fulfil the legal obligations for continual professional cover.

Changes have also taken place in the secondary care sector, with extended opening hours and 'out-of-hours' clinics introduced by many hospital pharmacies. The extent of these changes on the work patterns of hospital pharmacists is unclear, but is likely to increase the demand for pharmacists who are able and willing to work flexible hours.

There has been speculation that an increase in demand for pharmacists in the retail sector will create pressures in other branches of the profession. Local research studies have already highlighted the difficulties experienced in some areas of the UK in the recruitment of pharmacists into junior hospital posts (Royal Pharmaceutical Society of Great Britain 1996b). While the precise reasons for these problems are not clear, (though salary levels are likely to be a major factor), competition between the multiples for existing pharmacy labour resources, as well as between the community and hospital sectors, is only likely to exacerbate the problems.

Supply factors

Whilst commercial developments and changes within primary and secondary care have been emphasised as increasing *demand* for phar-

Supply	Demand
Increasing feminisation	Shift towards a primary care led NHS
Increasing 'Asianisation'	Increased patient through-put in hospitals
Age of practitioners	Increasing corporatisation
Retirement rates	Practice and professional developments
Career satisfaction	Organisational changes – longer hours
Part-time working	
Career motivation	
Changes to the pharmacy course	
Competition for posts	
Salary	

Table 2.2 Factors influencing supply of, and demand for, pharmacists

macists, concerns have also been noted which point to their inadequate *supply*. Aside from the more conspicuous factors that can affect the overall size of the workforce, such as new registrations, deaths, retirements, and removals from the register, other forces are likely to impact on workforce numbers. These factors, perhaps less obvious and immediate in terms of their impact on career motivation and practice patterns, arise from the demographic changes taking place within the pharmacy profession.

Women's entry into pharmacy and their impact on workforce issues

In all but four of the countries listed in Table 2.1, women comprise over half of the registered pharmacy workforce. The number of women pharmacists has increased over a relatively short period of time in the UK. The first UK workforce survey in 1964 reported that women represented 19% of registered pharmacists. By 1981 t hey constituted one third, and since then further increases have occurred at a rate of approximately 1% per year. According to the latest published survey (Royal Pharmaceutical Society of Great Britain 1996b) 47% of the UK pharmacy workforce are female.

In the UK, increasing female participation in paid employment has been an important factor in the growth of overall labour resources over the past thirty years, so the increasing prevalence of women in the pharmacy workforce is unsurprising. As in other labour markets, female employment in pharmacy has certain distinctive characteristics. For instance, female pharmacists, particularly married women with dependent children, are much more likely to be involved in part-time work, compared with men (Fanaeian *et al.* 1988), and although many women work in community pharmacy, they comprise the majority in hospital pharmacy. They also tend to be concentrated at the practitioner level and do not occupy senior positions in proportion to their number in the profession (Rees and Clarke 1990).

In UK pharmacy, this so-called '*feminisation*' process has led to concerns about workforce shortages. If women undertake the primary responsibility for child care in their families, inevitably they are unable to participate, full-time, in paid employment. Thus, it may be assumed that an increasing proportion of women pharmacists may reduce the size of the labour force, leading to a shortfall in the supply of pharmacists. However, researchers in Canada have challenged this assumption. Muzzin and colleagues (1994) speculate that female pharmacists are actually guaranteeing the survival of pharmacy. Because of their preference for employment in retail pharmacy in the larger corporate organisations, women are helping: '*to reorient pharmacy away from its business base and towards its chosen new professional jurisdiction of "patient counselling"*'. Muzzin *et al.* (1994) also point out that female pharmacists in Canada are more mobile than men, moving to geographical regions where staff shortages are greatest.

The growth in the number of women in pharmacy has led to some critical and theoretical sociological analyses exploring women's entry into pharmacy and into professional occupations generally. The concept of '*occupational segregation*', which refers to the way women are distributed through occupational categories compared with men, is central to this debate, as is the concept of '*vertical integration*'. Writing about UK pharmacy, Crompton and Sanderson (1990), whilst viewing the increased participation of women in the pharmacy workforce as one beneficial consequence of the rising qualification levels among girls, nevertheless argue that work patterns in pharmacy still reflect a '*gendered division of labour*'. To support this view, they cite women pharmacists' subordination to men in terms of job hierarchies and their concentration in stereotypical '*female*' niches and part-time work, which, although offering opportunities for flexible working, are perceived as bringing fewer rewards. Consequently, what appear better career opportunities for women are, in fact, simply an extension of women's disadvantage into new areas of work. This view is also associated with arguments that professions in which women participate are those in which material rewards have decreased and work has become routinised and de-skilled (Reskin and Roos 1987).

Looking at UK pharmacy, Bottero (1994) challenges this perspective, arguing that the increased prevalence of women in pharmacy coincided with a raising of educational entry requirements and with attempts to '*professionalise*' the pharmacist's role. The privileged positions held by many women in pharmacy are an indication of success, not subordination. Similar arguments have been put forward by Norris (1997) writing about New Zealand pharmacy. Norris argues that women's entry into pharmacy has coincided with an up-grading of the profession, which has seen pharmacy in New Zealand increase its science base and move from an apprenticeship entry model to one which requires higher education qualifications in order to secure a university place. Moreover, Norris (1997), in refuting the dominance of the secondary labour market thesis put forward by Crompton and Sanderson (1990), has also pointed out that while many women do work part-time, the majority nevertheless maintain a full-time commitment to their work. Both Bottero (1994) and Norris (1997) urge a more in-depth analysis of the pharmacy workforce. They suggest that '*feminisation*' is an inadequate description of the process that has occurred, not least because analyses of workforce change have tended to overlook the changing identity and motivations of male recruits into pharmacy, as well as age differences between men and women.

The increasing participation of ethnic minority groups in pharmacy

Until recently, the contribution to pharmacy of the UK's ethnic minority groups and the impact their presence is likely to have on wider workforce issues has been overlooked, although ethnic minority groups make up a significant proportion of the pharmacy workforce (Hassell *et al.* 1998). In a survey that included in the sample all 1991 pharmacy graduates, almost a quarter (23%) were from ethnic minority groups. Analysis of university applications and admissions data shows that the trend in entry rates is upward. Since 1990 when data on the ethnic background of applicants to higher education institutions were first recorded, ethnic minority applicants have made up an increasingly large proportion of all applicants and admissions to the 16 pharmacy schools throughout the UK. This proportion is much larger than for many other courses leading to a professional qualification (such as medicine, dentistry and law), and it is much larger than would be expected given their numbers in the UK population as a whole (Hassell 1997).

Applications to UK schools of pharmacy are made through the Universities and Colleges Admissions Service (UCAS). Using data supplied by UCAS, Table 2.3 compares the numbers and proportions of applications and admissions by ethnic group in 1990 and 1998. Just under two-fifths (39%) of applicants to pharmacy courses in 1990 were from students who classed themselves as belonging to an ethnic minority group, while students from an ethnic minority constituted 33% of actual admissions in the same year. By 1998, the proportion of ethnic minority applicants was 52%, while of those who secured a place, 44% were from an ethnic minority group.

This and other work on ethnic minority pharmacists has highlighted a number of important differences between white and ethnic minority pharmacists regarding career motivation, practice intentions, and employment patterns. Although ethnic minority group pharmacists are represented in all sectors of the profession, they are over-represented as independent business owners in the retail sector, and under-represented in managerial positions. While several ethnic groups are represented, members of the Indian ethnic group, most of whom are '*twice migrants*' from East Africa, predominate.

Even in the relatively short time that ethnic minority groups have become significantly represented in pharmacy, changes with respect to the ethnic profile of practitioners have taken place. Older ethnic minority pharmacists are mostly East African Indian, whose involvement largely reflects their cultural and socio-economic class background and the economic opportunities that were available for independent pharmacy business development shortly after their migration to this country. In seeking upward mobility after migration to the UK, they chose to enter a profession which provided them with opportunities to go into business for themselves. By so doing, they fulfilled a desire for status, a preference to remain independent and autonomous, and they made the best use of their ethnic resources and family expertise. As migrants, self-employment for the older Asian pharmacists is viewed as prestigious, and employment of any family labour in the business is viewed in relation to the long term benefits this provides for all the family, rather than in terms of any benefits it gives to the owner personally.

Younger ethnic minority pharmacists however, are beginning to diversify in terms of practice intentions, so that independent business is not as popular a choice as it was for their predecessors. Changing preferences among the younger groups in part reflect generational and ethnic group differences, as well as social class differences among the more recent ethnic minority recruits. Pakistanis as an ethnic minority group *per se*, are increasingly represented, as are ethnic minority women. Attributes such as autonomy and independence, which business ownership affords, are not as important for these two groups, and they have a greater tendency to want to work in hospital and corporate pharmacy settings. However, there is some evidence to suggest that experiences of racial discrimination may push them back into areas of practice where they are less likely to encounter prejudice. So while culture and personal preference explains the presence of many of the older East African Indians in the self-employed business sector, structural factors such as racial discrimination, may be playing a small part in pushing the younger ethnic minority pharmacists into self-employment.

These changes may have important implications for the pharmacy workforce. Ethnic minorities, some groups more than others, are certainly influenced by the perceived business opportunities in pharmacy. However, as we have seen, this is against a background of

Table 2.3 Number (and %) home applicants and accepted applicants to pharmacy 1990 and 1998 by ethnic group

Ethnic origin	1990		1998	
	Applicants	Accepted	Applicants	Accepted
White	2906 (59%)	711 (63%)	1848 (45%)	860 (52%)
Indian	929 (19%)	194 (17%)	815 (20%)	280 (17%)
Pakistani	396 (8%)	77 (7%)	568 (13.7%)	189 (11.5%)
Bangladeshi	56 (1.1%)	9 (0.8%)	87 (2.1%)	27 (1.6%)
Chinese	87 (1.8%)	11 (1%)	91 (2.2%)	43 (2.6%)
Other Asian	128 (2.6%)	31 (2.7%)	164 (4%)	63 (3.8%)
Black African	242 (4.9%)	31 (2.7%)	275 (6.7%)	75 (4.6%)
Black Caribbean			23 (0.6%)	7 (0.4%)
Black Other			24 (0.6%)	5 (0.3%)
Other	74 (1.5%)	18 (1.6%)	95 (2.3%)	37 (2.2%)
Unknown	113 (2.3%)	44 (3.9%)	145 (3.5%)	56 (3.4%)
All ethnic minority	1912 (39%)	371 (33%)	2142 (52%)	726 (44%)
Grand Total	4931	1126	4135	1642

falling opportunities for ownership, and increasing employee status. In addition, large shortfalls are expected in the future in the number of graduates filling hospital places (Royal Pharmaceutical Society of Great Britain 1996b). Thus, any reluctance on the part of the pharmacy profession to encourage diversification, or any reluctance among ethnic minority pharmacists, at an aggregate level, to enter hospital practice could have serious consequences for the health service in the future. Ethnic minority pharmacy graduates, indeed all graduates, may require more encouragement to move into sectors other than community pharmacy, particularly hospital pharmacy where a short-age of workforce is anticipated.

The success of such a strategy will largely depend on the pharmacy profession's willingness to accept any such movement into new practice areas by the ethnic minority pharmacists. It will also depend on increasing the awareness among white and ethnic minority groups of where the job opportunities in pharmacy are, and encouraging new recruits to consider a diversified range of career alternatives. Whether this happens is also likely to depend on salaries in hospital practice matching those in community pharmacy. Moreover, if ethnic minority pharmacists are experiencing discrimination in hospital and corporate settings, there is a case for encouraging employers to eliminate any disadvantages experienced by their staff.

Age and retirement

Another factor which will have an impact on the supply side of the pharmacy workforce equation is the age of existing practitioners. More than one third of all men on the UK register in 1994 were aged more than 55, compared with only 16% of the women. Many independent business owners, mostly men in their 50s, are selling their pharmacies to multiples and taking early retirement. Although often remaining as registered pharmacists, they may not return to work at all or may choose to work part-time for a number of years. If early retirement becomes widespread, then workforce supply may become even more problematic, especially if losses from the workforce are not matched by gains.

The significance of part-time work in workforce issues

Part-time work in pharmacy is usually discussed within the context of other studies, such as those concerning women in pharmacy, where it is seen as an important facet of women pharmacists' working lives. Indeed, in the labour market as a whole, part-time work is perceived as 'women's work', as five out of every six part-timers in Great Britain are female. Most of the literature on part-time work characterises it in this way, as 'women's work', where it is mostly viewed as 'marginal' (Myrdal and Klein 1956). It is often perceived as a 'trap' by means of which women are exploited as part of the secondary sector of the labour market, or of the reserve army of labour (Tam 1997). Other studies have focussed on part-time workers as being in some way different from full-time workers. There is reference to part-timers being, for example, less committed to their work (Hakim 1995). In general, part-time work is rarely considered as an issue in its own right, and furthermore, there is very little work on the nature of men's part-time working patterns.

Evidence suggests that pharmacy may be a special case. It represents a professional occupation, where, in terms of salary, work conditions and status, part-timers might be relatively less disadvantaged. It also differs in that a significant proportion of those who work part-time are male. Part-time work patterns are also extremely varied. A workforce survey conducted in 1978 differentiated between regular part-time work and casual or locum work (Royal Pharmaceutical Society of Great Britain 1980). A later survey undertaken in 1994 by the National Association of Women Pharmacists drew a distinction between employee and self-employed part-timers and between those working for independent or company pharmacies. A 'qualitative workforce' survey commissioned by the RPSGB in 1995 has highlighted some part-time work as an 'additional' occupation, that is, work done in addition to other work (Jefferson and Korabinski 1996).

An even greater variety of work patterns undertaken by part-time pharmacists has been described. They may work regular pre-arranged hours, or work at short notice. They may have one pattern of working, or a combination of several, and the patterns usually change over time as domestic circumstances and career aspirations change (Symonds 1998). There are also some gender-related differences regarding part-time work patterns. Men are more likely to be self-employed, to work for independent pharmacies or for a variety of types of pharmacy, and to work at short notice or have a mixture of working patterns. Women on the other hand, are more likely to be employees, to work for a multiple pharmacy chain, and to have pre-arranged work patterns. Symonds (1998) has also shown that the concepts of part-time work as either a 'bridge' or a 'trap', as described in previous employment studies (notably Tam 1997) were found to have some application to part-time work in community pharmacy. For some part-timers, their work is viewed as part of a long-term career plan which enables them to make the transition ('crossing the bridge') back into full-time work or into another occupation. Similarly, for older pharmacists approaching the end of their full-time career, part-time work is often seen as part of the 'winding down' process – a 'bridge' into retirement. However, where part-time work is seen as a 'career break', it is often perceived as a 'trap', which may have a disadvantageous effect on long-term career and promotion opportunities. On the other hand, this employment pattern does allow women, in particular, to pursue a '*practitioner*' career and to care for a family. For these pharmacists a return to full-time work may not be envisaged.

There is also a third concept of part-time work – as a '*balance*' – which can be applied in the particular case of pharmacy. Some part-time pharmacists stress the importance of having the freedom to choose where and when they work. They are most often self-employed pharmacists, rather than employees, and are taking advantage of the current favourable labour market conditions in pharmacy. They prioritise their different commitments: to family, to work, to study, to leisure pursuits and to community activities, describing this prioritisation as a '*balancing act*'. They generally express a high degree of satisfaction with their work pattern, seeing themselves as having the best of all worlds.

Factors previously mentioned, such as the legal requirements that necessitate the presence of a registered pharmacist on the pharmacy premises at all times, and the extended opening hours of many pharmacies, mean that pharmacies, especially in the community sector, may rely heavily on the services of part-time pharmacists. So whereas the general assumption is that part-time work reduces the supply of pharmacists, it may well be that part-time workers are actually filling a very real need.

Whilst research has shown that part-time workers have different and complex work patterns which are interpreted as having positive or negative outcomes for them as individuals, how part-time work is viewed by pharmacy employers has not yet been investigated. There are other occupations where workers taking a career break, or working part-time, are seen as creating a labour market '*problem*' with which managers have to deal. However, it may be that in the case of pharmacy, employers see part-time workers as a valuable and flexible labour supply with the ability to adapt to different work situations. They may see them as equally committed to their profession as full-time pharmacists, and fully justifying the investment that has been made in their training.

Other factors affecting supply

Other factors which affect the supply of pharmacists include the competition for posts, (both within different geographical locations and within professional '*specialties*'), the demands of training in a given specialty, and recruitment and retention policies in different practice areas. In the UK, problems associated with these policies have largely been attributed to pharmacists' job dissatisfaction due to factors intrinsic to the job, such as long hours, stress, and uncertainty over new working roles (Willett and Cooper 1996). High levels of staff turnover within community pharmacy in the USA have similarly been explained by the poor conditions under which pharmacists are expected to work. In one study of USA pharmacy practice, long hours and lack of help from support personnel were features of job dissatisfaction which led to the decisions of many pharmacists to leave their positions (Schulz and Baldwin 1990).

CONCLUSION

Despite workforce planning being fundamental to the continuing development of any profession, robust empirical and detailed evidence about pharmacy workforce issues is scarce, evidence varies between countries, theories explaining workforce changes are not uniform, and arguments about workforce shortages are by no means resolved. Nevertheless, several key features about the changing patterns of work and the demand for pharmacists, which have been highlighted here, have a potential bearing on the debate. Although pharmacist numbers have been increasing steadily, this trend may be threatened by moves towards earlier retirement, by the growth in part-time working, and by the increasing proportion of women on the register. Greater *'corporatisation'* has increased demand for pharmacists, and since hospital and community pharmacy must recruit from the same pool of graduates, competition between sectors is likely to exacerbate the problem.

Graduation, retirement and death are among the more obvious factors that alter the size of the pharmacy workforce. Others include: individual career preferences on leaving school, size of intake into schools of pharmacy, dissatisfaction with career choices, the likelihood of female pharmacists with dependent children working part-time for at least part of their working lives, and changes in the demand for pharmacists following a reduction in the number of independent pharmacies.

FURTHER READING

Bottero, W. (1994) The Changing Face of the Profession? Gender and Explanations of Women's Entry to Pharmacy. *Work, Employment and Society*, **6**, 329–346.

Hassell, K., Noyce, P. and Jesson, J. (1998) A comparative and historical account of ethnic minority participation in the pharmacy profession. *Work, Employment and Society* **12**, 245–271.

Tam, M. (1997) *Part-time Employment – A Bridge or a Trap?* Ashgate Avebury, London.

REFERENCES

Anderson, R.A., Bickle, K.R. and Wang, E. (1990) Pharmacy labour market assessment 1989. *Australian Journal of Pharmacy*, **71**, 492–501.

Bottero, W. (1994) The changing face of the profession? Gender and explanations of women's entry to pharmacy. *Work, Employment and Society*, **6**, 329–346.

Crompton, R. and Sanderson, K. (1990) *Gendered Jobs and Social Change*, Unwin Hyman Ltd., London.

Fanaeian, F., Jones, P.E. and Mottram, D.R. (1988) Women returning to pharmacy: a regional survey. *Pharmaceutical Journal*, **241**, R14.

Hassell, K., Noyce, P., Rogers, A., Harris, J. and Wilkinson, J. (1997) A pathway to the GP: the pharmaceutical 'consultation' as a first port of call in primary health care. *Family Practice*, **14**, 498–502.

Hakim, C. (1995) Five feminist myths about women's employment. *British Journal of Sociology*, **46**, 429–55.

Hassell, K. (1997) *An historical and comparative account of ethnic minority group participation in the pharmacy profession in the United Kingdom.* PhD Thesis (unpublished) University of Manchester.

Hassell, K., Noyce, P. and Jesson, J. (1998) A comparative and historical account of ethnic minority participation in the pharmacy profession. *Work, Employment and Society*, **12**, 245–271.

Jefferson, G.C. and Korabinski, A.A. (1996) *Report on the Qualitative Manpower Survey of the Home Register*, Royal Pharmaceutical Society of Great Britain, London.

Knapp, K.K. (1994) Pharmacy manpower: implications for pharmaceutical care and health care reform. *American Journal of Hospital Pharmacy*, **5**, 1212–1220.

Magirr, P. and Ottewill, R. (1995) Measuring the employee/contractor balance. *Pharmaceutical Journal*, **254**, 876–79.

Muzzin, L., Brown, G.P. and Hornosty, R.W. (1994) Consequences of feminisation of a profession: the case of Canadian Pharmacy. *Women and Health*, **21**, 39–56.

Myrdal, A. and Klein, V. (1956) *Women's Two Roles*, Routledge and Kegan Paul, London.

Norris, P. (1997) Gender and occupational change: women and retail pharmacy in New Zealand. *Australian and New Zealand Journal of Sociology*, **33**, 21–38.

Rees, J.A. and Clarke, D.J. (1990) Employment, career progression and mobility of recently registered male and female pharmacists. *Pharmaceutical Journal*, **245**, R30.

Reskin, B. and Roos, P. (1987) Status hierarchies and sex segregation. In: C. Bose and G. Spittz (Eds.) *Ingredients for Women's Employment Policy*. Suny, Albany, USA.

Royal Pharmaceutical Society of Great Britain (1980) Survey of part-time pharmacists. *Pharmaceutical Journal*, **224**, 44–45.

Royal Pharmaceutical Society of Great Britain (1996a) Survey of pharmacists, 1993 and 1994. *Pharmaceutical Journal*, **256**, 784–786.

Royal Pharmaceutical Society of Great Britain (1996b) Survey suggests hospital manpower shortages. *Pharmaceutical Journal*, **256**, 853.

Schulz, R.M and Baldwin, H.J. (1990) Chain pharmacists turnover. *Journal of Administrative and Social Pharmacy*, **7**, 26–33.

Symonds, B.S. (1998) *Part-time work in community pharmacy: a bridge, a trap, or a balance?* Ph.D. Thesis (unpublished) University of Nottingham.

Tam, M. (1997) *Part-time Employment – A Bridge or a Trap?* Ashgate Avebury, London.

Willett, V.J. and Cooper, C.L. (1996) Stress and job satisfaction in community pharmacy: a pilot study. *Pharmaceutical Journal*, **256**, 94–98.

Self-Assessment Questions

Question 1: List the factors which impact on the supply of, and demand for, pharmacists.

Question 2: What key changes in the workforce have taken place in the last few decades?

Question 3: In what different ways can part-time working be defined?

Question 4: Discuss the arguments for women's entry into pharmacy being linked with either the *'up-grading'* or *'down-grading'* of the profession.

KEY POINTS FOR ANSWERS

Question 1:

Supply factors include:

- Increasing proportions of women
- Increasing proportions of ethnic minority groups
- Age of practitioners
- Retirement rates
- Career satisfaction
- Career motivation
- Changes to the pharmacy curriculum
- Competition for posts
- Salary

Demand factors include:

- Shift towards primary care led health services
- Increased patient through-put in hospitals
- Increasing importance of large multiples
- Practice and professional developments
- Organisational changes, eg. longer hours

Question 2:

- More women
- Fewer men
- More ethnic minority groups
- Fewer independents
- More multiples

Question 3:

- Marginal or secondary employment
- Levels of commitment
- A '*Bridge*' to full-time work after career breaks
- A '*Trap*' when career opportunities and promotion prospects are adversely affected
- A '*Balance*' where the best of both worlds between family and work is achieved

Question 4:

Evidence in support of up-grading thesis:

- Increased educational qualifications
- Greater professionalisation
- Most women work full-time

Evidence in support of down-grading thesis:

- Presence of job hierarchies in which women are kept at practitioner levels
- Work has become routine
- Work has become de-skilled
- The presence of a secondary (i.e. part-time) labour market

3 Primary and Secondary Care Pharmacy

Catherine Duggan

INTRODUCTION	50
RECENT CHANGES IN HEALTH POLICY	50
PRESCRIBING ACROSS THE HEALTH CARE INTERFACE	50
The pharmacist's role in 'shared care'	51
The hospital pharmacist's role in patient care	51
The community pharmacist's role in patient care	52
Information transfer between the primary and secondary sector	53
Improving information transfer between hospital and community pharmacy	53
CONCLUSION	55
REFERENCES	55
SELF-ASSESSMENT QUESTIONS	56
KEY POINTS FOR ANSWERS	56

INTRODUCTION

This chapter describes the influences of health policy on the delivery of pharmaceutical care within community and hospital settings and the continuing development of seamless pharmaceutical care between these sectors. Whilst the focus is on pharmacy in the UK, reference is also made to comparable changes and influences on pharmacy in Europe, the USA, Canada and Australia.

In recent years, pharmacy, like other health professions, has undergone a change in the way it is practised as a consequence of technological advance and the changes in the nature of health care delivery. Changes in UK health policy beginning in the 1980s, including increased accountability of prescribers, the shifting emphasis towards disease prevention and self-medication, and a focus on primary care led health services. All have impacted on the delivery of primary and secondary pharmaceutical care.

RECENT CHANGES IN HEALTH POLICY

Since the inception of the National Health Service (NHS) in 1948, successive governments have struggled to balance the supply of, and demand for, health care. As medicines and technologies advance, and expectations of health increase, so too does the cost of meeting these demands. In the 1980s recommendations were made to increase the effectiveness of management within the NHS and to make general practitioners more accountable for the costs of the medicines they prescribed.

Legislation in 1990 imposed the principle of *'market forces'* on the provision of health care with separation of purchasers from providers of health care. Budget-holders (purchasers) included health authorities, general practitioners and private health care insurance companies. Suppliers (providers) included hospitals, private and voluntary care units (residential and non-residential care). Contracts and agreements were drawn up that itemised the costs of services, treatment levels and quality standards between the purchasers and providers. The so-called *'internal health care market system'* was in place.

PRESCRIBING ACROSS THE HEALTH CARE INTERFACE

At this time, new contracts increased accountability for prescribing and threatened the long established relationship between primary and secondary health care. General practitioners with constrained prescribing budgets were required to absorb the costs of expensive drugs such as erythropoietin, growth hormone, intravenous antibiotics for cystic fibrosis, ondansetron and fertility drugs prescribed at discharge by hospital specialists under the new arrangements – a practice described emotively as *'cost-dumping'* by general practitioners who were left to *'carry the costs'* in the community.

Guidance to ensure a smooth transfer of care for patients from hospital to their general practitioner was issued by the UK government in 1992. This proposed a *'shared care'* arrangement, whereby hospital consultants could notify general practitioners of any changes to a patient's diagnosis or drug therapy in adequate time, so that ongoing treatment is maintained following patient discharge.

The pharmacist's role in 'shared care'

Since the inception of shared care, pharmacists have been encouraged to develop guidelines for treatment in primary and secondary care, and provide expert pharmaceutical advice to inform the cost-effective delivery of expensive new therapies and 'lifestyle' drugs. These guidelines have numerous associated benefits such as cost-effective integration of primary and secondary prescribing, increased knowledge of newer therapies, and to provide support for general practitioners and community pharmacists with shared responsibilities for monitoring new therapies. However, the term *'shared care'* implied equal and shared responsibility for patients across the primary and secondary sectors, which could be contentious. To overcome this, the delivery of a consistent standard of care across the health care interface was renamed *'seamless care'*, defined as: *'... the desirable continuity in care delivery that a patient receives when they move back home from a hospital, requiring both health care sectors to work in unison rather than as separate entities'* (Barrett and Tomes 1992).

For seamless care to be achieved, effective communication between health care workers in both sectors is required. The Royal Pharmaceutical Society of Great Britain identified the concept of seamless care as an opportunity to explore the complementary roles of community and hospital pharmacists, which had hitherto developed largely in isolation of each other, and identify how they could best work together in the future (Royal Pharmaceutical Society of Great Britain 1992).

The hospital pharmacist's role in patient care

During the early 1980s, hospital pharmacists' responsibilities included taking drug histories, monitoring drug therapy and counselling patients. It was estimated that 15% of hospital admissions for elderly patients result from medication related problems including adverse drug reactions, drug interactions, inappropriate prescribing, and poor adherence to the prescribed regimen (Taylor and Chaduri 1992). Research published in the 1990s provided evidence for the additional roles of hospital pharmacists in addressing these problems. For instance, prescribing errors or omissions were reduced when pharmacists interviewed patients following hospital admission, and more appropriate medicines management resulted from increased treatment review by pharmacists (Cantrill and Clark 1992). In the USA, pharmacists were shown to prevent adverse drug reactions (Lin and Anderson 1997), whilst in Canada drug-related problems were reduced as a result of increased pharmaceutical care (Shalansky *et al.* 1996).

Hospital pharmacists increasingly provide drug advice, initiate prescribing, contribute to continuity of care, and are actively involved in discharge planning, as described later in this section. It has been suggested that as technicians assume a greater number of duties in the pharmacy, pharmacists will be able to devote more time to ensuring the delivery of seamless and effective pharmaceutical care (Dosaj and Mistry 1998).

Whilst hospital pharmacists in the UK have acknowledged their role in providing seamless pharmaceutical care across the health care interface, has a comparable role for community pharmacists been established?

The community pharmacist's role in patient care

Increasingly, community pharmacists are assuming the role of medicines' advisers and regularly assist patients in the management of their medication. These roles are enhanced by maintenance of computerised patient medication records (PMRs) and by the increasing deregulation of drugs available for over the counter (OTC) sale, which enables them to advise and treat a wider range of minor symptoms.

Legislation in 1990 recommended that appropriate information should be given to patients whenever possible, to explain therapy and give full and clear instructions. Subsequently, in 1995, UK pharmacists were required to counsel patients personally and ensure that prescription details were understood (Royal Pharmaceutical Society of Great Britain 1995). Likewise, patients throughout Europe and Scandinavia regularly seek more information from community pharmacists as they perceive them as accessible and appropriately qualified. Community pharmacists' activities have extended to encompass all issues of *'medicines management'*, including monitoring patient compliance, modifying drug therapy, communicating medication risk, counselling on the use of OTC drugs and medication review. In the USA, the development of programmes to deliver medical aid, benefited from community pharmacists' input and recommended that pharmaceutical care be incorporated into such aid programmes to ensure cost-effective use of the best available therapies.

Pharmacists' input into medicines management has been increasingly successful. For instance, pharmacists' interventions have resulted in safe and effective medicines use and reductions in drug-related morbidity. Furthermore, community pharmacy-based PMRs have been used to reduce drug-related problems resulting from incomplete drug-history taking on admission to a hospital, whilst pharmacy involvement in discharge summaries, has reduced prescribing errors. However, the transfer of information between hospital and community pharmacists, although desirable, is not routine. Three quarters of hospitals do not routinely supply written information for the patient's community pharmacist (Gray *et al.* 1996; Argyle and Newman 1996). Where communication has been established, both hospital and community pharmacists are enthusiastic about working together and the quality of patient care increases.

Information transfer between the primary and secondary sector

Problems were found to occur with medication following discharge from hospital and it has been suggested that approximately half of discharged elderly patients deviate from their prescribed drug regimen. Even when patients bring details of their symptoms and drugs to all consultations, discrepancies still occur, including changed doses, medicines being stopped or new ones started. Possible factors for these discrepancies include incomplete drug histories, continuation of drugs taken before admission, and changes in drug therapy not attributable to clinical decisions. A lack of information may also contribute to the incidence of these inconsistencies.

Effective communication between hospital and community sectors is essential to ensure that practitioners and patients are adequately informed about their discharge prescription and continuation treatment. Yet problems with supplies of prescribed drugs continue to be identified. For instance, elderly patients may not be issued with new prescriptions from their general practitioner following discharge, pre-admission supplies of prescribed medicines have been found in patients' homes, and medication discrepancies have been identified on admission to nursing homes (Burns *et al.* 1992). Overcoming these problems requires close liaison between hospital and community pharmacists, to ensure the effective transfer of drug-related information.

Improving information transfer between hospital and community pharmacy

Since the early 1990s, the provision of health care has shifted away from hospitals to the community. The successful provision of seamless care requires co-operation across all sectors of health care. Communication has been formalised between consultants and general practitioners, and although the pharmacists' role in seamless care is recognised, there has not traditionally been a formalised means of communication between hospital and community pharmacists.

Pharmacy discharge planning was thus initiated to formalise the provision of seamless pharmaceutical care as:

'... *the process whereby a patient is moved from one care environment to another with the assurance that all pharmaceutical requirements, including information, can be communicated and maintained in a safe, timely, efficient and user-friendly way*'   (Jackson *et al.* 1993).

The Royal Pharmaceutical Society of Great Britain recommended that there should be direct communication between hospital and community pharmacists, either by telephone or letter, but recognised that it would be difficult to implement such a system. There was a need for community support in continuing pharmaceutical care for elderly patients. Checklists for hospital pharmacists were designed to assess individual need and plan a programme of pharmaceutical care to facilitate the safe management of medicines (Coombes and Horne 1994). This formed a basis for pharmaceutical discharge planning, with the patient presenting the checklist at their community pharmacy to aid the smooth transfer of information.

The checklists initially formed the basis for pharmacy care plans, providing each identified patient with a visit from their community pharmacist once they had returned home, to ensure that all their pharmaceutical needs were met. The care plan was a means of communication between the two health care sectors. Such care plans were, however, specific for the elderly, labour-intensive and expensive to implement, but did provide a high standard of pharmaceutical care (Binyon 1994).

At this time a number of studies described the discrepancies between supplies of prescribed drugs following transfer of elderly patients from secondary to primary care, though these focussed on elderly patients who tend to be prescribed more drugs than other patient groups, and move in and out of hospital care more frequently. A study of general medical patients, investigated the incidence of such discrepancies in the supplies of prescribed drugs obtained by this patient group as they moved between hospital and community care. When community pharmacists were provided with information regarding drugs prescribed at discharge, the number of unintentional discrepancies observed in drug supplies was significantly reduced (Duggan *et al.* 1998). This study recommended that community pharmacists routinely received such information to reduce these problems following hospital discharge.

The concept of working together to improve patient care does not stop at pharmacists working with pharmacists across the health care interface but also has implications for inter-professional working: '*In a seamless service, organisational boundaries do not get in the way of care for patients ...*' (Department of Health 1997) ... '*a system of integrated care, based on partnership and driven by performance ...*' (Department of Health 1998).

In 1999, the UK Government initiated and implemented Primary Care Groups to shape services for patients by increasing multi-professional working within the primary care sector (see also Chapter 15). Such developments are not isolated to the UK. For instance, pharmacists in the USA are being urged to take part in the development of drug therapy guidelines for cost-effective quality care and to ensure the professions become integrated (Rough et al. 1996).

CONCLUSION

By giving community pharmacists information regarding drugs prescribed at discharge, they are able to be actively involved in the planning discharge process and reduce problems with prescribed drugs. Pharmacists, in both primary and secondary health care sectors, are able to capitalise on their drug knowledge base and, through interactions with the patients, ensure informed medicines management.

REFERENCES

Argyle, M. and Newman, C. (1996) An assessment of pharmacy discharge procedures and hospital communications with general practitioners. *Pharmaceutical Journal*, **256**, 903–905.

Barrett, C. and Tomes, J. (1992) Shared care: the way forward. *Hospital Update Plus*, 9–10.

Binyon, D. (1994) Pharmaceutical care: its impact on patient care and the hospital-community interface. *Pharmaceutical Journal*, **253**, 344–349.

Burns, J.A., Snedon, I., Lovell, M., McLean, A. and Martin, B.J. (1992) Elderly patients and their medication: a post discharge follow up study. *Age and Ageing*, **2**, 178–181.

Cantrill, J. and Clarke, C. (1992) Discharge counselling by pharmacists the need and the reality. *Hospital Pharmacy Practice*, **2**, 429–433.

Coombes, J. and Horne, R. (1994) A checklist for medication discharge planning. *Pharmaceutical Journal*, **253**, 161–163.

Department of Health (1997) *The National Health Service: a Service with Ambition*, HMSO, London.

Department of Health (1998) *The New NHS: Modern, Dependable*, HMSO, London.

Dosaj, R. and Mistry, R. (1998) The pharmacy technician in clinical services. *Hospital Pharmacist*, **5**, 26–28.

Duggan C., Feldman R., Hough J. and Bates I. (1998) Reducing adverse prescribing discrepancies following hospital discharge. *International Journal of Pharmacy Practice*, **6**, 77–82.

Gray, S.J., Gray, A.J. and Woolfrey, S. (1996) Community pharmacists and discharge medication advice to patients. *Pharmaceutical Journal*, **256 (suppl.)**, R27.

Jackson, C., Rowe, P. and Lea, R. (1993) Pharmacy discharge – a professional necessity for the 1990s. *Pharmaceutical Journal*, **250**, 58–59.

Lin, B. and Anderson, L.R. (1997) Role of the pharmacy department in the prevention of adverse drug events: survey of current practice. *Pharmacy Practice Management Quarterly*, **17**, 10–16.

Rough, T.B., Meek, P.D. and Thiekle, T.S. (1996) Pharmacy's role in the clinical practice guideline development process. *ASHP Annual Meeting*, **53 (June)**, MCS-2.

Royal Pharmaceutical Society of Great Britain (1995) New standard requires counseling by pharmacist. *Pharmaceutical Journal*, **254**, 833.

Royal Pharmaceutical Society of Great Britain (1992) Policy statement: pharmaceutical aspects of community care. *Pharmaceutical Journal*, **248**, 541–544.

Shalansky, S., Nakagawa, R. and Wee, A. (1996) Drug-related problems identified and resolved using pharmaceutical care. *Canadian Journal of Hospital Pharmacy*, **49**, 282–288.

Taylor, K. and Chaudhuri, M. (1992) Adverse drug reactions as a cause of hospital admissions. *Care of the Elderly*, **3**, 110–116.

SELF-ASSESSMENT QUESTIONS

Question 1: Discuss the barriers to successful seamless care and how these have been overcome.

Question 2: How does pharmaceutical care fit into the wider agenda of the NHS?

KEY POINTS FOR ANSWERS

Question 1:

Communication between professionals has been repeatedly identified as the main barrier for seamless care. This communication is particularly apparent when documenting the development of hospital and community pharmacy over the last decade. Each sector developed in isolation of the other. Drug-related problems were seen to occur as a result of poor levels of communication, as simple as the transfer of information, especially documenting the drugs prescribed to patients.

Developments included:

- Pharmacy checklists
- Pharmacy discharge planning
- Pharmaceutical care plans (especially for the elderly)
- Evidence-based approach to improving seamless pharmaceutical care
- Changing policy through evidence

Question 2:

The concept of working together to improve patient care does not stop at pharmacists working with pharmacists across the health care interface. This fits into the current and previous governments' commitment to increased multi-professional working.

The developments include:

- Local drive for quality through Primary Care Groups
- Promoting the unique role in the continuous standard of care patients receive
- Pharmacists are the health care professional who can ensure safe and appropriate medicines management
- Pharmacists must discard the notion of the hospital or community practitioner, whilst promoting the concept of pharmacist as *the* professional with medicines management expertise

The evidence:

- The unique positions of community and hospital pharmacists
- The interactive component of advising or informing patients about their medicines
- A concordant approach to understanding and informing patient behaviour towards prescribed drugs
- Pharmacists are increasingly integrated in primary and secondary health care teams

PART TWO

International Dimensions of Pharmacy Practice

4 Community Pharmacy in Europe

Foppe van Mil

INTRODUCTION	62
PHARMACY EDUCATION	62
HEALTH CARE SYSTEMS	63
Other providers of medicines	64
Availability of over the counter medicines	64
Professional protection	65
The size of pharmacies in Europe	65
The staffing of pharmacies in Europe	66
The range of products available from European pharmacies	66
The services provided in European pharmacies	67
Clinical pharmacy services	67
Pharmaceutical care	67
Diagnostic testing	68
Drug information to the public	68
Drug information to other professionals	69
CONCLUSION	69
ACKNOWLEDGEMENT	70
REFERENCES	70
SELF-ASSESSMENT QUESTIONS	70
KEY POINTS FOR ANSWERS	70

INTRODUCTION

In Europe, pharmacies are places where the public can get medicines. This however, is the only common denominator. In the past, pharmacy revolved around the manufacture and provision of medicines, rather than on those who consumed them. However, in the latter half of the twentieth century extemporaneous preparations largely disappeared in many European countries, such as Denmark, Greece, Portugal and Sweden. In the Netherlands they currently constitute 5.3% of all dispensed medicines. In the 1960s and 70s the focus of pharmacists' activities shifted towards an increased emphasis on the effects of medicines, namely clinical pharmacy. This change happened throughout Europe, although the pace of change differed between countries.

Pharmacies in Europe differ considerably in terms of size, staffing and the services provided, reflecting the independent development of health care across Europe. Before discussing these elements, this chapter will explore some of the factors which serve to explain these international variations.

The availability of medicines varies throughout Europe, due to differences in the registration procedures and policies of their pharmaceutical industries. However, the introduction of the European Agency for the Evaluation of Medical Products (EMEA) in 1993 will increasingly reduce this variation between countries belonging to the European Union, although national authorities still have some power under the so called decentralised procedure. The EMEA's new system for the licensing of medicinal products was introduced in 1995.

In most European countries only physicians, dentists and veterinary practitioners are permitted to prescribe medicines. However, Irish pharmacists have prescribing rights and in the UK it has been proposed that limited prescribing rights be extended to nurses and pharmacists (Crown 1999).

PHARMACY EDUCATION

Although there have been attempts to promote international cooperation and convergence, the content and duration of pharmacy courses vary greatly between countries. In most countries there has been a shift within the curriculum away from chemistry and biology, to a more clinical and social emphasis. The Scandinavian countries, the UK and the Netherlands were the first to incorporate clinical pharmacy into their curricula and Germany will probably include clinical pharmacy in the official pharmacy curriculum in 2000. There are however, still countries within Europe whose pharmacy education does not encompass clinical pharmacy. Many countries now also teach social pharmacy, including communication skills, as a separate subject area.

The duration of pharmacy courses varies between four and six years, with the average age of pharmacy graduates between 22 and 26 years. Subsequently, graduates undertake a further six months to four years of training before they are fully licensed as pharmacists. In some countries, some of those involved in the supply of medicines are not university educated. For example, some Scandinavian countries have *receptars*, who do not receive a university education, but have approximately the same rights as pharmacists. Receptars receive a two and a half year non-university training, which includes nine months' placement in a pharmacy. They can therefore be compared with the Dutch assistant-pharmacist. In the Netherlands, these assistant-pharmacists undertake a three year non-university education which includes a placement in a pharmacy. Both professions may only practice under (indirect) supervision of a pharmacist.

HEALTH CARE SYSTEMS

The national drug budgets in Europe vary between 9% (The Netherlands) and 26.4% (Portugal) of the national health care costs in the different countries. The high percentage in countries like Portugal and Spain (21%) can be explained by the relative low expenditures on health care in general. This also explains why some governments are more active in controlling drug costs than others. Nevertheless, the drug's budget is an important area for cost containment in most European countries. The cost of drug consumption, per capita, in 1998 varied between 400 Euros in Spain and 690 Euros in Switzerland. These differences are only partially due to different pricing systems but are mainly due to differences in consumption volume. Although the majority of European countries have a health care system wherein the rich support the poor, the systems for paying for medicines vary widely. This results in differences in the access of the population to drugs, depending on individual wealth and insurance systems. The UK is alone within Europe in having a National Health System (NHS) which has enabled health care costs, of which the drug budget is a part, to be controlled. Most other countries have a form of NHS for people with a low income, usually called a sick fund, and a private insurance system for people having a higher income. However, in some countries the state supports the insurance companies by paying part of their expenses. The method of remuneration in different countries is reflected in the administrative burden upon pharmacies. Co-payment systems vary throughout Europe. A co-payment is that part of the drug price paid by the patient. This can be a certain percentage, a stepped scale or a fixed sum. Whatever the patient has to pay to a pharmacist to obtain a medicine is regarded as the co-payment.

In many countries, e.g. the Netherlands and Denmark, the concept of co-payment has now been fully accepted. In Germany, the physicians' drug budgets are limited and they are being punished financially if they overspend their budgets. In other countries, such as

Hungary, Greece and the Netherlands, governments are trying to influence drug expenditure by stimulating pharmacotherapeutic discussions between physicians, pharmacists and sometimes hospital administrators.

Pharmacies are usually either independent or part of a chain. In Sweden the pharmacy system is different from the rest of Europe. In fact all Swedish pharmacies are owned by a '*company*', Apoteket (called Apoteksbolaget up until 1999). All community and hospital pharmacists are employees of this company. Although there have been attempts to break this 'company's' monopoly on drug-distribution, the issue is not scheduled to be addressed until 2001.

Other providers of medicines

In a number of European countries such as Austria, France, Iceland, the Netherlands and the UK, physicians may supply medicines to patients, usually in sparsely populated areas. The reason for this is that pharmacies in those areas are not commercially viable, and physicians are the most ready source of expertise about medicines. Often they are supported by pharmacists who compound preparations and occasionally supply drugs to the physician's pharmacy. However, in Switzerland dispensing doctors can also be found in cities and compete with pharmacists for their share of the drug-market.

Veterinary medicines are also sometimes dispensed through pharmacies, for instance in Finland, Iceland and Luxembourg. In other countries veterinarians dispense these drugs.

Although some attempts have been made to establish mail-order pharmacy in different European countries, this form of dispensing has not (yet) become popular, probably because Europe is relatively densely populated compared with the USA. Internet pharmacies have also not yet really penetrated the European market, although there are signals that some Europeans are starting to buy their medicines from internet companies. This applies especially to lifestyle drugs and alternative remedies.

Availability of over the counter medicines

Although Prescription Only Medicines (POM) are routinely supplied from pharmacies, the outlets for over the counter (OTC) medicines are varied. For a long time OTC medicines were only available from pharmacies, with the exception of the Netherlands and Germany where druggists (a person with a license obtained after a two-year part time non university education) were allowed to sell a limited assortment. The increasing pressure from the pharmaceutical industry in the 1990s has changed this situation. Many OTC medicines are now available in many countries through outlets, such as supermarkets and petrol/gas stations. Some Scandinavian and southern European countries still do not have this option with all medicines being sold through pharmacies, although change is imminent. In order to reduce drug costs, there has been a move to make some previously prescription only medicines available for sale. Consequently, the sale of OTC medicines from pharmacies and other outlets in some countries has increased (see also Chapters 9 and 10).

Professional protection

In the past, throughout Europe, only pharmacists could own a pharmacy (one pharmacy, one pharmacist). This is now changing, since governments want to introduce more competition in the distribution process for medicines, in anticipation that costs will be reduced.

In some countries, the government or pharmacy's professional body regulates the establishment/registration of a pharmacy. In the Scandinavian countries and the Netherlands the latter system resulted in relatively large pharmacies. In the Netherlands and Iceland this system has recently been abandoned. In Iceland this has resulted in smaller more competitive pharmacies, but in the Netherlands no similar effect has been observed. In Denmark and Norway the number of pharmacies is still restricted, and to become a pharmacy owner involves a rather complicated selection procedure, which ultimately benefits elderly pharmacists. However, in both countries, that system is under political pressure as well, and in Norway, will change in 2001.

The size of pharmacies in Europe

The size of pharmacies in Europe shows large differences (Table 4.1). In some countries, pharmacies serve relatively small populations (i.e. there are a large number of pharmacies serving a relatively small population), e.g. those in France and Spain, which on average, serve less than 3000 people, whilst in Greece an average pharmacy serves only 1900 people. By contrast, the average Danish pharmacy serves a population of nearly 18000, though in Denmark there are satellite pharmacies which are an organisational part of the main pharmacy.

Although there is a clear correlation between the number of clients and the average size, calculated as surface area of the pharmacy, it is remarkable that this average surface area also shows a large variation (Table 4.1).

The amount of time devoted to each customer in a pharmacy also shows variation between countries. If one only considers the prescriptions dispensed to clients per licensed staff member, then a staff member in Finland dispenses on average 24 prescriptions daily, in Great Britain 76, and in Spain 140 prescriptions per day. These numbers are a reflection of the internal organisation of pharmacies. In Finland for instance, the pharmacist often sits behind a desk when assisting the client. Packages are opened and tablets counted. All medicines are dispensed with an individual label. In Spain packages are never opened and the stock in the (small) pharmacies is limited.

Country	Average population	Average size in m²
Austria	7841	200
Croatia	7385	100
Denmark	17869	470
Finland	6599	104
France	2667	80
Germany	3883	165
Greece	1143	47
Hungary	4878	80
Iceland	5556	200
Italy	3563	60
Luxembourg	5429	120
Netherlands	10263	240
Norway	12760	270
Poland	6094	150
Portugal	3958	85
Spain	2075	70
Sweden	7368	300
Switzerland	4245	217

Table 4.1 Average size and population served by community pharmacies

The staffing of pharmacies in Europe

Depending on its size, a pharmacy may have one or as many as ten pharmacists. Where there are many pharmacists, there are usually few non-trained staff employed. In many countries, pharmacy staff members are licensed, the exceptions being Greece, Spain, France and the UK. These non-pharmacist staff members can perform some of the dispensing tasks in a pharmacy. Their education, however, shows a broad variation. Whereas in the Netherlands assistant-pharmacists are allowed to dispense drugs without the necessity of a pharmacist on the premises, in almost all other countries the pharmacist must be present and must supervise and control the dispensing process carried out by assistants or technicians. This supervisory role does not require the pharmacist to control all activities of a trained assistant, rather the pharmacist must have overall control of the pharmacy.

The range of products available from European pharmacies

In Europe, dispensing of prescribed medicines comprises approximately 80% of a pharmacy's financial turnover. However, in Switzerland this figure is only 50%. In some countries, pharmacies are heavily dependent on the sale of non-medical items such as cosmetics and food. In Croatia, Italy and Ireland such items add more than 20% to a pharmacy's turnover. Cosmetics are particularly important in Portugal, Great Britain and Ireland where they account for more than 10% of the turnover. OTC medicines constitute a large proportion (around 30%) of pharmacies' turnover in countries such as Sweden and Switzerland.

The place of alternative medicines (herbal and homeopathic drugs) in pharmacies varies, partially as a result of the historical developments in a particular country. In Germany and the Eastern European countries for example, they are much more prominent than in the Scandinavian countries, where they currently have a minimal place in health care.

The services provided in European pharmacies

Clinical pharmacy services

As pharmacists have embraced clinical pharmacy as a concept, their concern about adverse effects and drug interactions has increased and they have found a new role in the protection of patients from undesirable drug effects and drug-related problems. In most countries this role is poorly structured and involves performing retrospective drug use evaluations (see also Chapter 22). Prospective drug use evaluation, or medication surveillance, is not yet standard in Europe although it certainly is part of the Good Pharmacy Practice (GPP) concept in most countries.

Reliable medication surveillance can only be performed using a computer and when key patient related data such as indications and contraindications are accessible. Although the majority of community pharmacies in Europe are computerised, these systems were not originally developed for a clinical pharmacy function, but rather to enable the billing for the drugs dispensed and for labelling of medicines. Additionally, in most Scandinavian countries privacy laws prohibit pharmacists from keeping patient-data for an extended period of time on a computer.

Well-developed computerised medication surveillance can be found in the Netherlands, but even here the indications for drug use are not available to the pharmacist. In Iceland and Denmark concurrent drug use evaluation is always carried out when patients present a prescription in the pharmacy. However, in these countries essential patient data are also missing and, unlike in the Netherlands, patients in Iceland and Denmark do not always go to the same pharmacy. In Austria, Croatia, Poland and Sweden no medication data are kept in the pharmacy (see Chapter 22 for further details on medication surveillance methods) for the time being.

Pharmaceutical care

Around 1990 in many European countries the focus of the pharmacist's activities started to shift from the drug to the patient. This was due in part to the pharmaceutical care philosophy, developed first by Hepler and Strand (1990) in the USA. Currently, most countries are trying to incorporate pharmaceutical care into the pharmacy systems, stimulated by the national pharmacists' organisations and the International Pharmaceutical Federation (FIP). In practice many barriers to this implementation process are apparent throughout Europe as shown in Box 4.1. Universities and national pharmacists' organisations are now trying to address these barriers.

Pharmaceutical care has not yet been assimilated across Europe. No clear change in pharmaceutical practice can yet be noted in Italy, Greece and the former Eastern European countries. The opportunities for pharmaceutical care appear to be greatest in countries with large, well-equipped pharmacies such as those in Scandinavian countries and the Netherlands, where the time and money barriers are not major issues.

Box 4.1 The major barriers to implementing pharmaceutical care as identified in a study of the Pharmaceutical Care Network Europe (PCNE) conducted by the University of Groningen in 1998–99

- Lack of resources
- Lack of pharmacist's time
- The attitude and opinion of other health professionals
- Inadequate communication skills by pharmacists
- The health care structure in general

Another major barrier is where patients do not always visit the same pharmacy. In most countries except Greece, Iceland, the Netherlands, Norway and Switzerland less than 80% of the people visit the same pharmacy when they need medicines. Because care is by definition, a process over time, this is an important consideration.

Diagnostic testing

In the past, a wide range of diagnostic tests have been conducted in pharmacies. Urine tests, for example, are performed by almost all pharmacies in Denmark, Germany, Iceland, Spain and Switzerland, but not elsewhere. In the same countries plus Portugal and Italy, patients can go to almost any pharmacy for a blood-pressure test. Spain is the only European country in which the majority of pharmacies offer glucose testing. Although the performance of blood and urine tests in pharmacies was quite common at the beginning of the twentieth century, in most countries these activities are now performed by specialist laboratories.

Drug information to the public

Most pharmacies in Europe provide drug information to the public, although this has not always been the case. In many countries, physicians have long claimed the right to provide patients with drug information as they feared patients would become confused if they received such information from different sources. However, when the pharmaceutical industry began to inform the patient (because of liability issues) the situation changed. Patients often became upset when reading information leaflets in packages and sought other sources of information. In the 1970s pharmacotherapy was included in the pharmacy curriculum in most countries and consequently pharmacists have the knowledge to provide appropriate drug information to the public. The spontaneous provision of information from pharmacies is still limited. In Austria, Denmark, France, Germany, Greece, Poland, Portugal, and Switzerland, medicines are not labelled when dispensed. In most countries medicines are dispensed with special patient information leaflets, either from the pharmaceutical industry or from the pharmacy. However, this is still not routinely the case in Finland, France, Iceland, Ireland, Norway, Portugal, and the UK.

Drug information to other professionals

In some countries, pharmacists also provide drug information to other health professionals, especially general medical practitioners. This activity is still developing, and depends on an appropriate relationship between pharmacist and physician (see also Chapter 15). In Croatia, Greece, Ireland, Italy, Poland, Portugal and Switzerland, pharmacy organisations have reported that the relationships between the general practitioner and pharmacist are 'not so good'. However, governments are looking for pharmacists to influence prescribing patterns to achieve cost containment. In the Netherlands, for example, there are regular pharmacotherapeutic meetings between general practitioners and community pharmacists. All pharmacists and general practitioners attend regional or local meetings at least once every two months. Prescription data are used to analyse and influence general practitioners' prescribing behaviour (de Vries et al. 1999). In Norway, Germany and Switzerland, attempts are now being made to introduce a similar system.

CONCLUSION

Most pharmacies in Europe are moving towards a pharmaceutical care practice philosophy. Although it is still unclear what pharmaceutical care means in different countries, the patient is increasingly becoming the focus of pharmacists' attention. Concomitantly, clinical pharmacy has become increasingly important, as has the provision of information to patients and health professionals.

It is clear that throughout Europe, pharmacies are under financial pressure even though medicines are usually the cheapest treatment option available in health care. Governments are seeking to reduce their health care budgets, and in particular their drugs budget. Well educated pharmacists and influential pharmacists' organisations are required to inform these developments and facilitate the future development of pharmaceutical service delivery across Europe.

Acknowledgement

Most of the data in this chapter are derived from the results of an international questionnaire issued from the Department of Social Pharmacy and Pharmacoepidemiology, University of Groningen, in 1997, in cooperation with the Community Pharmacy section of the International Pharmaceutical Federation (FIP). Part of the results of this questionnaire have been published (van Mil, 2000).

References

Crown, J. (1999) *A Review of the Prescribing, Supply and Administration of Medicines*, Department of Health, London.

de Vries, D.S., van den Berg, P.B., Timmer, J.W., Reicher, A., Blijleven, W. and Tromp, T.F. (1999) Prescription data as a tool in pharmacotherapy audit (II). The development of an instrument. *Pharmacy World Science*, **21**, 85–90.

Hepler, C.D. and Strand, L.M. (1990) Opportunities and responsibilities in pharmaceutical care. *American Journal of Hospital Pharmacy*, **47**, 533–543.

van Mil,, J.W.F. (2000) Pharmaceutical care in world-wide perspective. In *Pharmaceutical Care, the Future of Pharmacy*. Zuidlaren. ISBN: 90-9013-367-4.

Self assessment questions

Question 1: What major factors can you identify which influence pharmacy practice in the different European countries?

Question 2: What kind of differences can you recognise in the products available in pharmacies over Europe?

Question 3: What would be the influence of the staff size of a pharmacy on professional possibilities, and what outcome(s) would the staff size possibly affect?

Key points for answers

Question 1: Pharmacy education and health care systems

Question 2: There is a large variation in the availability of non-medical articles and herbal remedies

Question 3: e.g. time available to serve a client, chances for pharmaceutical care, chances for the provision of additional services. The outcome affected will be patient satisfaction and possibly also clinical outcomes

5 Pharmacy in North America

Joaquima Serradell and Albert Wertheimer

INTRODUCTION	72
THE US HEALTH CARE SYSTEM	73
PHARMACEUTICALS	74
MANAGED CARE	75
MANAGED CARE PHARMACY	76
Formularies	76
Co-payments	76
DRUG DISTRIBUTION SYSTEM	77
PHARMACY PERSONNEL	78
CANADA AND MEXICO	78
CONCLUSION	79
FURTHER READING	79
REFERENCES	79
SELF-ASSESSMENT QUESTIONS	79
KEY POINTS FOR ANSWERS	80

INTRODUCTION

In the USA there are fundamentally two types of health care system. The privatised health care system, encompassing 80% of the population, is financed by premium payments. The other system, covering 20% of the population, is financed by the government schemes: Medicare and Medicaid. In the Medicare system free inpatient medicines and hospital treatment are provided to those aged 65 and over and the disabled. It excludes several types of treatment and nursing homes. The Medicaid programme provides medical cover for poor people aged under 65 years who cannot afford to pay insurance premiums. In the privatised systems, a premium is paid based not on the ability to pay but on the services required and the probability of being sick. With insurance schemes a health premium is paid to an insurance company and the individual is free to go to any doctor or hospital for treatment. Insurance companies pay the bill. This has the disadvantage of high costs for the insurance company as there is no direct control on the provider of health care. In health maintenance organisations (HMOs) the health insurance company and the provider of health care have a contract with each other. The individual is restricted to the doctors and hospitals nominated by the insurance company. HMOs have subsequently become managed care organisations (MCOs) (see later).

Health care in the USA is provided by a range of differing organisations (see Box 5.1).

Box 5.1 Organisations providing health care in the USA

- Private, not for profit (e.g. Blue Cross/Shield)
- Voluntary not for profit (e.g. religious groups, industrial unions and co-operatives)
- Federal Government systems (e.g. Veterans Administration, Indian health services, prisons, etc.)
- State and Local Government services (e.g. State university medical schools, etc.)
- Academic Medical Centers, attached to their teaching hospitals and speciality clinics

Pharmacy as a component of the overall health care system must be compatible with it. Growing expenditure on pharmaceuticals over the last decades has motivated employers, insurers and managed care organisations to better manage this cost. Between 1980 and 1990 prescription expenditures grew by an average of 9% per year, with prescription prices outpacing nearly all other goods and services during the same period, the total prescription drug expenditures reached $93.4 billion in 1998.

The US pharmaceuticals market is comprised of several sub-markets. There is the conventional fee-for-service sector where there are usually only two parties, the prescriber and the patient. Here, a branded drug product is usually prescribed, free from any formulary or other controls. The patient pays for such medications out of their own pocket, or in some cases, is partly or wholly reimbursed by an indemnity health insurer. A second market is the institutional one, including hospitals, long-term care facilities, governmental facilities, prisons, the military, and veterans care centres. Most often, these large buyers make purchase decisions based upon annual tenders or solicited bids and use generic products wherever possible.

A third market is the managed care market where branded and generic products are used, based upon negotiations between manufacturers and managed care organisations, regarding price, rebates and market share requirements. If an HMO was able to guarantee that a particular product would maintain 90% of its therapeutic category sales, that HMO would be able to purchase that product for its patients at a lower price than an HMO guaranteeing a market share of 60%.

THE US HEALTH CARE SYSTEM

It might be more accurate to describe the US health care environment as a non-system. Unlike the UK, where an overwhelming majority of care is provided, and paid for, by a single organisation, the National Health Service, in the USA, there exist simultaneously, a number of systems that do not routinely communicate with each other. This can lead to inefficiencies, duplication, and ultimately, increased costs. This has a historical basis. The founders of the USA escaped religious and other persecution and believed in *'small government'* that would do only what people could not do for themselves.

The different religious groups established their own hospitals to care for their own communities as well as to provide for the poor. This was accomplished independently of what was happening or being planned by other religious denominations. The military services created a health care system of ambulatory sites and hospitals to take care of their members, and dependants. The Veterans Administration established a network of hospitals and clinics to serve those no longer in the military services. Medical faculties provide care at major university sites to generate revenue, to provide patients for teaching and research purposes and to offer their expertise in difficult and complex situations. Cities and counties have established hospitals, originally for treatment of the poor, and to compete with other urban areas, to attract industry, jobs and people interested in having services nearby. Prisons have health services, and there are student health facilities at colleges, nursing homes and mental health care centres. There is also another huge establishment, the *'for profit'* chains of hospitals, long-term care facilities, and emergency care centres.

PHARMACEUTICALS

There has been food and drug legislation in the USA since 1906. While it originally dealt with adulteration and mis-labelling of products, it has gradually evolved into the Food and Drug Administration (FDA), that today regulates food, drugs, cosmetics, medical devices and radiation emitting equipment. There are only two categories of pharmaceuticals:

- Those which require a prescription from a duly licensed practitioner (physician, dentist, veterinarian, osteopath or optometrist). Some pharmaceuticals (i.e. controlled substances) are controlled more carefully than others
- Those which may be sold anywhere, without any professional supervision

The latter group may be sold in any type of store, vending machines, door-to-door, mail order, and are typically found at gasoline stations, hotel gift shops and convenience grocery markets.

The FDA evaluates safety and efficacy only. Price is a separate matter for the manufacturer to determine and for the marketplace to evaluate. The FDA approves the label and in particular, the claims made for the product. It is not necessary to ask for advance approval of marketing and advertising materials since the manufacturer knows the limits of what claims have been approved. The FDA monitors the media and has the ability to stop advertising that does not portray a fair balance between benefits and risks, or activities that exceed the approved claims. A recent phenomenon in the USA is *direct to consumer* advertising of drug products requiring prescription. A manufacturer might advertise to the public on television or in print that: *'It is no longer necessary to suffer from your allergies. Effective medication is now available. Ask your physician to prescribe XYZ Tablets for you.'* The FDA also monitors this.

Over the counter (OTC) medicines include antihistamines for allergies and as hypnotics, topical steroid creams and ointments, topical antibiotic agents, H_2 antagonists for ulcers, hair restorers, phenylpropanolamine as a decongestant and dieting aid and dextromethorphan as a cough suppressant. In addition, there are many thousands of preparations that have been available OTC for many years such as aspirin, some non-steroidal anti-inflammatory drugs (NSAIDs), antacids, wart removers, laxatives, vitamins and minerals.

Until the mid-1960s, a pharmacy transaction was a two-party interaction. The first party, the patient, brought a prescription to the pharmacy. The second party, the pharmacist, dispensed medication and charged a fee to the patient, who paid that bill. Sometimes, that patient would have indemnity health insurance and would submit the receipt for the prescription to the insurance company for eventual reimbursement. In the mid-1960s, the government Medicaid program was introduced. This included outpatient prescribed drugs for these unable to pay for their own medication. At the same time, some trade unions obtained prescription drug benefit coverage, adding to their coverage of hospital and doctor services.

It is often said that: *'He who pays gets to call the shots.'* This is equally true with a drug benefit. Certain events occur in the USA that are not permitted in other countries. The payer establishes a network of retail pharmacies which agree to discount the dispensing fee. A typical scenario would be where the usual and customary pharmacy dispensing fee is $5.00 and where an insurer visits pharmacies, saying that the workers of Zoom Motorworks will have a new medical insurance plan that includes prescribed medicine. They are to print a directory of pharmacies where these prescriptions may be dispensed at a co-payment fee of only $2.00 per prescription. Your shop can be in that directory if you agree to accept a dispensing fee of $3.00. In such a case, you collect the $2.00 from the patient and $1.00, plus the ingredients cost from the health insurance company (Navarro and Wertheimer 1996).

The pharmacist appreciates that $3.00 is lower than the customary payment, but may agree on the basis that an increased number of customers will visit the shop, some of whom will also purchase additional merchandise while waiting for the prescription to be dispensed.

MANAGED CARE

Health insurers had little choice other than to reimburse for services rendered. However, this was not acceptable for progressive, pro-active firms that wanted to have a say about care, and not only pay the bills retrospectively.

In the mid to late 1970s, some health insurers evolved into Health Maintenance Organizations (HMOs). They managed care as well as costs, established utilisation review procedures, case management and cost control efforts and made contracts with physicians, hospitals and pharmacies that would offer discounts based on their bargaining power. Just as they set up their own network of community pharmacies, they sought discounts at local hospitals and sent all of their patients to those one or two hospitals offering them the lowest prices. For instance, they might ask for bids from ophthalmologists for cataract removal procedures. If the going rate was $2000, they would accept an offer of $1500 from one clinic for a two-year contract for ALL of their patients requiring cataract removal. In two years, the bidding process would begin again, and those ophthalmologists who were excluded for the past two years could be expected to be aggressive bidders, perhaps opening offers at $1200 this time around.

HMOs subsequently became managed care organisations (MCOs). They were able to compare the cost of prescribing, number of patients seen, etc., for different locations. Just as they limited the number of ophthalmologists, they also limited the number of pharmacies, and controlled the variety and selection of drugs they would pay for. This was accomplished through the use of a formulary, a booklet listing all the prescription medicines for which the MCO would pay.

MANAGED CARE PHARMACY

Managed care organisations place limitations on each of the participants in the health system. Patients have some incentives and disincentives to influence their choices and have to face some limitations. Physicians have limitations on what they can prescribe and pharmacists have constraints on their pricing and on what items they can expect to be paid for. Let us examine these instruments of cost containment and quality assurance.

Formularies

There are two basic types of formularies: positive and negative. Positive formularies are vastly more popular for a number of reasons. They are inclusive and specify which drugs are eligible for reimbursement. If the practitioner does not find the beta blocker required in the formulary, the beta blocker section will present acceptable alternative agents in that category. The positive formulary gives control to the publisher. If it is not listed, it is not paid for. A negative formulary is exclusive and lists drugs not covered. There is a constant battle to use a positive formulary, which lists each new product as it is marketed, hence excluding the product until enough information is available or until such time that the formulary committee can discuss it and make a decision. A negative formulary is a never ending endeavour and must be revised almost constantly.

Formularies serve several purposes. They may be used as an instrument to eliminate inferior, less effective or more dangerous items. They can be a tool to contain costs by including only the least costly items in each category or those found to be optimally cost-effective. And they may be used as a revenue source. Some managed care organisations ask a fee from manufacturers to have drugs listed in the formulary. There are business negotiations undertaken routinely where an additional discount is offered to MCOs if a specified product achieves a certain market share.

Co-payments

Co-payments are fees charged to the patient at the time of dispensing. There have traditionally been two co-payment levels; one for drugs in the formulary and one for non-listed medications. A typical co-payment for a covered drug varies from $6.00 to $12.00. The co-payment for non-formulary items can be $20.00 to $35.00 or more and would serve as a strong incentive for the patient to authorise the dispensing of the cheaper medication. This was the conventional system, but a new feature is being added widely around the country – the use of a third co-payment level. The third level is usually the least expensive if the patient is willing to accept generic (multi-source) medications. Here, the generic drug might have a $4.00 co-payment; the branded formulary-approved item $8 per dispensing act, and the non-formulary medication might require a payment of $35, for a one-month supply (Wertheimer and Navarro 1998).

Prior authorisation is used as an interim step. Often it is used as a utilisation management tool until a formal formulary decision is made. Providers might have to telephone the MCO and describe the rationale for the new or authorisation-requiring drug. The mere fact that a telephone call is required usually serves as a deterrent to its use. Prior authorisation is seen as reasonable for drugs with a high liability due to off-label (i.e. unconventional) usage.

A patient brings his or her plan membership card and the prescription to any pharmacy participating in the network of community pharmacies. The pharmacist enters the patient identification information and the prescription data into the computer and instantly receives a message from the Pharmacy Benefit Management (PBM) company or directly from the MCO. Patient eligibility is checked, the co-payment rate is provided to the dispensing pharmacist and a drug utilisation review (DUR) process is initiated. If the drug is contraindicated with other drugs used by that patient, dispensed at any network pharmacy, a message is sent to the dispensing pharmacist, alerting the pharmacist to the situation. Similarly, if a sugar-containing syrup is prescribed for a diabetic patient, that would be called to the attention of the pharmacist.

Not visible to the pharmacist or patient are the data gathering functions of the computer system. It is typical for PBMs to track the percentage formulary compliance of the physicians, percentage generic drug use, cost per patient, average cost per prescription, total cost for prescribed drugs, compared to other physicians within the same category and location.

DRUG DISTRIBUTION SYSTEM

The vast majority of prescription medicines are dispensed through community pharmacies, with a growing percentage through large corporate chains, pharmacies located in supermarkets and from mail service pharmacies. Recently, internet based pharmacies have emerged, though these generally use a mail service pharmacy to deliver drugs. While their market share is currently small, it is expected to grow rapidly due to its convenience, speed and price advantages.

PHARMACY PERSONNEL

Pharmacists attend university for a six-year program leading to the Doctor of Pharmacy (Pharm. D.) degree. This usually comprises two years in general studies followed by four years at a pharmacy faculty. After the university requirements are satisfied, a state licensure examination is sat. Each of the 50 states conducts its own examination.

It is common to see the pharmacist assisted by a certified technician or assistant. Technicians are most widely used in hospitals, and in the mail service pharmacy areas. State laws usually regulate the maximum number of assistants who may be supervised by one pharmacist. In the future we will see an increasing incidence of robotics and automation within pharmacies.

CANADA AND MEXICO

Canada has a type of national health insurance program, operated through each of the provinces and territories. Essentially everyone is covered. Fees are established centrally and there is a combination of public and private institutions, which work side-by-side. Benefit design varies slightly from province to province. The provincial governments determine their own formularies. Virtually all Canadian residents are included in the plan. The same drugs as in the United States are marketed by the same multinational firms within the Canadian market.

Mexico is more difficult to characterise since three systems operate independently and in parallel. A large social security system operates that provides care for the poor. Another huge system provides care for government employees and some employees of government-owned firms. Both of these groups have formularies and other utilisation controls. There is also a robust and rapidly expanding private sector made up of fee-for-service care and the newly emerging managed care and indemnity health insurance market places.

Unlike its sister North American nations, one may walk into a Mexican pharmacy and purchase over the counter nearly all drugs with the exception of narcotics and scheduled, abusable products. The personnel at pharmacies are usually minimally educated lay people. Prices are frequently half of those in the USA or Canada. Mexico also shares one positive feature with Europe, not seen in the USA or in Canada: pre-packaged medicines. In the US, the pharmacist dispenses a prescription for 36 or 45 or 90 tablets by counting that number of tablets from a bottle of 500 or 1000 tablets.

CONCLUSION

Pharmacy is practised differently in every region of North America reflecting different social, political, economic, historical and financial traits, customs and traditions. It is impossible to say which systems are *'right'*. Likewise, it is would be over simplistic to state which systems are *'best'*. Some are more efficient or more controlled, but the basic question is whether the drugs/pharmacy sector can satisfy local expectations and remain compatible with changes and improvements in the overall health care delivery system.

All three of these systems are vastly different from the health care delivery characteristics seen in other countries and yet they appear to function adequately. It remains an intriguing question as to whether certain system features might have universal benefit and be applicable elsewhere.

FURTHER READING

Fincham, J.E. and Wertheimer, A.I. (1998) *Pharmacy and the US Health Care System* (2nd Edn.), Haworth Press, New York.

Health in the Americas (1998 Edition) Pan American Health Organization, Washington.

Raffel, M.W. (1980) *The US Health System: Origins and Functions*, Wiley, New York.

Health Statistics from the Americas (1998 Edition) Pan American Health Organization, Washington.

Wertheimer, A.I. and Smith, M.C. (1989) *Pharmacy Practice: Social and Behavioural Aspects*, Williams and Wilkins, Baltimore.

REFERENCES

Navarro, R. and Wertheimer, A.I. (1996) *Managing the Pharmacy Benefit*, Emron, Warren, New Jersey, p 53.

Wertheimer, A.I. and Navarro, R. (1998) *Managed Care Pharmacy: Principles and Practices*, Haworth, New York, pp 318–20.

SELF-ASSESSMENT QUESTIONS

Question 1: Describe the structure of the US health care system.

Question 2: What are the different categories of drugs sold in the USA?

Question 3: Why did indemnity health insurance firms move to become Managed Care Organisations (MCOs)?

Question 4: What are the advantages of a positive formulary over a negative one?

Question 5: Describe the US Medicaid and Medicare programs.

KEY POINTS FOR ANSWERS

Question 1: A *'non-system'* comprising a large number of parallel and often duplicative service providers, having little communication with each other, from governments, religions, for profit firms, etc.

Question 2: Two general categories:

- Over the counter (OTC) drugs – can be sold at *any* site: pharmacies, gift shops, vending machines, mail order, door-to-door, grocery stores, etc. Copious label information negates the need for any professional supervision.
- Prescription drugs – can only be sold pursuant to a practioner's order. Prescription orders can be telephoned, faxed or e-mailed to the pharmacy, except for controlled (abusable) substances, where additional controls are in place.

Question 3: Indemnity health insurance (reimbursing) firms cannot manage, influence or control what they do not know about until after the fact. MCOs can dictate what services will be used by patients and from where they will be obtained.

Question 4:

- A positive formulary does not include items (including new drugs) until action is taken to list them
- A negative formulary is always behind newly introduced products that can arise without warning

Question 5:

- Medicaid is a welfare type program for persons who qualify as being medically indigent
- Medicare, operated by Federal Government, is a health insurance program for the elderly, independent of wealth or income. Workers pay premiums during their working years to the Federal Government

Pharmacy in Developing Countries

Felicity Smith

INTRODUCTION	82
HEALTH IN DEVELOPING COUNTRIES	82
Patterns of morbidity and mortality	82
Determinants of health	83
THE PLACE OF PHARMACY	85
DRUG USE AND POLICY	88
WHO Action Programme on Essential Drugs	88
Drug donations	90
Problems of irrational use	90
Self-medication and cultural perspectives	92
Pluralism in health care	93
THE PHARMACEUTICAL INDUSTRY	94
Orphan drugs	94
Counterfeit products	95
PHARMACY EDUCATION AND SERVICES	95
CONCLUSION	96
FURTHER READING	97
REFERENCES	98
SELF-ASSESSMENT QUESTIONS	100
KEY POINTS FOR ANSWERS	100

INTRODUCTION

The United Nations (UN) classifies countries into developed (or industrial) and developing, based on their level of economic and industrial
development. A sub-group of developing countries are designated as
least developed countries (LDCs). These are countries with very low
per capita income. Based on this classification, in 1998, of 179 countries,
50 were classified as industrial and 129 as developing of which 48 were
designated as LDCs. Despite this classification, there are countries
which possess some features typical of developed and other characteristics typical of developing countries. For example, countries in the
Middle East, have been described as being neither exclusively developed or developing, but 'in-between' with wide variations of wealth
(Stephen 1992).

The classification by the UN corresponds to many important
national features of the political, social and economic profile of a
country. These features are reflected in the resources available for
health care, the provision and delivery of health services, the health
status of the population, as well as the role of health professionals and
patterns of drug use. Many of the poorest developing countries are
hampered in their endeavours to improve the economic, social and
health status of their populations, because of having to service vast
debts to industrialised countries.

The World Health Organisation (WHO) has identified particular
problems in developing countries in relation to the supply and use of
drugs. In response to these difficulties, the WHO believes that
pharmacists can make an important contribution in health care, by
promoting the safe and appropriate use of medicines (World Health
Organisation 1988a).

This chapter will discuss the delivery of pharmacy services in the
context of political, economic and social outlooks of developing countries, patterns of health problems and wider health service policy
objectives and provision. The roles of pharmacists and the practice of
pharmacy should reflect the specific health needs and health care
problems of developing countries. Although, there are differences
between developing countries, there are also many similarities which
result in common issues for pharmacy services.

HEALTH IN DEVELOPING COUNTRIES

Patterns of morbidity and mortality

There are striking differences in the morbidity – the distribution of
disease in a population – and mortality patterns – the distribution of
deaths as a proportion of the total population – between developed
and developing countries (see Box 6.1). Although many developing
countries are experiencing changes in morbidity and mortality

In 1997, approximately 43% of an estimated total of 40 million deaths in developing countries were due to infectious and parasitic diseases. In developed countries this was the cause of only 1% of (a total of 12 million) deaths. Circulatory disease is a major cause of mortality in developed countries (46% of deaths in 1998), although this has begun to decline. What is notable is that in developing countries deaths from circulatory disease (although still accounting for lower proportions of deaths than in developed countries) increased from 17% to 24% in the period 1990–1997 (World Health Organisation 1998).

towards patterns generally associated with developed countries, nevertheless, in developing countries, diarrhoea, malnutrition, malaria, HIV infection, tuberculosis and other tropical infectious diseases persist as major health problems. The patterns of morbidity and mortality will be important determinants of the drugs required, and pharmacy services should be geared to the health needs of the country.

There are marked differences in the population structures of industrialised and developing countries, with developing countries having higher proportions of younger people. However, as in industrialised countries, the populations of developing countries are also ageing, which will have implications for health care needs and provision. Despite this, infant mortality remains high. In the least developed countries, in 1995, 40% of deaths were children under 5 years. Although this is projected to fall as these populations age, it is still projected that in 2025, 23% of deaths will be in this age group (World Health Organisation 1998).

In many developing countries mortality and morbidity rates, health status and health care provision vary significantly between urban and rural areas. In general, access to amenities such as clean water, sanitation facilities and health care are better in urban areas.

Determinants of health

The relationship between poverty and health, both between and within countries, is widely acknowledged. Many people believe that poor health and poverty are so closely linked that major improvements in the health status of the world's poorest people cannot be realised without addressing the underlying political, economic and socioeconomic factors. The low levels of economic development and the lack of finance is reflected in the extent and quality of infrastructure, education, housing, transport, social support, enforcement of law, nutrition, etc, all of which affect health status, and the ability of governments and health professionals to provide appropriate services to address the health needs of their populations. In favouring primary health care, the WHO identified the need for an approach to health care which emphasises low-technology, preventative services rather than high-technology curative care, with community-based provision, based on local resources and services, targeted at local priorities and needs.

A landmark in the development of health policy was the International Conference on Primary Health Care which took place in Alma-Ata in 1978. This conference called for a new approach to health and health care that would lead to a more equitable distribution of health care resources, and emphasised that primary health care would be the most effective means of achieving this. States were invited to formulate, strengthen and/or implement strategies to achieve a goal of *'health for all by the year 2000'*. Many countries did so. In the subsequent decades, some countries achieved vast improvements in the health status of their populations. However, in many LDCs difficulties in providing basic health services to many population groups persist.

The WHO, in promoting primary health care to address the extreme health problems in developing countries, recognised that these problems were a result of complex interactions between political, social, economic, environmental and lifestyle factors; and that they needed to be tackled as such. For example, the lack of access to clean water is a major health hazard for many people. In many developing countries, especially in Africa, there is a high prevalence of water-borne infectious disease. Schistosomiasis (bilharzia) is transmitted as a result of faecal or urinary contamination of water in which people bathe. There are an estimated 300–500 million cases of malaria annually and between 1.5–2.5 million deaths, most of which occur in sub-Saharan Africa (WHO 1998). Dehydration from diarrhoea as a result of gastrointestinal infestation is a common cause of death among young children.

Health status is inextricably linked to the role and opportunities of women in society. Investment in the education of women is seen as an important factor, both as a mark of, and in promoting, political, economic and social development in society. In the LDCs, in 1995, an estimated 51% were believed to be illiterate, the majority of whom were women (UNESCO figures quoted in World Health Organisation 1998). In most households and societies, informal health carers are predominantly women. Thus, the increased emphasis on the education of girls and women, both contributes to health care indirectly though promoting socio-economic development, and directly as a result of informal carers being in a position to understand more about health problems and the use of drugs and other therapies. It is to women that information about health and medicines should principally be targeted. Illiteracy, especially among women, has major implications for the provision of pharmacy services in developing countries.

Although many health problems in developing countries are rooted in poverty and low levels of development, it is clear that problems cannot be addressed by the health sector alone. Problems are often compounded by a lack of high quality facilities and professional services (including pharmacy services) where they are most needed. Drug therapy exists for many of the most prevalent health problems in developing countries. However, as a result of wider problems, these drugs are often not available when needed, and although pharmacists could assume an important role in providing guidance on their use, they too are often in short supply.

THE PLACE OF PHARMACY

Health care world-wide is a mixture of public and private provision. Pharmacists may be formally integrated within a national or public system or they may exist as independent practitioners alongside other professionals or organisations providing health care. In some countries, a public or a private system predominates, in others different systems exist side by side. Even in countries in which most health care is financed by private individuals (by direct payment or voluntary insurance) and/or provided by commercial or voluntary organisations, some public sector involvement is usual. In general, public sector provision provides at least a basic service for the poorest people in society, for whom health care would otherwise be inaccessible. Similarly, in countries with health services funded from general taxation or compulsory insurance, some health care is invariably purchased by individuals from private organisations.

In many of the poorest countries, publicly provided health care is often inadequate to meet the basic needs of the population, even though a high proportion of the population may depend on it for their care. Health insurance schemes exist in many developing countries. These are not generally comprehensive, being either private voluntary schemes in which people opt to pay a premium and in return receive specified services as required, or public sector schemes which are commonly restricted to specific sectors of the population. For example, in Egypt, the Government Health Insurance is available to public sector workers.

In many developing countries, a private health care market, funded by private individuals (or voluntary insurance contributions) and provided by private practitioners or institutions, exists independently from the public sector. As in any market, the services provided in the private sector are generally those for which purchasers are able and willing to pay. It is generally the most affluent individuals in any society who are able and willing to purchase health care privately. Thus, the services provided in the private sector are largely geared to their perceived needs. In developing countries, urban populations tend to be wealthier. Consequently, health professionals often prefer to work in cities, and private sector health care tends to be concentrated in urban rather than rural areas.

Within developing countries there are often huge discrepancies in wealth, health and access to health care. Again, these often follow the urban-rural divide: hospitals, well-equipped clinics and private health facilities being more accessible in the urban areas. The more wealthy people in developing countries are often keen for resources to be directed to high-technology curative services of a standard that approaches those of industrialised countries. Directing health personnel and resources to primary care in the poorer rural areas requires a tough political will, and has perhaps limited the achievements of primary health care in many countries. In discussing health care in the Arab world, Stephen (1992) describes how politicians, particularly in developing countries, are pressurised by the educated urban classes and the majority of the medical profession to promote high-technology hospital-based services, rather than focusing on primary health care initiatives designed to improve the health status of poorer people in the rural areas.

Drugs account for a significant proportion of health expenditure. Many developing countries are unable to find sufficient funds to ensure continuous supplies of essential drugs to remote areas. In some publicly funded facilities, consumers are expected to make some payment on using a particular service; these contributions are termed co-payments, e.g. prescription charges or contributions to the costs of drug therapy.

Charging for health care, including drugs, may deter people in need of services or therapy from using them. This may be particularly detrimental when long-term drug use is important for successful therapy, when symptoms may subside before the end of a course of therapy, and for people with very low incomes. However, co-payments also provide the health sector with a much needed source of finance.

A system of co-payments was the basis of the Bamako Initiative of the United Nations Children's Fund (UNICEF). The proposal was that UNICEF would provide essential drugs for use in primary care maternal and child health clinics on the condition that charges would be made for drugs and services, and the resulting income spent on health workers' salaries or other aspects of primary care services. Not surprisingly, the proposal was controversial. It was criticised on both ethical grounds, e.g. charging sick and poor people for essential medicines, difficulties in operating the scheme and deciding what to charge, especially as some drugs were donated at no cost to the governments (Kanji et al. 1992) (See Box 6.2).

The Bamako Initiative, involving co-payments for drugs became incorporated into pharmaceutical policy at primary care level in many developing countries. It is believed by many to have provided positive benefits as a means of promoting essential drugs programmes and community participation in primary health care.

It is common for pharmacists in the public sector, or those employed by a hospital or health care organisation, to receive a salary

Box 6.2 Examples of the impact of the Bamako Initiative

Pharmacists in the community however, are generally private practitioners. Pharmacists' incomes are usually largely obtained directly from the public through the sale of pharmaceuticals and other products, and to a lesser extent by payments through health agencies or insurance companies. Additional services which may be provided (e.g. administration of injections, consultation, interpretation of medical reports) are often not remunerated. There has been much debate on the advantages and disadvantages of different methods of payment. Many people believe that remuneration should seek to achieve optimal professional practice (and many payment systems in industrialised countries have been devised and modified to achieve specific health care objectives). In a system in which pharmacists' income is derived from the sales of medicines, they have a financial incentive to sell expensive products, irrespective of whether or not this is the most appropriate response to an individual's health needs. In discussing this issue, Cederlof and Tomson (1995) cite research which demonstrated that interventions to influence selling behaviour of drug retailers, which resulted in no financial losses to the retailer, were more likely to be successful than those which had a negative impact on their income. They considered ways in which financial incentives for pharmacists to provide essential rather than non-essential drugs could be incorporated into health policy.

As with other private health care facilities in developing countries, pharmacies are generally concentrated in the urban areas, where there is a market for drugs and hence an income for the pharmacists and their staff. Thus, the urban-rural divide in many developing countries, extends to pharmacy services (professionals being more numerous in cities) and the availability of drugs (usually a wider range and more dependable supplies in urban areas). However, problems of irrational drug use in urban areas in developing countries are also well documented.

Fees for private primary medical care are determined by doctors. The costs of care and patients' perceptions of their health needs will influence the extent of their use of medical services. To avoid costs of medical consultation, many people are believed to go direct to a pharmacy for medication. Thus, pharmacies may fulfill a health need for people who cannot afford to see a doctor, or where there is no medical practitioner available.

There is a positive correlation between a country's health expenditure per person and its wealth. This trend is reflected in expenditure on drugs. Per capita drug consumption in developed countries has been estimated at 10 times that of developing countries (World Health Organisation 1988b). Drugs may account for a high proportion of the health budget, e.g. in Egypt, Morocco and Yemen, up to 70% of health spending is on pharmaceuticals (most of it through private financing) (World Health Organisation 1998). It has also been shown that poor households spend a higher proportion of their income on drugs than rich ones (Mills and Lee 1993).

It is easy to assume that the principal determinants of drug use relate to health problems and health status, i.e. that patterns of drug use will reflect a country's health needs. However, differences in drug use between countries are subject to a wide range of political, economic and other factors. For example, drug policy (e.g. whether or not a country has a national drug policy in operation) and its regulation will influence which drugs are on the market. The availability of products will be affected by the country's infrastructure and transport. The health care system will determine whether or not consultations with professionals, as well as drug therapy, are free at the point of use and to whom; people's ability to pay may determine their consumption. The accessibility of health professionals to the public will have an impact on the extent of self-medication and the appropriateness of drug use. Education and information for professionals will affect the quality of prescribing, advice-giving and non-prescription drug recommendations. In many developing countries 'Western' medicine exists alongside other traditions of care. These social and cultural contexts will also affect health-seeking behaviours and drug use (see also Chapter 7).

Two major problems of supply and use of drugs in developing countries commonly highlighted, are the non-availability of essential drugs to many people and irrational use of both prescribed and non-prescription medicines.

WHO action programme on essential drugs

In reviewing the world drug situation in the 1980s, the WHO estimated that of 5 billion people in the world, between 1.3 and 2.5 million, the majority of whom lived in developing countries, had little or no regular access to essential drugs (World Health Organisation 1988b). In an effort to improve the availability of medicines, the WHO devised the Essential Drugs List, comprising around 300 products, which is updated approximately every 3 years. The WHO estimated that approximately 200 to 300 drug products should be sufficient to address the health care needs of the majority of the populations in developing countries, and the Essential Drugs List is intended as a model from which individual countries draw up their own list to comprise drugs which *satisfy the health care needs of the majority of the population and should therefore be available at all times in adequate amounts and in appropriate dosage forms*' (World Health Organisation 1998).

The Action Programme on Essential Drugs was introduced in 1981 to promote the development of national drug policies and essential drugs lists. The WHO advocates that every country should have a national drug policy that provides a framework for an adequate supply of safe and effective drugs of established quality, at an affordable price, which are properly prescribed and used. The programme was established to provide operational support to countries developing national drugs policies (World Health Organisation 1992). The WHO recognises that problems such as the lack of resources, poor infrastructure, shortages of skilled personnel, difficulties of planning and enforcing policy and the economic crisis have resulted in limited success of programmes. Although large numbers of people are still without regular access to essential drugs, the WHO reports that the situation has improved (World Health Organisation 1998).

Many developing countries, including over 80% of African countries have a national drug policy. Although many were initially devised to make available essential drugs, they also aim at rationalising the use of drugs through better information, prescription and compliance (Health Action International 1997) (Box 6.3).

In Bangladesh, prior to the introduction of a national drug policy, the drugs market was described as being *'flooded'* with products which were believed not to be appropriate to the people's health needs such as many tonics, vitamin mixtures, cough and cold remedies, blood alkalizers and many other undesirable products which accounted for a third of expenditure on drugs, whilst essential drugs were mainly imported and in short supply (Quadir *et al.* 1993). A national drug policy was introduced to address these problems. However its success was hindered internally as a result of inadequate resources for implementation, a lack of trained health personnel, antagonism from within the medical professional who feared restrictions on their prescribing; and by opposition of drug companies who feared that these developments and recommendations from the WHO, if they were more extensively applied in developing countries, would threaten their commercial interests (Rolt 1985; Quadir *et al.* 1993).

The introduction of a national formulary in Zambia was reported to have improved the availability of essential drugs and provided a foundation for rational prescribing (Baker 1984). A report of the Essential Drugs Programme in Tanzania, identified a need to improve local production, quality assurance, inspection, intersectoral linkages and active local participation in shouldering the financial burden to ensure the programme's sustainability and self-reliance (Munishi 1991).

Box 6.3 Examples of national drug policies

Drug donations

Many developing countries, in an effort to meet the needs of their populations, have received drug donations from other countries. However, concerns have been expressed about the suitability of these products. Many instances have been reported of donations of products of poor quality (sometimes unacceptable for use in the donor country), products that have expired or are near to their expiry date, or inappropriate to the needs of the population. Guidelines have now been devised by the WHO in collaboration with other organisations, summarised in Box 6.4.

Box 6.4 Guidelines for drug donations (World Health Organisation 1999)

Drug donations should:

- Be guided by close communication with recipients regarding their needs
- Be included in national lists of essential drugs
- Be of assured quality
- Comply with quality standard in both donor and recipient countries
- Be in appropriate form, quantities, presentation
- Have appropriate labelling, packaging and shelf-life

Problems of irrational use

Irrational drug use refers to the prescribing and/or consumption of ineffective, unsuitable, sub-optimal and/or unsafe pharmaceutical products. Many researchers have highlighted the incidence and prevalence of irrational drug use in developing countries. They have explored associated factors and attempted to explain some of the structures of, and processes in, the delivery of care, from the perspectives of both health professionals and consumers, that lead to irrational use. Fabricant and Hirschhorn (1987) assert that the use of conventional pharmaceuticals is based on a rational-scientific model, but that in practice drugs are distributed, prescribed and used in highly irrational ways.

Many features in patterns of drug use have been found to be common to developing countries. These include inappropriate treatment with unsuitable products, extensive practice of poly-pharmacy, due to both wide use of combination products and multiple prescriptions, frequent injections and use of coloured preparations and vitamins (Laing, 1990). Drug use in Uganda, which displays many features typical of developing countries, has been characterised by extensive poly-pharmacy, frequent demands for injections, overuse of antibiotics, self-medication without adequate knowledge and information, misuse of drugs and the ability to pay as the main criterion for providers to give drugs without a prescription (Health Action International 1997).

The wide availability of 'prescription' medicines without a prescription has been documented in many developing countries. Products can be purchased from pharmacies when available, but in rural areas there are often no pharmacists. People are forced to rely on untrained personnel, obtaining drugs from other drug stores or through hawkers and peddlers. Many researchers have identified the co-existence of formal (legal) and informal (outside legal or professional control) sectors for the distribution of medicines in developing countries. Van der Geest (1991) describes how the formal and informal sectors in Cameroon are closely interwoven. For example, he cites instances such as the supply of medicines to official institutions being offered for sale on the '*informal circuit*'. Van der Geest recognises the potential for inappropriate drug use as a result of distribution through the informal sector, but he also points out that the informal sector has a role in the provision of drugs to rural populations who would otherwise go without.

Irrational drug use is not confined to the informal sector. A number of descriptive studies have examined prescribing practices of medical practitioners and advice-giving and recommendations from pharmacies (Box 6.5).

A survey of drugs supplied by medical practitioners in the public and private sectors and from private pharmacies in India, analysed drug supply in relation to patients' presenting complaints. The findings revealed extensive use of drugs including many instances of questionable prescribing and sales. There are many influences on prescribing which include the quality of information available to the practitioner, the expectations and wishes of clients, the costs of different treatment options etc. The author in this study concluded that a rational drugs policy and/or essential drugs list would be useless unless accompanied by an improvement in the continuing education of doctors and pharmacists, and a reduction in the commercial pressures to prescribe and supply unnecessary drugs (Greenhalgh 1987).

Observation of 62 general practitioners and 28 paediatricians in Karachi, Pakistan, managing childhood diarrhoea, reported inadequate use of oral rehydration therapy and over-prescribing of antibacterials, antidiarrhoeals and antiamoebics (Nizami *et al.* 1996). Concerns have also been expressed about the quality of counter-prescribing for childhood diarrhoea as well as other health problems in pharmacies.

Problems of resistance resulting from overuse of antibiotics are of concern in industrialised and developing countries. However, in developing countries, problems are believed to be greater. Researchers have attributed inappropriate use to both irrational prescribing by medical practitioners as well as the wide availability, and use by individuals, of medicines purchased without a prescription (Greenhalgh 1987; Calva 1996).

Box 6.5 Examples of irrational drug use

Poor people spend a higher a proportion of their income on drugs. In promoting rational use by advising appropriately, pharmacists may be able to reduce purchases of unnecessary and inappropriate products (Box 6.6).

Many researchers have been critical of pharmacists and their staff (trained and untrained) for selling pharmaceuticals without

Box 6.6 Inappropriate drug purchases (Cederlof and Tomson 1995)

questioning or advising clients on the suitability of products. In many urban areas, retail pharmacies are numerous. Pharmacists have an important role in promoting safe and appropriate use of products. A number of features of pharmacies in developing countries which contribute to their prominence as a source of health advice have been identified (Box 6.7).

- Ease of access
- Availability of medicines
- No waiting
- Convenience of (long) hours of opening
- Cheaper products
- Availability of credit or the option to buy drugs in small amounts

Box 6.7 Features of pharmacies as sources of health advice (Goel *et al.* 1996)

In many rural areas in developing countries, pharmacists are scarce and pharmaceutical services are denied to these populations. It has been reported that 80% of the population of Tanzania do not have access to pharmaceutical services and that the East African country of Eritrea is served by a total of 53 pharmacists (Health Action International 1997).

Self-medication and cultural perspectives

People's understanding and use of medicines is not only restricted to the pharmacological and therapeutic properties, but will also be influenced by their social and cultural circumstances, views and perceptions of their health problems, expectations of health care and beliefs regarding the role and effects of medicines.

Pharmaceutical anthropology is a discipline which seeks to explore the social and cultural contexts in which medicines are produced, exchanged and consumed (van der Geest and Whyte 1988). The promotion of rational drug use will only be successful if policies are devised that take into account relevant political, economic, social and cultural priorities and contexts. Also, within industrialised countries differences between population groups with different cultural backgrounds, distinct perspectives on health, health care and drug use have been identified.

Pluralism in health care

Just as the co-existence of formal and informal sectors have been identified in the distribution of 'Western' drug products, in many developing countries traditional and 'Western' medical practices also operate side by side.

China is the only country in the world where traditional Chinese medicine (TCM) and 'Western' medicine are practised alongside each other at every level of the health care system (Hesketh and Zhu 1997). It is estimated that 40% of health care is based on TCM. Collaboration between the systems is illustrated by the fact that 40% of drugs prescribed in Western medicine hospitals are traditional and a similar proportion prescribed in TCM hospitals are Western. At a local level, practitioners may prescribe both TCM and Western medicine. TCM and Western medicine each have their own schools of medicine and pharmacy, hospitals and research institutes. In addition colleges of Western medicine also include training in TCM.

Many developing countries have experienced periods of colonisation by the industrial nations. Western medicine, introduced by the colonial powers for the benefit of immigrant personnel, would exist alongside existing traditions of care, gradually becoming more pervasive. Banerji (1974) traces the development of health services in India from the period prior to British rule. Focussing on political and economic changes, he illustrates how a Western health care system, including education, was imposed to serve the perceived needs of the British immigrants and 'privileged' Indians, and eventually dominated formal health care. He questions whether, at the time of the introduction of Western health care this was superior to the existing systems.

The importing and imposition of Western systems in developing countries has had a major impact on patterns of drug use, pharmacy services and professional education. In many developing countries Western medicine has remained more concentrated in urban areas, whilst other traditions of medical care have persisted and are more widely practised in rural areas. It would be expected that when two or more systems operate side by side, that each may influence the development of the other. Many authors have described how different health care systems, whilst remaining distinct, have incorporated practices from other traditions. Regarding the use of drugs, instances in which Western drugs have become part of the armamentarium of traditional practitioners and cases of indigenous remedies being incorporated in Western practice have been documented. Furthermore, people seeking care move between these different health care systems according to factors such as traditions of help-seeking in the society, perceived needs, perspectives on the roles of different health personnel or healers, beliefs regarding the appropriateness of particular courses of action, the availability of practitioners, and the success of therapy.

Drug companies with the largest worldwide market shares are concentrated in small number of developed countries. However, some developing countries produce a relatively high proportion of drug products for domestic consumption. For example, local drug production in Egypt, Iran, Morocco and Pakistan covers more than 80% of total drug consumption. However, others (especially those in Africa) produce very little and depend on foreign imports (World Health Organisation 1988b).

Considerable controversy surrounds the issue of the extent to which the operations of the drug companies in developing countries are an appropriate response to the health needs of the populations. Many authors have been critical of operations of the pharmaceutical industry. For example, local production of pharmaceuticals does not necessarily focus on the country's needs, or fall in line with their national drugs policies or assist in the provision of essential drugs (World Health Organisation 1988b). Some locally produced drugs on the market in Egypt are products for which the efficacy, safety or appropriateness are questioned in many industrialised countries. The marketing of substandard drugs (e.g. with inadequate levels of active ingredients) produced by local companies in Bangladesh has been reported, with a call for the stricter application of the national drug policy, in particular in regard to the issue of licences and sanctions against firms breaking the law (Roy 1994).

The practices of drug companies in promotion and marketing have been criticised by many authors and practitioners. Researchers have uncovered evidence of varying standards in marketing and information provided about drugs. For example, promotional material distributed in developing countries may include wider indications and less comprehensive information regarding the side-effect profile, whilst drugs will often be more expensive in the poorer countries.

From the point of view of pharmacists practising in developing countries, promotional material from drug companies is often their main source of product information. In developed countries, not only are impartial sources of information more accessible, but promotional material itself will be more reliable and comprehensive. In developing countries there are commonly high proportions of company representatives per medical practitioner and government controls regarding marketing and availability of pharmaceuticals are frequently less effective than in industrialised countries (Lexchin 1995).

Orphan drugs

The motive of drug companies in producing new pharmaceutical products is the maximisation of profits. The most profitable products will be those for which consumers are able and willing to pay. The pharmaceutical industry has always claimed that as a result of the financial investment required for successful research and development, new products will be costly to the consumer. Thus, the pharmaceutical industry is less inclined to invest extensively in products for which the market is limited in terms of health needs or available finance for purchasing. The term *'orphan drug'* is used to refer to products for which there is a health need, but for which, because of the lack of purchasing power of potential consumers, the industry would be unlikely to recoup the research and development costs.

Counterfeit products

Production and distribution of counterfeit medicines is acknowledged to be a problem in many developing countries. Counterfeit medicines have been defined as *'medicinal products which have been deliberately or fraudulently mislabeled with respect to identity and/or source'*. They may include products with the correct ingredients, wrong ingredients, without active ingredients, with insufficient active ingredients or with fake packaging (Dickinson and Davidson 1993). In a survey of experiences with counterfeit products, respondents from developing countries (especially LDCs) were more likely than those in developed countries to report that circulation of these products was a problem. Respondents in developing countries were also likely to report that the problems were significant or substantial, whereas those in developed countries would describe them as insignificant. The problems reported in developed countries related to prescription medicines, whereas respondents in developing countries reported significant or substantial problems with both prescription and non-prescription medicines. A lack of quality control, corruption and ineffective enforcement of current laws were identified as factors which made these problems difficult to address. Researchers have emphasised the need for continuing vigilance among pharmacists and the benefits of distributing medicines through pharmacies.

PHARMACY EDUCATION AND SERVICES

Not all developing countries have their own schools of pharmacy, but depend on pharmacists educated elsewhere. In those that do have their own schools, many do not have sufficient practising pharmacists for their needs. This may be because pharmacists choose to work in countries other than their own. For example, Egypt is acknowledged as an exporter of health personnel, including pharmacists, to neighbouring oil-rich countries in the Middle East as well as to the USA, Canada and countries in Western Europe. Migration from developing to developed countries is more common than vice versa. Of pharmacists who choose to stay in their own country a high proportion remain in the cities, thus the distribution of professionals within developing countries is very uneven.

To contribute to the health needs of their own countries, pharmacists' education must be relevant to the health care frameworks and outlook of the government and the population. Pharmacy education in China includes both Western and traditional Chinese medicine. The education of health professionals in many developing countries was based on that in industrialised countries (especially in cases in which there is a historic link, e.g. former colonies). For instance, the University of Ife which is the oldest pharmacy education institution in Nigeria initiated a pharmacy degree programme in 1963. The curriculum was substantially modelled on those of the pharmacy schools in Britain at the time (Erhun and Rahman 1989). Pharmacy education is continually evolving and schools inevitably look to other institutions when planning and developing courses in an effort to ensure the provision of high quality education comparable to that elsewhere.

Universities are generally located in the large cities. Their students will necessarily be people who have had educational opportunities that are not available to the majority of the population. They may have limited contact or understanding of the life and problems of rural areas. Graduate health professionals do not necessarily possess the most relevant knowledge and skills for addressing health problems in these areas. Having undertaken university education similar to that offered in industrialised nations, students may feel that their aspirations are unlikely to be realised in poor rural areas, even though the health needs there may be greater.

CONCLUSION

There are many features of pharmacy services that are common to developing countries, and a number of significant differences between developed and developing countries have been identified. These include being less well-equipped educationally, professionally, technologically and economically; lacking pharmaceutical expertise, accepted codes of practice, enforceable legislation with adequate finance; lacking a developed infrastructure, pure water supply, sewage treatment, waste disposal, sources of power and local sources of suitable equipment; facing greater health problems, tropical diseases, inadequate nutrition; and lacking strong government health policy (Richards 1990).

The provision and delivery of pharmacy services must be viewed in the light of the political and economic frameworks in which they operate, and the social and cultural contexts in which services are perceived and used. The WHO has recognised the potential contribution that pharmacists could make to the health care of people in developing countries (World Health Organisation 1988a). The WHO also emphasises the importance of pharmacy education that is designed to equip pharmacists for their future roles in hospitals and the community. Their document, Good Pharmacy Practice (World Health Organisation 1996) states the need for health promotion, disease prevention, supply and use of prescribed medicines, influencing prescribing and rational use of medicines. The potential contribution of pharmacists extends to all levels of planning and provision of services.

At a health and drug policy level, pharmacists must be aware of political and economic factors, and their impact on the provision and delivery of drugs and pharmaceutical services. Decisions regarding health care will always be made in the context of wider policy objectives and the political priorities of the government. Thus, in South Africa, during the period of apartheid, health care provision to different racial groups reflected government policy.

Health care in most developing countries is hampered by a lack of finance to support a comprehensive and high quality service. Many of the poorest countries are forced to direct a high proportion of their national income to repayment of debts to industrialised countries. Economic considerations also operate on a micro-economic level in which individual pharmacists may be influenced by financial incentives to sell products which are not the most suitable for a person's needs. Financial considerations may also play an important part in an individual's decision regarding whether to consult a doctor or go directly to a pharmacy to obtain drug therapy. Purchases of part-packets or individual tablets are also common among people on low incomes in developing countries.

Research into irrational drug use has uncovered many examples of questionable prescribing practices. In many developing countries, pharmacists are in private practice and there is little documentation on formal links between them and prescribers. Should the political and professional frameworks exist, the training of pharmacists should equip them to gradually assume more prominent roles in facilitating good prescribing.

In developing countries, most drugs are supplied without a prescription. In the supply of medicines, the pharmacist may be the only health professional in a position to ensure the appropriateness of further supplies of a prescribed medicine, or advise on the management of a common ailment. Self-medication with pharmaceutical products is common practice in developing countries. In societies in which both traditional and Western medical practices operate, people often perceive benefits of, and resort to Western pharmaceutical products. In advising people on the management of health problems and the appropriate use of drugs, health professionals must ensure that their advice is relevant to the concerns and perspectives of the individuals they serve.

FURTHER READING

Gray, A. (Ed.) (1993) *World Health and Disease*, Open University Press, Buckingham.

van der Geest, S. and Whyte, S.R. (Ed.) (1991) *The Context of Medicines in Developing Countries: Studies in Pharmaceutical Anthropology*, Het Spinhus Publishers, Amsterdam.

Webster, C. (Ed.) (1993) *Caring for Health: History and Diversity*, Open University Press, Buckingham.

World Health Organisation (1998) *The World Health Report 1998: Life in the 21st Century – a Vision for All*, World Health Organisation, Geneva.

REFERENCES

Baker, P. (1984) The introduction of limited list prescribing in Zambia. *Journal of Social and Administrative Pharmacy*, **4**, 187–191.

Banerji, D. (1974) Social and cultural foundations of health services systems. *Economic and Political Weekly*, **August**, 1333–1346.

Calva, J. (1996) Antibiotic use in a periurban community in Mexico: a household and drugstore survey. *Social Science and Medicine*, **42**, 1121–1128.

Cederlof, C. and Tomson, G. (1995) Private pharmacies and the health sector reform in developing countries – professionals and commercial highlights. *Journal of Social and Administrative Pharmacy*, **12**, 101–111.

Chaulagai, C.N. (1995) Community financing for essential drugs in Nepal. *World Health Forum*, **16**, 92–95.

Dickinson, R. and Davidson, A.W. (1993) Counterfeit medicines: a joint survey by the Commonwealth Pharmaceutical Association and the International Pharmacy Federation. *International Pharmacy Journal*, **7**, 65–70.

Erhun, W.O. and Rahman, A.W. (1989) Comparative appraisal of the pharmacy curricula at a Nigerian university. *Journal of Social and Administrative Pharmacy*, **6**, 92–98.

Fabricant, S.J. and Hirschhorn, N. (1987) Deranged distribution, perverse prescription, unprotected use: the irrationality of pharmaceuticals in the developing world. *Health Policy and Planning*, **2**, 204–213.

Goel, P., Ross-Degnan, D., Berman, P. and Soumerai, S. (1996) Retail pharmacies in developing countries: a behaviour and intervention framework. *Social Science and Medicine*, **42**, 1155–1161.

Greenhalgh, T. (1987) Drug prescription and self-medication in India: an exploratory survey. *Social Science and Medicine*, **25**, 307–318.

Habiyambere, V. and Wertheimer, A.I. (1993) Essential drugs should be accessible to all people. *World Health Forum*, **14**, 140–143.

Health Action International (1997) *Fragile Economies, Flooded Markets: Networking for Rational Drug Use in East Africa*, Health Action International, Amsterdam.

Hesketh, T. and Zhu, W.X. (1997) Traditional Chinese medicine: one country, two systems. *British Medical Journal*, **315**, 115–117.

Kanji, N., Hardon, A., Harnmeijer, J.W., Mamdani, M. and Walt, G. (1992) *Drugs Policy in Developing Countries*, Zed Books Ltd, London.

Laing, R.O. (1990) Rational drug use: an unsolved problem. *Tropical Doctor*, **20**, 101–103.

Lexchin, J. (1995) *Deception by Design: Pharmaceutical Promotion in the Third World*, Consumers' International, Penang.

Mills, A. and Lee, K. (Eds.) (1993) *Health Economic Research in Developing Countries*, Oxford University Press, Oxford.

Munishi, G.K. (1991) The development of the essential drugs programme and implications for self-reliance in Tanzania. *Journal of Clinical Epidemiology*, **44** (suppl.ii), 7S–14S.

Nizami, S.Q., Khan, I.A and Bhutta, Z.A. (1996) Drug prescribing practices of general practitioners and paediatricians for childhood diarrhoea in Pakistan. *Social Science and Medicine*, **42**, 1133–1139.

Quadir, M.A, Rumore, M.M. and Faroque, A.B.M. (1993) The National Drug Policy of Bangladesh 1982–1993. *Journal of Social and Administrative Pharmacy*, **10**, 1–14.

Richards, R.M.E. (1990) Developing pharmacy in developing countries. *International Pharmacy Journal*, **1**, 19–24.

Rolt, F. (1985) *Pills, Policies and Profits*, War on Want, London.

Roy, J. (1994) The menace of substandard drugs. *World Health Forum*, **15**, 406–407.

Stephen, W.J. (1992) *Primary Health Care in the Arab World*, Somerset House, Somerset.

van der Geest, S. (1991) The articulation of formal and informal medicine distribution in south Cameroon. In S. van der Geest and S.R. Whyte (Eds.) *The Context of Medicines in Developing Countries: Studies in Pharmaceutical Anthropology*, Het Spinhus Publishers, Amsterdam.

van der Geest, S. and Whyte, S.R. (Eds.) (1991) *The Context of Medicines in Developing Countries: Studies in Pharmaceutical Anthropology*, Het Spinhus Publishers, Amsterdam.

World Health Organisation (1988a) *The Role of the Pharmacist in the Health Care System*, World Health Organisation, Geneva.

World Health Organisation (1988b) *The World Drug Situation*, World Health Organisation, Geneva.

World Health Organisation (1992) *Essential Drugs: Action for Equity*, World Health Organisation, Geneva.

World Health Organisation (1996) *Good Pharmacy Practice: Guidelines in Community and Hospital Pharmacy Settings*, World Health Organisation, Geneva.

World Health Organisation (1998) *The World Health Report 1998: Life in the 21st Century – a Vision for All*, World Health Organisation, Geneva.

World Health Organisation (1999) *Guidelines for Drug Donations*, World Health Organisation, Geneva.

SELF-ASSESSMENT QUESTIONS

Question 1: Outline ways in which health problems in developing countries differ from those in industrialised countries.

Question 2: What features distinguish a) health care systems and b) patterns of drug use in developed and developing countries? What implications may this have for pharmacy services?

Question 3: What role has the WHO organisation had in improving access to drugs and rationalising drug use in developing countries?

Question 4: Describe the development of pharmacy to address the health care needs of, and respond to the problems of drug use, in developing countries.

KEY POINTS FOR ANSWERS

Question 1: Patterns of mortality and morbidity, in particular infectious disease. These should be viewed in the context of the determinants of health.

Question 2:

a) Health care systems: Patterns of public and private provision, quality of care, coverage in particular between urban and rural areas.

b) Drug use: Patterns of production and consumption, in some cases a reflection of morbidity patterns. Lack of availability of essential drugs especially in rural areas, availability for purchase without a prescription of a wide range of products in many developing countries.

Also cultural perspectives, patterns of self-medication, pluralism in health care.

Question 3:   The WHO Action programme on essential drugs, tackling problems of inappropriate marketing and use and to promote access to essential drugs for increasing proportion of population in developing countries.

Question 4:   Pharmacy services are part of the political, economic and cultural frameworks in which their health care systems operate. Pharmacists have to respond to inappropriate drug marketing, counterfeit products, lack of availability of essential drugs, poor coverage of health services, lack of purchasing power among the poorest people. In many developing countries (in particular in the rural areas) there is a shortage of appropriately trained pharmacists.

PART THREE

Health, Illness and Medicines Use

7 The Social Context of Health and Illness

Sarah Nettleton

INTRODUCTION	106
LAY HEALTH KNOWLEDGE	108
Why study lay health knowledge?	108
Defining health	109
Health maintenance and disease prevention	110
Lay views of medicines and drugs	111
THE EXPERIENCE OF ILLNESS	113
The sick role	113
Access to the sick role	114
Lay legitimization of the sick role	115
SELF-HELP GROUPS	116
PROFESSIONAL-PATIENT RELATIONSHIPS	117
CONCLUSION	118
FURTHER READING	119
REFERENCES	119
SELF-ASSESSMENT QUESTIONS	120
KEY POINTS FOR ANSWERS	120

INTRODUCTION

This chapter will explore the changing nature of contemporary society by first highlighting some of the salient features of our current social context. It will then focus more specifically on people's understanding of health and their experiences of illness. Finally, the implications of these for interactions between health professionals and patients will be discussed.

There are a number of characteristic features of modern society that are salient to the understanding of health knowledge and health practice. First, the changing nature of the disease burden. The latter half of the twentieth century saw a move from predominantly acute, life-threatening infectious diseases to chronic, and sometimes non-life-threatening conditions such as cancer, cardiovascular disease, diabetes and asthma. Life expectancy is also increasing and these chronic conditions are more prevalent in an aging population. However, although we are living longer there are signs that we are experiencing increasingly high levels of morbidity. Concomitantly, in addressing ill health there has been a shifting emphasis from intervention to surveillance (e.g. screening), and from curing to caring. By definition, chronic conditions are not amenable to successful intervention and so medicine is limited to ameliorative responses.

The changing nature of the disease burden and the amelioration of symptoms has occurred alongside the growing emphasis on the prevention of illness and promotion of health. The causes of contemporary disease burdens have changed and are now considered to be largely preventable. Hence the emphasis on screening for early intervention, and the growing preoccupation with so called 'lifestyle' factors such as smoking, diet, stress, alcohol. The health services' response to physical and mental ill-health are increasingly community rather than hospital-based. The responses to ill-health are facilitated by technological changes – not least the growth in information technological which enables screening and the surveillance of 'at risk' populations. However, the main determinants of poor health in the Western world are poverty and social inequalities (see Chapter 8).

The growth of information communications technologies (ICTs) is one of the major changes in contemporary society. The rate of change is fast. Indeed, the rapidity of change is said, by some commentators, to be one of the key features of modern society (Giddens 1991; 1999) This is especially the case in relation to a process termed *globalization* The process is typified by the internet, wherein time and space become contracted. For example, information on health and illness can be accessed almost instantly by the public and professionals alike. See the hypothetical example in Box 7.1.

A further change in contemporary society is that formal 'expert' knowledge is being challenged. Those hitherto regarded as experts – such as scientists and health professionals are increasingly subject to challenge. This process has intensified with the 'crises' surrounding

Box 7.1 An example of the public's access to health information

issues such as BSE and the debate on genetically modified food. Increasingly experience, trial and error, and having *gone through it* seem to carry as much authority or legitimacy as the codified knowledge of the 'expert'. The pharmacist, the doctor, the counsellor, the social worker, the nurse, the health visitor are not the only sources of advice and information. The fact that professionals have been schooled in a particular way and have a body of codified knowledge is not enough. For example, people may ask the pharmacist about a particular drug regimen, but then turn to the internet to check out the suitability of a drug and its possible adverse effects. Medical sociologists have argued for some time that the public possess expertise about their own health and illness. Nowadays though, people are increasingly aware of their own expertise and are willing to share it. The growth of self help groups is an illustration of this.

The internet is commonly used to access information, on just about everything, and can be accessed in a variety of ways, for example, locating *websites* set up to provide information on particular conditions. Or it may involve making contact with other people who have a shared experience of a given condition via *newsgroups*. There are currently thousands of different newsgroups and publically accessible discussion lists and there are literally millions of web pages. People may use these to access information on topics such as health, illness and how to treat various ailments and diseases, or seek advice about an illness which they are currently suffering from. Box 7.2 contains an example of a *thread* (i.e. a set of exchanges) from a *newsgroup*.

In addition to the World Wide Web there is a growing range of other information sources, for example the proliferation of health and fitness magazines and the health and lifestyles programmes on television. There is also an increasing diversity of types of health care – the growth of alternative medicine being perhaps the most obvious example. Thus, patients are not passive recipients of health care and health advice; increasingly they are discerning consumers and users of health care.

Given the way that rapid social change impinges on everyday life, it is imperative that health practitioners have some appreciation of the

Box 7.2 An example of a thread from a newsgroup on the Internet

social context in which they function. These changes also point to the fact that all modern day practitioners should have some understanding of the nature and complexity of people's views about health and illness. Sociological studies of ideas about health and illness can throw some light on these.

LAY HEALTH KNOWLEDGE

Why study lay health knowledge?

The sociological study of lay (i.e. non-professional) health knowledge is of value to health care practice in a number of ways. First, the findings can contribute to an understanding of professional-patient interactions, in that they can provide an insight into lay conceptualisations which might otherwise be treated as simply 'incorrect' knowledge by professionals. Second, an understanding of people's ideas about health maintenance and disease prevention are crucial to the effectiveness of health education and health promotion pro-grammes. Third, the study of health beliefs may contribute to our knowledge of *informal* health care. Most health care work is carried out by lay people either in the form of self-care or caring for relatives and friends. Finally, lay knowledge is not static: people's knowledge, ideas and beliefs are constantly changing and are shaped by the social milieu of their lives.

Defining health

It is customary to distinguish between both *negative* and *positive* definitions of health and *functional* and *experiential* definitions. The medical view of health – *the absence of disease* – is clearly negative. By contrast an example of a positive definition is that offered by the World Health Organisation (WHO): *a state of complete physical, mental and social well-being*. A functional definition implies the ability to par-ticipate in normal social roles (see below) and this may be contrasted with an experiential definition which takes sense of self (i.e. ideas about who '*I am*' as a person) into account. Another approach to defining health is via the examination of people's perceptions of the concept. For example, in a study of elderly people in Aberdeen, Williams (1983) identified, from his interview data, three lay concepts of health:

- Health as the absence of disease
- Health as a dimension of strength, weakness and exhaustion
- Health as functional fitness

Empirical studies have found that people's ideas are likely to incorpor-ate a number of these dimensions. However, there is evidence to suggest some relationship between types of beliefs and social circum-stances. For example, Cornwell (1984) found that the gender-depen-dent division of labour impacted upon women's response to illness. Whilst men could take time off work women could not. As one partic-ipant in the study notes:

'*Men, they are like babies. You don't know what I put up with from him. Women, they get on with it ... I'd say woman have more aches and pains than men, but, as I say, when you've got a family, you will find a women will work till she's dropping. But she'll do what she's got to do and then she'll say, "Right, I'm off to bed". Whereas its alright for a man. If he's ill he's got nothing to do, he just lies there doesn't he?*'

Moreover, this experience appears to transcend '*race*'. In her study of Pathan mothers living in Britain, Currer (1986) reports participants as stating that '*we do not have time to be ill. I have not been ill at all ... whether we are well or ill, happy or unhappy, we do our work*'. Clearly then, definitions of health are related to the structure of people's everyday lives. The relationship between beliefs and structural location should not, however, be overstated. For example, in a comparative study of middle and working class women, Calnan (1987) did not find clear distinctions between the classes.

Health maintenance and disease prevention

Ideas about the maintenance of health are separated in lay logic from ideas about the prevention of disease. Calnan (1987) states that health and disease are not direct opposites:

'lay ideas about health maintenance were more coherent than ... ideas about disease prevention. This suggested that people, irrespective of their social class, operate with a range of definitions of health that are not simply connected. Thus promoting health and preventing disease are not direct opposites, that is, positives and negatives, and while women had clear recipes about how to maintain health, they did not necessarily feel they were applicable to disease prevention'.

Whilst people consider that diet, exercise, rest and relaxation might contribute to maintaining health, it does not follow that such activities will *prevent* the onset of illness or disease. Ideas about disease causation tend to emphasise biological rather than behavioural factors. For example, Blaxter (1983) found that the working class women she interviewed considered the most common causes of disease to be infection, hereditary factors and agents of the environment.

There are diseases to which certain types of people are presumed to be more susceptible than others. Heart disease provides the classic example where people with certain temperaments, who are overweight and who are obsessively active are considered as being most likely to be susceptible. These ideas reflect medical epidemiology which has identified type A and type B behaviours as being more or less prone to heart disease. Thus, people are able to identify heart disease *'candidates'* based on information given by health educators i.e. those who eat saturated fats, do not do any exercise and who are hyperactive. However, as Davison *et al.* (1991) point out people collectively develop a *'lay epidemiology'* which recognises that not all candidates have heart attacks whilst some do, and this must therefore be due to chance. Health promoters, keen to present unequivocal, simplified and straightforward messages, fail to address these anomalies and so underestimate the sophistication of lay thinking. Davison goes on to point out that it *'is ironic that such evidently fatalistic cultural concepts should be given more rather than less explanatory power by the activities of modern health education, whose stated goals lie in the opposite direction'.*

There appears to be a moral dimension to health. In Cornwell's study, people were keen to present themselves as being healthy, and initial statements on health status often bore no relation to their medical histories. For example, one woman described herself as healthy and lucky in that she had good health and yet:

'Kathleen's medical history included having such bad eyesight as a child that she was expected to be blind by the age of twenty, lung disease including tuberculosis in her late teens, a miscarriage, a thyroid deficiency which requires permanent medication, and six years prior to interviews, a hysterectomy' (Cornwell 1984).

As well as an insistence on good health and a scorn of hypochondriacs and malingerers the analysis of *'public accounts'* revealed a necessity to be able to prove the *'otherness'* of illness as a separate thing that happened to the person and was not something for which they could be held responsible.

Lay views of medicines and drugs

The rich and complex nature of people's views is evident in accounts of their use of medicines which have been either prescribed by general practitioners or bought over the counter. In those countries where Western bio-medicine is dominant, two contrasting images of drugs appear to prevail (Morgan 1996). On the one hand, medicines are seen positively as being *cures, miracles, remedies* and *effective treatments*. On the other hand, they are seen as being *harmful, dangerous* and may be *ineffective* or have *bad side effects*. Such images are evident in the media for example, tales of *wonder drugs* and *medical disasters* are fairly commonplace in the newspapers and on television. Research into people's ideas and use of drugs has found evidence of both these positive and negative views of drugs, although they do appear to be more tempered and considered than those that appear in the media.

Based on an analysis of 30 qualitative interviews with men and women from a range of social backgrounds in London, Britten (1996) was able to classify her interview transcripts into what she termed *orthodox* and *unorthodox* accounts (Box 7.3).

Aspects of these orthodox and unorthodox views can be discerned in Morgan's (1996) study of 'White' and Afro-Caribbean patients' use of anti-hypertensive drugs. From interviews carried out with 30 'White' and 30 Afro-Carribean men and women who had being prescribed such drugs for at least a year, the researchers learned how different people managed and used their drugs in different ways. They identified three different types of responses to this drug regimen. There where what they labelled as *'stable'* adherents (16 'White' and 8 Afro-Caribbean) those who took the medicines as prescribed, and who did not express any major worries or concerns about taking their tablets. Two further groups identified were: the *'problematic'* adherents (10 'White' and '4 Afro-Caribbean'); and those who *did not take the drugs as prescribed* (two 'White' and 18 Afro-Caribbean). These people were concerned about the actual or possible adverse effects of the drugs. They expressed concerns such as not wanting to become dependent on drugs, and were anxious about the potential of long term addiction. Some made use of alternative remedies such as herbal treatments. The

Box 7.3 Orthodox and unorthodox accounts of medicines (Britten 1996)

extent to which these concerns led people to either reduce their dosage or to stop taking the drugs altogether was linked to their assessment as to the seriousness of their condition, and to the benefits of taking the medicines. Amongst those Afro-Caribbean patients who had concerns about the drugs, the most common response was to take the drugs irregularly, taking them as and when they felt they needed them and in response to their blood pressure levels. They were less likely than the White patients therefore to stop altogether. Those groups who had concerns about the long term use of these drugs mirrored the responses of the unorthodox group identified by Britten (1996). As with this unorthodox group they were also more likely to use alternative, traditional remedies which were considered to be more *'natural'*.

These studies capture the views of some men and women living in London in the 1990s. It is important to remember that they will be shaped by their social and historical context. The Afro-Caribbean men and women in Morgan's study (1996) were born in the Caribbean. It is possible that the children's generation might hold different views. This is true of course for any social group. For example, as we saw at the beginning of this chapter, at a time when there is more and more information on aspects of health, illness, treatments and so on, people's perceptions and responses to the administration and use of medicines is likely to change. Practitioners must invariably be sensitive to such changes and be able to acknowledge and respond to the views of their patients or clients.

THE EXPERIENCE OF ILLNESS

Bio-physical changes have significant social consequences. Illness reminds us that the *'normal'* functioning of our minds and bodies is central to social action and interaction. In this respect the study of illness throws light on the nature of the interaction between the body, the individual and society. If we cannot rely on our bodies to function *'normally'* then our interaction with the social world becomes perilous; our dependency on others may increase and, in turn, our sense of self may be challenged. To illustrate, the onset of rheumatoid arthritis can result in a severe restriction of bodily movements, this may mean that the sufferer becomes dependent upon others to perform tasks previously carried out by him or herself. As discussed above, there is a moral and cultural dimension to this. Within a culture which emphasises independence and self-reliance, for example, a condition which limits that which previously had been presumed to be *'normal'* functioning, can be threatening to the sufferer's self-esteem. Essentially then, chronic illness can impact upon a person's daily living, their social relationships, their identity (the view that others hold of them) and their sense of self (their private view of themselves). It is on these experiences of illness that sociologists have focussed their attention. Responses to illness then, are not simply determined by either the nature of biophysical symptoms or individual motivations, but are shaped and imbued by the social, cultural and ideological context of an individual's biography. Thus, illness is at once both a very personal and a very public phenomenon.

The sick role

Illness is often related to one's capacity to work and/or fulfil one's social obligations. However, the presence of illness must be sanctioned by the medical profession. This forms the central premise of Parsons' (1951) concept of the *sick role*. Parsons makes a distinction between the biological basis of illness and its social basis and argues that to be sick is a socially, as well as a biologically, altered state. Thus, the sick role proscribes a set of rights and obligations, these are that a person who is sick cannot be expected to fulfil normal social obligations and is not held responsible for their illness. In turn, however, the sick role obliges that the sick person should want to get well, and to this end, must seek and co-operate with technically competent medical help. It appears that this 'role' is acknowledged within the lay discourse of Western societies as can be seen by the comments made in interviews cited by Herzlich and Pierret (1987): *'When one is sick, one obviously tries to get better as soon as possible. Personally, I do everything I can, I try to do my utmost to be cured as quickly as possible … I would be a good patient come to think of it.'*

The sick role therefore indicates that the person who makes an effort to get well will be granted a social status, as Herzlich and Pierret (1987) again explain:

*'To be **sick** in today's society has ceased to designate a purely biological state and come to define a status, or even a group identity. It is becoming more and more evident that we perceive the reality of illness in these terms, for we tend to identify our neighbour as a "diabetic", almost in the same manner as we identify him [sic] as "a professor", or "a mason". To be "sick" henceforth constitutes one of the central categories of social perception.'*

Thus, illness may become part of the identity of the sufferer and this is especially significant, as we shall see, for those with long term illnesses.

The concept of the sick role as described by Parsons is an ideal type and therefore does not necessarily correspond with empirical reality. Indeed a moment's reflection on our own experiences is likely to bring to mind circumstances where the sick role did not apply. For example, we might have symptoms but refuse to seek out professional help or we might feel ill but carry on with activities which may make our condition worse. Furthermore, as discussed above, the patient may not rely solely on the advice and information given by the doctor, but may be effective in seeking out his or her own information and developing his or her own expertise. However, the sick role is a useful concept with which to assess actual illness behaviours and experiences. Studies such as these reveal the range and complexity of illness behaviours. Let us take two examples of divergence from the ideal. First the issue of *'accessing'* the sick role and second, the issue of other people *'legitimizing'* the sick role.

Access to the sick role

If a person adopts the sick role when they feel ill they have an obligation to get well and this first requires that they seek medical advice. However most people, most of the time, do not go the doctor when they are ill. Indeed prevalence studies have revealed that most symptoms are never seen by practitioners (Hannay 1980) – there is a *symptom iceberg*. Certainly most of the time, if people have a cold, bad back pain or a bout of hayfever they probably would not want to bother their general practitioner. Conversely if they did, general practitioners would get rather irritated as one of the main sources of exasperation with their work is patients who present with trivia conditions. However, it is not only trivial symptoms that fail to reach health professionals, studies have also found that people suffering from extreme pain do not necessarily seek help.

People do not respond to the biophysical aspects of symptoms, but rather to the meaning of those symptoms. Many '*common*' ailments, for example, stomach pains, headaches or a stiff neck, may be '*explained away*' or be '*normalised*'. They may be attributed to circumstances such as working late at night, eating too much strong cheese or sitting in a draft. If these ailments do turn out to be manifestations of a more serious illness it may take some time for this to be recognised. Thus accessing the sick role can take a long time.

Lay legitimization of the sick role

Legitimacy of access to the sick role can be compounded by moral evaluations. This may even occur when someone has received confirmation of sick role status from a health professional. For example, the credibility of a medical diagnosis may well be undermined for those who are only mildly affected by a disease or those who have remissions. As a respondent in Robinson's (1988) study of multiple sclerosis articulates:

'*Some people can't understand why I'm in a wheelchair sometimes and not other times ... with some as long as I look cheerful and say I'm feeling fine they can cope with me but if I say I don't feel well they ignore the remark, or say I **look** well! I feel that some of them think I'm being lazy or giving up if I'm in a wheelchair, and they are inclined to talk right over my head to my pusher*' (emphasis in original).

Conditions such as chronic pain, which do not fit in to any medical category and are idiopathic, i.e. they have no identifiable cause, are especially problematic for sufferers. We have seen that entering the sick role is more complex than the original concept suggests, as meanings and perceptions interfere with the process. Finally, there are also pragmatic constraints which prevent the straightforward acquisition of a sick status. For example, it may be impossible to be relieved of normal social duties if these involve caring for others and/or the general running of the household. Graham (1984) points out:

'*While a mother is quick to identify and respond to symptoms of illness and disability in others, she appears less assiduous in monitoring her own health. Her role in caring for others appears to blunt her sensitivity to her own needs. Being ill makes it difficult for individuals to maintain their normal social roles and responsibilities: since the mother's roles and responsibilities are particularly indispensable, mothers are reluctant to be ill*'.

During recent decades the scientific literature has tended to locate the causes of disease in features of people's personalities. If the personality is the source of illness, for example if the stressful or anxious person is more likely to get coronary heart disease or cancer, then this can have significant implications for the sufferer's sense of self, the reactions of others and the ability to overcome the illness.

The sick role then, constitutes a culturally specific, ideal, typical response to illness. The reality of everyday life however is more complex than the concept itself suggests. The interpretation of symptoms, the decision to seek help, the conferring of rights and expectations to the sick person are mediated by the social and cultural environment. A key dimension of the sick role is that it is incumbent on the sick person to make every effort to get well. Clearly this might be inappropriate for those people who are chronically ill. Help may come not just from professionals but friends, relatives and others who share common experiences.

SELF-HELP GROUPS

It is evident that patients are not simply passive *recipients* of care but they, and their relatives and friends, are also *providers* of that care – a fact that has long been recognised by sociologists of health and illness. Thus, lay people develop considerable amounts of expertise and knowledge which may even surpass that of the so-called 'experts' within the medical profession. This knowledge and experience may be shared amongst those people who suffer from the same illness. Self-help groups have been set up, sometimes at the instigation of, and sometimes in opposition to, the medical profession, to provide informal support for those people with certain conditions, to educate people more generally about a particular disease, to support relevant research, and to lobby for changes. Self-help groups concerned with illness are, arguably, a relatively new phenomenon and form *'part of the larger protest movement'* that is becoming evident in contemporary Western societies. These processes are likely to be accelerated within the context of the information society.

Self-help groups provide support on both *individual* and *collective* levels. For their individual members they may offer emotional support and may be invaluable during the early stages of a person's illness career to overcome social isolation and loneliness. As many members have expertise in the provision of care, practical assistance may also be available. The ability to provide this level of support may contribute to the positive identity of people who are sick. This is also facilitated by a sense of solidarity which can be achieved amongst those who share a common problem. At the collective level the establishment of solidarity amongst a self-help group may result in the pursuit of change at a political level. It can result in the mobilisation of those concerned to become more active consumers of care and engage in activities which are aimed at overcoming prejudice and discrimination.

Continuing the theme of change, it is argued here that the nature of relationships between lay people and experts has changed during the last few decades. Growth of lay knowledge, legitimacy of experience and declining faith in *'experts'* are likely to impact on professional and patient or client interactions. The professional-patient relationship, once characterised as a meeting between the knowledgeable expert and the ignorant lay person, is now more appropriately, and more accurately, described as a *'meeting between experts'* (Tuckett *et al.* 1985). The fact that people are encouraged to take responsibility for their own health and are more knowledgeable about factors which influence their health status adds to this view. Many illnesses today are associated with social and behavioural factors and these are matters which are becoming *'common knowledge'*. Consultations are increasingly likely to include discussions about lifestyle choices and not just focus on writing prescriptions for specific pathological conditions.

Research indicates that practitioners have often neglected to take the patient's view seriously and this has been identified as a serious limitation of contemporary formal health care. This is important because as we have seen, most people are able to develop sophisticated accounts about health and illness. The social science literature has revealed that lay people want to, can, and do play an important part in interactions with trained health care workers, and the quality of interaction impacts upon the outcomes of health care. Such outcomes might include the extent to which a patient recovers from an illness for which he or she has been treated, or the level of satisfaction with the health care provided.

Patients then, may have more knowledge about their condition than health care professionals. People often accumulate expertise about their own bodies and come to have a special knowledge of their experience of health and illness. It is thus frustrating if the practitioner does not want to acknowledge the patient's view. One woman who was describing the difficulties she had in making the doctor listen to her put it thus: *'I've lived with this body for seventy odd years. If I don't know when its not working properly I don't know who does'* (Sidell 1992).

At a time when behavioural factors are increasingly being recognised as the antecedents of many illnesses, value judgements may be made as to the patient's culpability for their illness. This can result in patients' feeling guilty about their symptoms. Value judgements may also be made about the suitability of treatment. For example, in the summer of 1993, much controversy was generated in the UK media, as a result of decisions taken by some medical consultants not to administer tests and carry out coronary bypass surgery on people who continued to smoke. They argued that the resources should not be spent on people if they smoke as they have little chance of recovery. Decisions such as these are considered by many to be value judgements rather than purely clinical decisions. The debate, which focussed on the need to ration resources and direct them to those cases who will benefit most, highlights the extent to which responses to individual patients are likely to vary according to the economic and political context in which they are made.

Patients who are not satisfied with their interactions may deal with conflicts in a number of ways. For example, they may formally complain about a practitioner. In recent years there has been a significant increase in complaints made within the National Health Service. It has been suggested however, that there may still be an iceberg of dissatisfaction because although many more people are complaining about health professionals, especially doctors, most people do not know how to complain.

For those people who do complain about primary health care practitioners, two concerns are particularly prevalent. First, the manner of practitioners and, second, difficulties in convincing them of the seriousness of a patient's condition for whom a visit is being requested. The ability to be supportive and empathetic to patients is also recognised by lay people to be an essential quality of health professionals. For example, one patient, in a letter of complaint, wrote: '*It would seem that Dr X lacks some of the qualities that will give his patients feelings of trust and understanding, qualities **which I feel are essential** for a good GP*' (Nettleton and Harding 1994). Further, lay people do not always accept the clinical decisions of '*experts*' uncritically. Indeed, another complainant cited in the same study reported how, after being prescribed a particular drug, she looked it up in the British National Formulary, and finding no reference to her condition, did not collect the medication.

Patients then, are not simply *passive* recipients of care, but are *active* participants in the processes of health care work. The relationship between professionals and patients is likely to be enhanced if practitioners are able to recognise and encourage patients to be involved. As patients and clients have access to ever more information this point is likely to become especially salient.

CONCLUSION

For most people, interactions with health professionals form their main encounters with health care services, and prescribed medicines are the most common form of treatment in Western medicine. People's knowledge and ideas about their treatments and how they actually *experience* health and illness will be contingent on the social context in which they live out their lives. This chapter has indicated that the social context is constantly changing, and the current pace of change is very rapid indeed. This is not least because of the growing proliferation of knowledge and information that people have available to them. Thus lay people bring to their encounters with professionals considerable amounts of knowledge, information and expertise which may be derived from the wide range of sources, be it their own personal experience, or a specialist *website* on the internet. During the last few decades the contribution that lay people make to the nature of interactions has been acknowledged, and it has been suggested that their participation has increased. This increasingly active role played by the clients, patients or lay people may be emblematic of wider social transformations such as: a decline in faith in *'experts'*; a questioning of modern scientific knowledge; the emergence of a consumer culture; and the formation of an information society.

FURTHER READING

Albrecht, G.L., Fitzpatrick, R. and Scrimshaw, S. (2000) *The Handbook of Social Studies in Health and Medicine*, Sage, London.

Harding, G., Nettleton, S.J. and Taylor, K.M.G. (1990) *Sociology for Pharmacists: an Introduction*, Macmillan, Basingstoke.

Hardy, M. (1998) *The Social Context of Health*, Open University Press, Buckingham.

Nettleton, S.J. (1995) *The Sociology of Health and Illness*, Polity Press, Cambridge.

REFERENCES

Blaxter, M. (1983) The cause of disease: women talking. *Social Science and Medicine*, **17**, 59–69.

Britten, N. (1996) Lay views on drugs and medicines: orthodox and unorthodox accounts. In: S. Williams and M. Calnan (Eds.) *Modern Medicine: Lay Perspectives and Experiences*, UCL Press, London.

Calnan, M. (1987) *Health and Illness: The Lay Perspective*, Tavistock, London.

Cornwell, J. (1984) *Hard Earned Lives: Accounts of Health and Illness from East London*, Tavistock, London.

Currer, C. (1986) Concepts of mental well- and ill-being: the case of Pathan mothers in Britain. In: C. Currer and M. Stacey (Eds.) *Concepts of Health, Illness and Disease: a Comparative Perspective*, Berg, Lemington Spa.

Davison, C., Davey Smith, G. and Frankel, S. (1991) Lay epidemiology and the prevention paradox: the implications of coronary candidacy for health education. *Sociology of Health and Illness*, **13**, 1–19.

Giddens, A. (1991) *Modernity and Self-Identity: Self and Society in the Late Modern Age*, Polity Press, Cambridge.

Giddens, A. (1999) The Runaway World *The Reith Lectures 1999* BBC Radio 4 http://news.bbc.co.uk/hi/english/static/events/reith_99/default.htm

Graham, H. (1984) *Women, Health and the Family*, Harvester Wheatsheaf, Brighton.

Hannay, D.R. (1980) *The Symptom Iceberg: A Study of Community Health*, Routledge and Kegan Paul, London.

Herzlich, C. and Pierret, J. (1987) *Illness and Self in Society*, Johns Hopkins University Press, Baltimore.

Morgan, M. (1996) Perceptions and use of anti-hypertensive drugs amongst cultural groups. In: Williams, S. and Calnan, M. (Eds.) *Modern Medicine: Lay Perspectives and Experiences*, UCL Press, London.

Nettleton, S. and Harding, G. (1994) Protesting patients: a study of complaints made to a family health service authority. *Sociology of Health and Illness*, **16**, 38–61.

Parsons, T. (1951) *The Social System* Glencoe, Free Press, London.

Robinson, I. (1988) Reconstructing lives: negotiating the meaning of multiple sclerosis. In: R. Anderson and M. Bury (Eds.) *Living with Chronic Illness: The Experiences of Patients and their Families*, Unwin Hyman, London.

Tuckett, D. Boutlon, M. Olson, C. and Williams, A. (1985) *Meetings Between Experts*, Tavistock, London.

Williams, R. (1983) Concepts of health: an analysis of lay logic. *Sociology*, **17**, 185–204.

SELF-ASSESSMENT QUESTIONS

Question 1: Identify at least four reasons why pharmacists should have an understanding of lay knowledge.

Question 2: In what ways can changes to the social context affect everyday pharmacy practice?

Question 3: In what ways is illness a socially altered state as well as a biologically altered state?

KEY POINTS FOR ANSWERS

Question 1:

- Informs professional-patient interactions
- Informs why people take actions to maintain health and the actions they take when ill
- Understanding informal health care
- Ideas on health are always changing and are linked to wider social changes

Question 2:

- People have access to new types of information
- People are experiencing different types of illness
- Social circumstances affect why people seek help
- Social circumstances affect how people follow professional advice
- Social context affects health status, e.g. living conditions are linked to diseases such as asthma

Question 3:

- The body may not function to meet social requirements
- Illness affects social relationships
- Illness may result in absence from work and changes to other social roles
- Illness may be perceived as having a moral dimension

Inequalities in Health and Health Care

Mark Exworthy

INTRODUCTION	124
WHAT ARE HEALTH INEQUALITIES?	124
Health inequalities – a brief history of the UK policy context since the 1970s	125
EVIDENCE OF AND EXPLANATIONS FOR HEALTH INEQUALITIES	126
Summary of health inequality evidence from key reports and studies	126
The Black Report	126
The Acheson Report	127
Saving Lives: Our Healthier Nation	128
Medical practice variations	128
Medicines and health care inequalities	129
Explanations of health inequalities	130
Cultural and behavioural explanations	131
Social (or natural) selection explanations	131
Structural explanations	131
THE POLICY RESPONSE TO HEALTH INEQUALITIES	132
CONCLUSION	135
ACKNOWLEDGEMENT	136
FURTHER SOURCES OF INFORMATION	136
REFERENCES	137
SELF-ASSESSMENT QUESTIONS	138
KEY POINTS FOR ANSWERS	138

INTRODUCTION

This chapter provides an introduction to health inequalities by examining the various definitions of health inequalities, documenting and explaining the research evidence on the state of health inequalities in the late 1990s, and by reviewing the ways in which the National Health Service (NHS) in the UK is responding to them. The chapter also makes some conclusions about the likely success of current strategies for reducing inequalities.

WHAT ARE HEALTH INEQUALITIES?

Health inequalities has become such a commonplace term in policy and practice that it seems somewhat strange to begin the chapter by clarifying the term itself. However, unless the term is clarified, the way in which research evidence is interpreted and policies are implemented, will be less than optimal. Clarity is required in three main ways.

First, although the term health inequalities is widely used, there is some debate as to whether it should refer only to inequalities in health or to inequalities in health care as well. The former would refer to health status and health outcomes in measures of morbidity and mortality, for example. The latter would refer to health service provision in, for example, measures of activity and distribution of health care practitioners. This chapter uses health inequalities to mean inequalities in both health and health care.

Second, inequalities need to be defined in terms of certain parameters and norms, that is, equal x for equal y. In terms of health *per se*, it has been defined according to equal outcomes (that is, health) for equal (demographic) need, whereas in terms of health care, it has usually been in terms of equal *access* (to services) for equal *need*. Such definitions have been termed the *'who and what'* questions; equal what for whom? The *'who'* questions refer to age, gender, ethnicity, social class and geography whilst *'what'* refers to expenditure, provision, access, use and outcome. Under the equal x for equal y formula for defining inequality, studies are beset by difficulties in measurement such as the classification of social class (based upon occupation), the criteria for access (whether social, physical or cultural), and the geographical unit of analysis (e.g. neighbourhood, district, city or county).

Third, health care inequalities have generally not had much connection with medical practice variations. This is an oversight since these variations (which are considered below) concern the ways in which health service practitioners practise, diagnose and treat (or refer) which can, in themselves, be forms of health care inequalities or contribute to wider patterns of inequalities in terms of, say, access, provision or use. In this chapter, the standard notation of medical practice variations is used rather than medical practice inequalities.

Health inequalities – a brief history of the UK policy context since the 1970s

The election of the Labour government in May 1997 was accompanied by, among other things, a commitment to tackle social exclusion and reduce the *health gap* (between the most and least healthy members of society), a term often used by policy-makers to refer to health inequalities. This was evident in the government's plans for reforms of the NHS (Department of Health 1997), the creation of the Social Exclusion Unit (based in the Cabinet Office) in 1997 and the commissioning of an independent inquiry into inequalities in health published in 1998.

Under various previous governments, the policy emphasis was placed on an individual-approach based upon choices of lifestyles rather than socio-economic determinants of health. The issue and term health inequalities had been dismissed in favour of what was termed *health variations*. The term *'variations'* was supposed to be less politically controversial by giving less emphasis to the structural factors (such as the state of the economy or government funding) underlying health inequalities. Health variations were considered different to medical practice variations. The Conservative government did, towards the end of its office institute a number of policy measures which pointed towards a different approach. For example, the *'Health of the Nation'* document (Department of Health 1992) was a strategy for health (as opposed to health care) for England. The document emphasised the need for monitoring health variations but did not include measures to reduce them. Also, a sub-group of the Chief Medical Officer's Health of the Nation working group was charged with reviewing *'health variations'*. This marked the return of health variations/inequalities to the national policy agenda.

One of the most significant landmarks in health inequalities history was the publication of the Black Report (1980). Although the then Labour government commissioned it, it was published by the incoming Conservative government. However, recommendations concerning income re-distribution and affirmative government action as ways of reducing inequalities were unpalatable messages for Conservatives. Its political importance was heightened by the decision to publish the report on the Friday before a Bank Holiday weekend, a traditional device to '*side-line*' an issue. Moreover, only a limited number of copies were published. Paradoxically, this had the effect of galvanising proponents of the research: it was subsequently published some time later, although the full impact of the Black Report's findings upon policy remains somewhat uncertain given the hostile political environment at that time and for some years afterwards.

Summary of health inequality evidence from key reports and studies

The evidence relating to the causes and manifestations of health inequalities has been accumulating for many years and there is now a reasonably detailed picture of the impact of such inequalities in different places, over time and in different socio-demographic groups. Whilst the impact of *health care* inequalities upon *health* inequalities remains one of several areas yet to be fully investigated, a number of research projects are currently ongoing, which will remedy some of the gaps in knowledge about health inequalities in its widest sense. This section provides a summary of the main studies and attempts to show the broad parameters of the inequalities *'problem.'*

The Black Report

The Black Report (1980) described the pattern of health inequalities according to occupational class, sex, geography (by region), ethnicity and housing tenure in terms of mortality and morbidity (illness) by social class. It considered the trend of inequality patterns over time and made some international comparisons. It also addressed inequality in terms of the *'availability and use of health services'*, equating to provision, access and use in the terminology employed here.

A clear pattern emerged in which unskilled classes (social class V) had mortality rates 2.5 times those of professional classes (social class I) (Table 8.1). This pattern was consistent between men and women. The pattern is often called the social class gradient and is perhaps the most widely cited health inequality.

This pattern is replicated in geographical variations. The Black Report compared death rates (SMRs, standardised mortality rates) by English and Welsh regions. There is a clear north-south division in these figures, with more southerly regions experiencing lower than expected mortality rates (Table 8.2).

Table 8.1 Death rates by sex and social class (15–64 years; rates per 1,000 population in England and Wales, 1971). Source: Black Report (1980)

Social class	Men	Women
I – professional (e.g. lawyer, pharmacist)	3.98	2.15
II – intermediate (e.g. teacher)	5.54	2.85
IIIN – skilled non-manual (e.g. shop assistant)	5.80	2.76
IIIM – skilled manual (e.g. bus driver)	6.08	3.41
IV – partly skilled (e.g. farm labourer)	7.96	4.27
V – unskilled (e.g. cleaner)	9.88	5.31

Standard region	SMR by age	SMR by age and class
Northern, Yorkshire & Humberside	113	113
North West	106	105
East Midlands	116	116
West Midlands	96	94
East Anglia	105	104
South East	90	90
South West	93	93
Wales (South)	114	117
Wales (North)	110	113
England and Wales	**100**	**100**

As the England and Wales average is 100, Standardised Mortality Rates above 100 imply a greater than expected mortality rate and vice versa.

Table 8.2 Regional variations in mortality in England and Wales. Source: Black Report (1980)

The Acheson Report

An Inquiry, commissioned by the Labour government in 1997 and chaired by Sir Donald Acheson, was charged with reviewing the latest information on health inequalities and identifying priority areas for future policy development. The report was divided into '*the current position*' on inequalities and (eleven) priority areas for policy development; the focus here is on the former.

The Acheson Report highlighted the trends over time which show a decline in mortality rates for gender and social class groups and yet the differentials between them have persisted or even increased. For example, the ratio of (male) mortality rates for social classes IV and V to classes I and II in 1976–81 was 1.53 whilst the ratio in 1986–92 had increased to 1.68 (Table 8.3).

The Acheson Report examined five specific causes of death and made comparisons between different social class. The broad social class gradient was persistent throughout these different causes and had remained despite a general decline in mortality rates. This is illustrated by deaths from lung cancer (Table 8.4).

Social class	1976–81		1981–85		1986–92	
	Men	Women	Men	Women	Men	Women
I/II	621	338	539	344	455	270
III Non-manual	860	371	658	387	484	305
III Manual	802	467	691	396	624	356
IV/V	951	508	824	445	764	418

Rates per 100,000 for England and Wales, age-standardised.

Table 8.3 Mortality rates (all causes) for men and women (aged 35–64), by social class, over time. Source: Acheson Report (1998)

Table 8.4 SMRs for lung cancer in England and Wales by social class, for men, aged 20–64. Source: Acheson Report (1998)

Social class	1970–72	1979–83	1991–93
I – professional	41	26	17
II – managerial & technical	52	39	24
IIIN – skilled, non-manual	63	47	34
IIIM – skilled manual	90	72	54
IV – partly skilled	93	76	52
V – unskilled	109	108	82
England and Wales	73	60	39

Rates are per 100,000

This summary of the evidence presented in the Black and Acheson reports is intended to provide an overview of the parameters of health inequalities generally. It would be difficult to do justice to the volume of evidence that currently exists. For example, there are 529 references in the Acheson Report. The reader is therefore directed to the reference list and contact list at the end of the chapter to explore these sources.

Saving Lives: Our Healthier Nation

The government's public health White Paper, *Saving Lives: Our Healthier Nation*, published in July 1999 (Department of Health 1999) is considered to be the formal response to the Acheson Report. The White Paper highlights health inequalities by presenting some further evidence (see Box 8.1).

Box 8.1 Evidence of health inequalities (Department of Health 1999)

In 1900, 24% of deaths were among those aged 65 years and above, and 25% died aged less than 1 year. By 1997, 84% of deaths were among those aged 65 years and above and only 4% of deaths were among those aged less than 45. This general improvement of the overall health of the population is contrasted with rising health inequality. In 1930–32, the ratio of mortality between social class I and V was 1.2 whilst in 1991–93, this ratio had risen to 2.9.

The White Paper is consistent with earlier government policy in stating that it attempts to deal with health inequality by tackling '*in the round all the things that make people ill*' and by pursuing '*partnerships between the various local and regional organisations ... to reduce health inequalities*'. Controversially, the White Paper did not set targets for the reductions in health inequality; a notable omission given the government's emphasis on performance management and assessment.

Medical practice variations

The distinction between health inequalities and health care inequalities is evident in medical practice variations. Despite the image of modern health care as based upon scientific knowledge, research has revealed variations in the ways in which health professionals practise. However, it is axiomatic that professional work (such as in health care), is bound to generate differences in the ways in which practitioners act. Yet studies have shown that these variations persist when differences in health care need are taken into account. As such, *'medical practice variations'* are often considered to be synonymous with health care inequalities (Bevan 1990).

Medical practice variations are evident at all levels – between countries, within countries and across small areas such as between different hospitals and practitioners. Andersen and Mooney (1990) report on studies, which examined seven surgical procedures in the USA, UK and Norway. The degree of variation in this inter and intra-country study differed for each procedure. A five-fold difference within countries was found for tonsillectomy, whereas appendectomy and hernia repair had consistently low levels of variation. By contrast, hysterectomy and prostatectomy had moderate levels of variation. The variations between countries seemed relatively stable across all three countries, which is significant in terms of explanations.

Explaining these *'variations'* (or inequalities) is notoriously difficult and has generated a research sector of its own. As these variations focus on the health care (rather than health *per se*), it is reasonable to look at the health care system for explanations. Andersen and Mooney (1990) highlight two possible explanations. One is what economists call *'supplier-induced demand'*. In health care, the patient is heavily dependent upon the practitioner to undertake the course of action which is in their best interests. This dependence generates demands for more resources (such as interventions in the form of surgery or drugs) which would be unknown to the patient. These demands will vary according to the resources available to practitioners, thereby generating variations in rates of surgery or prescribing. A second explanation lies in the legacy of procedures being common without being sufficiently evaluated. However, this explanation raises a conundrum in the sense that the aims of some health care interventions are often equivocal, for instance, some practitioners might disagree as to the best course of action for a patient.

Resulting from these two explanations is the notion that some variations may indeed be legitimate differences but also, as Bevan (1990) argues *'the very existence of such [medical practice] variations is an indication of geographical inequities'*. Whilst ensuring the equitable provision of health care resources, practitioners and managers need to promote the continuous evaluation of day-to-day practices which should include an assessment of the impact on equity, inequality and variations.

Medicines and health care inequalities

By definition, examples of inequalities in terms of pharmacy focus on health care inequalities relating to service provision and fall into the area of medical practice variations. The pharmacy evidence selected for this chapter is oriented towards primary care but many issues also apply to secondary care.

Majeed *et al.* (1996) considered factors that might affect prescribing variations between general medical practices. Their unit of variation was the mean net ingredient cost per patient and the study included 131 practices in southwest London. They found that about one third of the variation in prescribing costs could be explained using routine data, including age and other census characteristics as well as practice characteristics. This means that two-thirds of the variation was due to other factors such as general practitioners' knowledge and preferences. Healey and colleagues (1994) conducted a similar study. Their aim was to determine the implication of variations in general practitioner prescribing behaviour for the determination of prescribing budgets. They concluded that:

'97% of the variation in practice prescribing costs can be explained by differences in practice list size, the proportion of patients aged 65 years and over, the proportion of patients living in "deprived areas" and whether or not the practice qualifies for "inducement payments"'.

Weighted capitation formulae based on such factors are, in their view, justified. Linking prescribing behaviour to organisational factors was the purpose of a study by Houghton and Gilthorpe (1998) in 263 Birmingham practices. In particular, they focused on the impact of general practitioner fundholding. They found that fundholders spent less and prescribed fewer items than non-fundholders even though prescribing activity was steadily increasing.

The conclusion of such evidence suggests that information on clinical effectiveness is not being used sufficiently. Although medical care is *'variable and uncertain'* (Bunker 1990), health care inequalities persist. The positive responses to such evidence by practitioners have often been to establish confidential and educational system of data feedback; negative responses have ignored or dismissed the evidence (McColl *et al.* 1998). The positive responses have had some success (Keller *et al.* 1996; Centre for Reviews and Dissemination 1998). The sub-optimal use of evidence has implications for resource allocation; practices not adopting the *'best evidence'* may be at a financial disadvantage.

Explanations of health inequalities

Whilst identifying the manifestations of health and health care inequalities is difficult in itself, it is arguably more difficult to explain such patterns. Indeed it is a contentious issue. However, three broad explanations can be identified, although the role of each in any one particular example of inequality might vary. Since no single explanation will suffice, many studies are now involved in isolating the contribution of each explanatory factor in the overall inequality picture.

Cultural and behavioural explanations

The focus in these explanations is mainly upon the individual's choice of lifestyle. Thus, individuals' *'reckless'* or *'irresponsible'* behaviour may have inimical consequences upon their health. For instance, excessive amounts of drinking, smoking or eating may be detrimental to their health. Whilst some point to the lack of education or understanding of these impacts upon an individual's lifestyle, others argue that it is an individual's free will to pursue such a lifestyle. However, the choice that individuals face is constrained by their circumstances which are primarily shaped by their socio-economic situation. Thus, an unemployed person has much tighter constraints in terms of the options they have for pursing a *'healthy'* lifestyle. Access to shops selling cheap, good quality foods may be limited by the lack of transport. Alternatively, the housing market may operate in such a way that only poor quality, damp housing is available. The cultural norms of particular social groups or social classes influence the type of lifestyle that individuals pursue. Rates of smoking, for example, are higher among manual and unskilled occupational groups.

Understanding behaviour in this cultural context makes a clear link between the structural explanations (discussed later) and individual lifestyles. As such the two explanations are clearly inter-related but the nature of that relationship is not yet fully understood.

Social (or natural) selection explanations

These explanations suggest that individuals with certain characteristics drift into lower social classes and thereby receive fewer economic rewards (such as lower salaries). As well as problems of identifying cause and effect, this thesis suffers from a lack of conclusive evidence to support it. It is unclear whether the bio-genetic composition of individuals alone would merit such a conclusion, although social processes such as the job and housing markets help generate a finely graded social system.

Structural explanations

These explanations focus on the structure of society and the material living conditions. They highlight the connection between socio-economic processes of employment, government expenditure and the impact upon health. At one level, this involves the link between hazardous occupations (such as coal-mining) and individual health, but it points more broadly to more endemic processes of an individual's chances to secure adequate housing, a balanced diet, gainful employment (among other things) so as to enable them to participate fully in society. Despite rising living standards and generally improving levels of health in the UK, there are areas of high deprivation and poverty that are clearly associated with income inequality. This form of inequality reflects not only the level of income earned, but also the net income taking into account benefits and taxation. The persistence of areas of deprivation points to the continuation of forces encouraging income inequality. Redistribution in the form of government taxation and expenditure is one way in which such inequality may be reduced, but its effects are moderated by the workings of a capitalist, market-based economy.

Although many social divisions are becoming less clear-cut than once they were (in part, due to the changing nature of employment and the increased participation of women in the workforce) and living standards are rising, the general pattern of health inequalities remains. Several commentators, notably Wilkinson (1996), have sought to explain the persistent social class gradient in health inequalities. Wilkinson examined the degree of income inequality in various countries and concluded that the overall level of wealth (or poverty) was not a significant factor in explaining health inequalities, but rather the difference between the richest and poorest. Thus, income inequalities are related to health inequalities. Moreover, those societies with lower income inequalities had higher levels of 'social capital' which translated through unspecified mechanisms into the level of health. Others have sought to operationalise Wilkinson's thesis by examining the mechanisms of social capital within societies. Social capital refers to the social solidarity between citizens promoting feelings of well-being and social cohesion or inclusion – the systems and processes by which individuals feel part of society. This may be manifest in terms of turnout at elections, participation in social groups (e.g. sports clubs), voluntary organisations or church attendance, or donations to charity. One problem of the social capital thesis is establishing the precise connection between health and these multifarious types of social capital; the causal mechanisms are not so clear-cut.

THE POLICY RESPONSE TO HEALTH INEQUALITIES

As demonstrated, health and health care inequalities are complex and deep-rooted phenomena that lie beyond the scope of health care systems alone, and thus are not simply amenable to remedy by government interventions. Indeed the social determinants of health lie well beyond health care interventions. It involves the interaction between age, sex and constitutional (genetic) factors and individual lifestyle factors, social and community networks and general socio-economic, cultural and environmental conditions (Dahlgren and Whitehead 1991). As such, health services can play only a small role in tackling health inequalities, but in certain ways these roles may still be important (Benzeval et al. 1995). This is manifested, for example, by the Acheson Report which devotes only nine pages to the role of the health service in reducing health inequalities, but 68 pages to factors such as tax and benefits, education, housing, employment, environment, pollution and transport.

The current UK Government has placed great emphasis on tackling health inequalities by pursuing a more integrated approach called *joined-up government* at national and local levels. Partnerships across governmental departments and across local agencies are the main way by which the government thinks health inequalities will be reduced. It is claimed that joined-up solutions (i.e. partnership) are the solution to complex problems (i.e. health inequalities) (Exworthy and Powell 1999). The Health Action Zone initiative is a prime example of this policy (see below). Though appealing as a concept, partnerships suffer from difficulties that are inherent in multi-agency working. For example, different forms of local accountability and different professional practices often undermine attempts to integrate the actions of health and social services. Nationally, the efforts of say the NHS, to ensure the equitable access to services may be undermined by efficiency considerations of the Treasury.

Notwithstanding these caveats, the NHS can make a significant contribution to promoting equity and reducing health and especially health care inequality. The existence of the NHS with a reasonable degree of access and services (mostly) free at the point of delivery is arguably, in itself, a major contribution to ensuring a reasonable degree of access to health services for the whole population. (Co-payments for prescriptions are one exception to this). By contrast, more than 40 million Americans are without health insurance. In this sense, the NHS through its very existence, rather than any specific initiative, moderates the impact of health inequalities (caused by structural factors).

Beyond the NHS as a concept, there are specific areas of NHS activity which have implications for reducing health inequalities and promoting equity. The NHS is established on a local structure of health authorities (HAs, or boards), NHS trusts and Primary Care Groups (PCGs). There are currently 100 HAs in England, which determine the health needs of the population for which they are geographically responsible. They do this by means of a Health Improvement Programme (HImP), a strategic document which sets out the shape and direction of services locally. This document will, for example shape the decisions in commissioning services from NHS Trusts. The Trusts, hospitals and community health service organisations provide the services which the commissioners deem necessary. There are service and financial frameworks which act as '*contracts*' between the commissioner (purchaser) and the provider. Primary Care Groups were introduced in England by the Labour government, elected in May 1997 (different terms and structures were introduced in Scotland, Wales and Northern Ireland). These primary care associations have three roles:

- to improve the health of the population
- to commission secondary care services
- to develop primary and community health services

They fulfil these roles in conjunction with the HImP. PGCs operate at four levels, from advisory bodies (working under the umbrella of the HA) to fully-fledged Trusts (independent of the HA).

Health Action Zones (HAZs) were another initiative introduced in 1997. These area-based schemes, involving mainly public agencies, have been given greater flexibility in meeting the needs of their particular populations. They are 'experiments' in inter-agency partnerships and subject to national and local evaluation.

Health Authorities, due to reforms implemented in 1998, are now responsible for developing local partnerships through a HImP, and local authority agencies and PCGs are required to commit themselves to the HImP. However, the HImP is but one issue for HAs as they support the development of PCGs and promote clinical governance, among many others. Though PCGs illustrate a form of decentralisation, which may foster greater diversity (and possibly inequality) as they respond to local needs, the HImP is designed to avoid a fragmentation that was apparent under GP fundholding. Despite the development of primary care through PCGs, difficulties remain in primary care. For example, recruitment of staff to deprived areas is still problematic. However, the NHS (Primary Care) Bill, passed in the final days of the Conservative government in 1997, enables HAs to introduce an option for the employment of salaried general practitioners who would be contracted to provide a specific range of services.

Specific actions that HAs can take, and have taken, include an explicit recognition of the scale and nature of local health, the development of local inter-agency strategies (often called 'healthy alliances'), the development of an equitable allocation of resources within its territory, and the creation of particular initiatives to assist specific groups or areas (Benzeval 1999). In addition, all agencies can review the impact that their own policies and practices are having upon health and health care inequalities. This might include the use of comparative data, thereby including a consideration of medical practice variations. This 'equity audit' monitors the impact of policies upon inequality and highlights areas for action.

Equity of access to services (one of the 'what' questions identified earlier) was mentioned by the Acheson Report as an important area for the NHS to address. One of the prime difficulties of ensuring such equity is defining health need. Adjustments have to be made for case mix (the 'mix' of patient needs in terms of severity or complexity). The goal of 'equal access for equal need' is thus problematic. The Acheson Report identified the tension or trade-off between ensuring equity of access and the critical mass (in the number of staff or procedures conducted) that some services require in order to encourage the best outcomes. Hence equity of access and equity of outcome may conflict especially when clinical and cost-effectiveness are also considered. However, the 'inverse care law' (Hart 1971) states that those individuals with the greatest health needs have the least access to services, thereby stressing the likelihood that equity of access is not always promoted

As such, it has an intuitive appeal and some evidence to support it, but it suffers from a lack of precision and contradictory evidence.

The Acheson Report stressed equity of access to the extent that it should be a governing principle of the NHS. Though clarifying the access issue, it also places emphasis on an *equitable allocation of NHS resources.* It is important that NHS agencies place particular stress on securing these types of equity. Whilst equity of (health) outcomes may be beyond the immediate scope of the NHS, equity of resource allocation and of access are within its remit. Improvements can thus be made but need to be monitored.

CONCLUSION

Benzeval (1999) summarises the evidence of health inequality thus: *'The weight of evidence seems to suggest that it is the cumulative effect of people's material and social circumstances that are the most important determinants of health inequalities'.*

The current state of change in NHS policy, especially with regard to health and health care inequalities, is in such flux that it is premature to predict the outcome of the initiatives mentioned here. However, some factors can be identified which might impinge upon the *'success'* of the policy initiatives.

A number of factors are essential for policies towards health inequalities and health care inequalities to be effective. A far from exhaustive list is shown in Box 8.2.

If governments are serious about making significant and lasting progress in reducing inequality, these factors also need to be accompanied by a degree of income redistribution.

Health inequality is beyond the scope of health services alone. Partnerships are essential but extremely difficult to achieve. Also, other policy pressures are likely to impinge and, as mentioned previously, trade-offs are inevitable. In order to be serious about reducing inequalities, policy-makers need to be clear about the timescales (i.e. which proposals should be tackled first and when might change be evident?) and the costs of their proposals (i.e. what are the opportunity costs of pursing this proposal?). This was one of the most serious criticisms levelled against the Acheson Report. Its

Box 8.2 Essential factors for effective policies to reduce health and health care inequalities

- Clarity of objectives in inequality policies; that is, clarity of 'who' and 'what'
- Inclusion of equity and reducing inequality as governing principles in the day-to-day work of practitioners and agencies
- Strong incentives for partnership to overcome traditional resistance at both government department and local agency levels
- Wider structural reform, including equity considerations in education, employment, transport and nutrition
- Measures to monitor and assess progress towards reducing inequality

recommendations were neither given priority order nor costed. In short, it is not sufficient to simply present the evidence about inequalities; it must also be backed up by an understanding and commitment to policy change that recognises the demands that practitioners and policy-makers face.

ACKNOWLEDGEMENT

This chapter draws on research undertaken for the Health Variations Programme of the Economic and Social Research Council (ESRC) (Award no.L128251039). I am grateful to Lee Berney (LSE Health, London School of Economics) and Caron Weeks (Southampton General Hospital and East Southampton PCG) who commented on a draft of this chapter.

FURTHER SOURCES OF INFORMATION

Centre for the Analysis of Social Exclusion (CASE), London School of Economics:
Discussion papers and summaries are available free of charge via the Internet:
www.lse.ac.uk/case
Department of Health / NHS Executive:
The DOH publishes new reports and documents on their web-site:
www.doh.gov.uk
This site includes the Acheson Report and the Public Health White Paper, which may be down-loaded.
Economic and Social Research Council (ESRC) – Health Variations Programme:
This site contains summaries for projects examining various aspects of health inequalities in the UK:
www.lancs.ac.uk/users/apsocsci/hvp.htm
International Society for Equity and Health:
This international group promotes equity in health:
www.iseqh.org
LSE Health, London School of Economics:
A research centre specialising in health policy and health economics with particular expertise in issues of equity and inequality in the UK and Europe. The site contains summaries of current and recent projects and useful links:
www.lse.ac.uk/Depts/lse_health/res_projects/.htm
UK Health Equity Network:
A network of researchers, practitioners and policy makers formed in 2000. It aims to facilitate debate and exchange between research and policy / practice:
www.ukhen.org.uk

References

Acheson, D. (Chair) (1998) *Independent Inquiry Into Inequalities in Health*, The Stationery Office, London.

Andersen, T.F. and Mooney, G. (Eds.) (1990) *The Challenge of Medical Practice Variations*, Macmillan, London.

Benzeval, M., Judge, K. and Whitehead, M. (Eds.) (1995) *Tackling Inequalities in Health: An Agenda for Action*, King's Fund, London.

Benzeval, M. (1999) Tackling inequalities in health: public policy action. In: S. Griffiths and D.J. Hunter (Eds.) *Perspectives in Public Health*, Radcliffe Medical Press, Abingdon, pp 34–46.

Black, D. (Chair) (1980) *Inequalities in Health: Report of a Research Working Group*, Department of Health and Social Security, London.

Bunker, J. (1990) Variations in hospital admissions and the appropriateness of care: American pre-occupations? *British Medical Journal*, **301**, 531–532.

Centre for Reviews and Dissemination (1999) Getting evidence into practice. *Effective Health Care*, **5**, University of York, York.

Dahlgren, G. and Whitehead, M. (1991) *Policies and Strategies to Promote Social Equity in Health*, Institute of Futures Studies, Stockholm.

Department of Health (1992) *Health of the Nation. A Strategy for Health in England*, HMSO, London.

Department of Health (1995) *Variations in Health: What can the Department of Health and the NHS do?* HMSO, London.

Department of Health (1997) *The New NHS: Modern, Dependable*, The Stationery Office, London.

Department of Health (1998) *Our Healthier Nation*, The Stationery Office, London.

Department of Health (1999) *Saving Lives: Our Healthier Nation*, The Stationery Office, London.

Exworthy, M. and Powell, M. (1999) *Joined-up solutions to address health inequalities: a model of policy failure*? Paper presented to the Social Policy Association Conference, Health Policy at the Millennium, London School of Economics, London.

Hart, J.T. (1971) The inverse care law. *Lancet*, **i**, 405–412.

Healey, T., Yule, B. and Reid, J. (1994) Variations in general practice prescribing: costs and implications for budget setting. *Health Economics*, **3**, 47–56.

Houghton, G. and Gilthorpe, M. (1998) Variations in general practice prescribing: a multi-level model approach to determine the impact of practice characteristics including fundholding and training status. *Journal of Clinical Effectiveness*, **3**, 75–79.

Keller, R.B., Chapin, A.M. and Soule, D.N. (1996) Informed inquiry into practice variations: the Maine Medical Assessment Foundation. *Quality Assurance in Health Care*, **2**, 69–75.

Majeed, A., Cook, D. and Evans, N. (1996) Variations in general practice prescribing costs: implications for setting and monitoring prescribing budgets. *Health Trends*, **28**, 52–55.

McColl, A., Roderick, P., Gabbay, J., Smith, H. and Moore, M. (1998) Performance indicators for primary care groups: an evidence based approach. *British Medical Journal*, **317**, 1354–1360.

Wilkinson, R.G. (1996) *Unhealthy Societies: From Inequality to Well-being*, Routledge, London.

SELF-ASSESSMENT QUESTIONS

Question 1:   What do health inequalities mean to you? In devising policies, what would you address first?

Question 2:   How does the press define health inequalities? Examine recent newspapers to assess how the causes and effects of health inequalities are interpreted.

KEY POINTS FOR ANSWERS

Question 1:   Consider the following:

- Access to general practitioner surgeries (in terms of time geography/location, cultural)
- Sickness rates by age and sex
- Health outcomes (e.g. mortality rates)
- Expenditure patterns between acute and primary care services
- Distribution of pharmacists between one area and another

Question 2:   Consider whether they explain the causes by:

- Individual explanations
- Structural explanations
- Genetic pre-disposition
- Combination of all these

9 The Supply and Consumption of Over the Counter Drugs

Ian Bates

INTRODUCTION	140
THE LAW	140
ETHICS	141
Personal autonomy	141
Non-maleficence	142
Beneficence	142
DRUG DEREGULATION	142
DRUG ADVERTISING	145
CONCLUSION	147
FURTHER READING	147
WEBSITE	148
REFERENCES	148
SELF-ASSESSMENT QUESTIONS	148
KEY POINTS FOR ANSWERS	148

INTRODUCTION

A core function of pharmacists is to supply drugs to the public in exchange for money. This retailing activity differs from other types of selling. Selling medicines requires expertise and knowledge of these products, in order to prevent harm. However, so does selling motor bikes or life insurance policies, the mis-selling of which could potentially cause physical or financial harm. Pharmacists assume medicines are conceptually different from other consumer products. In this chapter, some issues relating to the sale of medicines will be examined.

THE LAW

Virtually all countries have specific legal restrictions relating to the supply of drugs to the public. The term *'drug'* is taken here to include a raw drug compound, a formulation of a drug, or any other chemical which may be classified as a *'poison'* according to any particular legal system (for the purposes of this chapter, herbal preparations or vitamins are not included). There is a basic distinction between drugs which can only be supplied via a legal order from a recognised prescriber (usually a registered medical practitioner or dentist) and those which can be sold directly to the public, without a consultation with a doctor or dentist. In the latter case, this sale can usually only be performed by a registered pharmacist, within a registered pharmacy. In the UK, there is an additional legal status for some drugs, such as common analgesics or anti-cough products in defined, small quantities, which may be sold direct to the public without the presence of a pharmacist. The usual situation, in the majority of European countries, is that many types of drug may be sold, by a pharmacist, from a pharmacy (see also Chapter 4). A legalised monopoly. The purpose here is not to detail all the legal specifications (there are many adequate texts on pharmacy law) but to set the scene, and speculate on trends. For instance, in the UK, some types of *'medicinal product'* may now be prescribed by registered nurses working from a doctor's surgery. Likewise, there is a concerted movement towards pharmacists being able to prescribe certain drugs (Crown 1999). Supplying prescribed drugs on the orders of a practitioner is a regulated activity. Supplying drugs (legally) without a prescription is also regulated, though to a lesser extent, but these drugs carry the term *'deregulated drugs'*, or are more commonly called over the counter (OTC) medicines. One exception to the pharmacy only restriction on the sale of deregulated drugs is in the USA, where this particular legal category does not exist. Here, deregulated drugs may be sold virtually anywhere, a freedom apparently denied to the rest of the world.

ETHICS

Restrictions and regulations on the supply of drugs to the general population can be viewed as an essentially paternalistic function. Controlling the public's access to medicines has a rational basis: drugs are potentially dangerous chemicals, and pharmacists and doctors possess specialist knowledge, ensuring the safe and appropriate supply of medicines. However, this presents an ethical dilemma. Although some client-pharmacist consultations do not result in the sale of a drug, many do, and there is clear potential for commercial and ethical conflict. Clients have to purchase drugs through pharmacists, who in turn rely on their sale to earn a living (see also Chapter 12).

In recent years, medical paternalism (i.e. the doctor/pharmacist *knows best*) has come to be seen as anachronistic, being viewed as limiting freedom through regulation, however good the intention. This tends to infringe on an individual's autonomy, which together with beneficence and non-maleficence, is commonly held to be a cornerstone of ethical thinking (see also Chapter 13). Increasing the personal autonomy of individuals has been a feature of many reforms, both commercial and medical, in recent times. Governments and those who control health systems have been at pains to implement strategies for increasing personal autonomy, which is generally held to be a good thing (despite sceptics who claim that the hidden motives of this movement are to reduce welfare costs).

Personal autonomy

The following section of this chapter will describe the expanding OTC market, a result of deliberate drug deregulation by governments, a primary purpose of which is to increase individuals' choice of medicines, hence enabling greater autonomy in self care. However, accepting greater autonomy necessitates greater responsibility for one's actions and choices. This in turn requires that appropriate information and education is available to consumers, and that pharmacists are able and willing to provide this.

Here again is a potential ethical conflict. The most appropriate information a pharmacist could provide for a client might theoretically result in the sale of a generic formulation of a drug. For many of the available non-prescription drugs, there is little or no evidence to suggest that a commercial brand of, say, ibuprofen, is any more or less efficacious than a cheaper generic equivalent. The latter will however, have smaller trading margins, resulting in reduced income for the pharmacist.

Non-maleficence

Non-maleficence, the second principle of bioethics, means '*do no harm*' and the supply of medicines should be an activity with minimal risk to individual consumers. It is worth noting that there is little evidence that many OTC medicines, particularly more '*traditional*' formulations (for example expectorant cough preparations) are any more effective than placebo. These products tend not to have serious adverse effects but it should be considered whether selling such a medicine is ethical in terms of non-maleficence. However, it should be noted that many customers ask for these more traditional medicines, and seem to derive some psychological, if not physiological benefit.

Beneficence

Beneficence is doing good, or our best to help others. In one context this may involve not selling to a consumer the drugs requested. Selling drugs which do not have any proven value is also contrary to this principle. Thus, commercial trading in the context of health raises issues of biomedical ethics.

DRUG DEREGULATION

The value of the market for OTC medicines has been steadily expanding, with large increases in the last decade due to more deregulation procedures being adopted by many countries (Figures 9.1 and 9.2). It is likely that this policy will continue. Why have we seen this extraordinary rise in the number and range of drugs now available without a prescription? Some of the increase in individual countries can be partly explained in terms of the harmonisation of medicine regulations across the European Union, but there are other reasons why governments and agencies are promoting this policy (Box 9.1).

Many governments see drug deregulation as an opportunity to reduce state-financed drug costs, especially in those countries with welfare based health systems. The assumption is that encouraging an increase in consumer purchase of OTC drugs will be associated with a reduction in the tax-supported (prescribed) drugs bill: a reasonable assumption, but one for which there is little direct evidence at present. It is also assumed that this will lead to efficiency gains, with a reduction in the number of consultations with prescribers, i.e. it is assumed that the greater availability and purchase of OTC drugs means fewer medical consultations for '*minor*' illness. Again, there is no direct evidence for this but pharmaceutical organisations point out that consulting a pharmacist is free of charge and use this fact to argue for increased responsibilities and roles for pharmacists in primary care sectors (at no extra for government-funded health care).

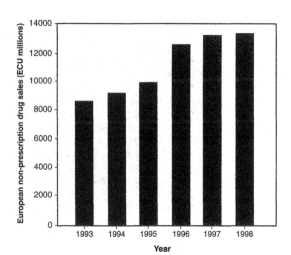

Figure 9.1 Total European sales of non-prescription drugs (Source: Association of the European Self-Medication Industry 1999)

Deregulating medicines will lead to increased independence and autonomy for patients. Many governments strongly emphasise the increased personal responsibility for health, commensurate with such a policy. Once again, there is little evidence to support this concept. Nobody has asked the population if they really want this increased autonomy; how far it should go, or if people actually prefer a form of benign paternalism when it comes to their choice of drugs.

From the viewpoint of the pharmaceutical industry, an expanded direct market for drug products will lead to increased sales (Figure 9.1), which the industry asserts, will in turn lead to increased wealth and investment in drug research and development programmes (and increased dividends for shareholders).

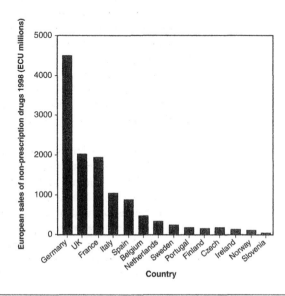

Figure 9.2 European sales of non-prescription drugs by country (Source: Association of the European Self-Medication Industry 1999)

Box 9.1 Reasons and implications of drug deregulation

The medical profession, in general, regard drug deregulation to be a welcome development. However, in some health care systems where doctors are paid per patient visit or per capita (for instance with some third party-funded health care systems), increased OTC sales could result in loss of income for these doctors, as patients will tend to self medicate (or consult a pharmacist) rather than visit a doctor. On the other hand, where doctors are not paid according to how many patients they see (as in most welfare type health care systems) there is no financial disincentive for drug deregulation from their perspective. There are some considerations that are not so obvious. For instance, some patients may be unwilling to accept a doctor's recommendation for the purchase of an OTC medicine instead of a written prescription (for products which may be free or at a reduced charge) and to assume that all patients want greater autonomy and empowerment may be erroneous.

Unsurprisingly, pharmacists generally welcome the deregulation policy with the corresponding access to a wider range of effective drugs for OTC recommendation. Deregulation will lead to increased sales and therefore increased income. However, pharmacists are not paid for the associated information, advice and counselling. It may also lead to a reduction in dispensing fees associated with any reduction in doctors' prescribing. Deregulation policies do represent an opportunity to increase the professional status and public standing of pharmacists, perhaps through better collaborative practice between prescribing doctors and pharmacists. The adoption of joint prescribing guidelines, which includes OTC drugs, is one such example (see also Chapter 15).

The general public are the '*consumers*' of health care. As alluded to earlier, some individuals want increased choice, which may translate as easier access to health care professionals and self medication. However, care is required to guard against the possibility of obtaining wrong or inappropriate information and advice about drugs and drug products. Encouraging more autonomy and self-medication through increased access to symptomatic drugs could potentially mask more serious underlying pathologies. Manufacturers claim that responsible advertising and information will minimise this risk, but as with many of the issues described above, there is little evidence on which to base this claim.

It may be argued that although the policy of drug deregulation continues, interpretation of this policy and the motivation of the groups concerned varies. Politicians see deregulation as a means of cost containment for national drug bills, increasing the responsibility for self-health care. Consumers have wider choice and greater autonomy and perhaps better access to medicines and information (through pharmacies). Medical practitioners may have more time for treating serious illness, and pharmacists will see an increase in sales and a wider range of illness and medicines from which to counter prescribe. Conversely, however, continued deregulation may lead to inappropriate use of more potent drugs and medicines, more undisclosed symptoms and illness and perhaps a greater risk of adverse drug events. However, there is little doubt that increased consumption of medicines has occurred over the last few years and at least part of this increase can be explained by the increase in activity of manufacturers, in particular OTC drug advertising.

DRUG ADVERTISING

The growth of the self-medication market across Europe, fuelled by deregulation polices, has led to a corresponding rise in the amount of direct-to-the-public advertising of drug products. Direct-to-public advertising of prescription only medicines is not permitted in Europe, in contrast to the situation in the USA where direct-to-public advertising for prescription only products has risen greatly in recent years. It is unlikely that any society with a welfare-based health system would be comfortable with pharmaceutical companies advertising regulated drug products direct to the consumer. However, some manufacturers have claimed that this form of advertising has benefits imparting health education and awareness. Advertising regulations usually state that advertisements should be disease-specific and enhance consumer education, or that warnings and precautions associated with drug use should be explained. In reality, this usually takes the form of 'small print', in language that has very little meaning to the typical consumer. How this is expected to increase consumer education is unclear. What is evident, is that all advertisements for prescription products are designed to increase the prescribing of them. Selling products is the basis of any manufacturing industry, as is maximising profits and bonuses for shareholders (the responsibility of company executives is fundamentally towards their shareholders). The pharmaceutical industry justify this free market behaviour by pointing out that they are responsible for much of the original research and development that goes into drug design and manufacture, which in turn enriches global health care. This is true, but only to those systems or individuals who can afford it. Where this advertising practice is allowed, we rarely see direct-to-public advertising of generic or cheap drug alternatives almost always the latest 'me-too' products (i.e. products very similar to those already on the market).

Consumer advertising of non-prescription drugs is a different matter. Here, the decision to purchase rests with the consumer. The state, taxpayers, prescribers or third parties are not directly involved Producing OTC drug advertisements is a complicated branch of advertising because of the ethics and legislation involved. Generally, it is considered that consumers should be protected from improper advertising. Some countries, such as the UK, have a mix of legal control (for instance general consumer law to protect consumers) and voluntary industry-monitored vetting of OTC drug advertisements. If advertisements are not produced according to the relevant code of ethics, the drug industry regulatory bodies or authorities may intervene. In the UK this has not happened for many years because of a pre-vetting system, which refers back any unsuitable advertising copy before publication. Pre-vetting is not in operation in some other European countries, although there are authorised government agencies to control OTC drug advertising.

In general, drug law relating to the advertising of OTC drugs to the public tends to prohibit misrepresentation of claims and tries to protect the lay-person in the situation of 'unequal information'. Knowledge about the use of drugs, appropriate and inappropriate, is a specialist subject (which is one reason why pharmacy is a university entry profession) and this particular economic market is unlike other consumer markets (see Chapter 23). Doctors and pharmacists are expected to use their knowledge about drugs to protect the public from unsubstantiated claims. The law surrounding advertisements for OTC drugs have similar principles in many EU countries. For instance information should not be outdated or leave essential things unstated whilst the reference to some conditions, such as tuberculosis, venereal diseases or cancer is not permitted.

If advertisers are not misleading or unfair in their descriptions and portrayals of OTC drugs intended for the public, does advertising actually work? There is surprisingly little available evidence. One point of view is that manufacturers would not spend vast amounts of money advertising products if they thought the process did not work. It might also be argued that not advertising (when all your competitors do) is a risk not worth taking. It has already been indicated that the drug market, both for prescription and OTC drugs, is distinguished from other markets by asymmetry of information. Since some drugs are allowed to be directly purchased by consumers (i.e. OTC drugs) it could also be argued that advertising plays an important role in reducing the information gap between professionals and consumers. Advertising may be of significant importance for both consumers and manufacturers, particularly for newer drugs which may have undergone recent deregulation from prescription only to OTC. Advertising of OTC drugs can thus be justified on the grounds that it will inform the public about newly available medicines and facilitate consumer choice. This is a classical view of marketing – the supply of drugs adapts to demand for medication. An alternative, postmodern, view of marketing theory reverses this relationship between product and consumer, arguing that advertising can create the demand in order to meet supply. In many areas of marketing, advertising itself has almost become the reason to advertise, with *'creativity'* and *'re-branding'* becoming more synonymous with the advertisement than the product on offer. Such developments are reflected by the plethora of televised national and international *'award ceremonies'* where self-aggrandising prizes are presented for the creativity of advertisements, in a direct emulation of the performance arts.

CONCLUSION

The increasing immediacy of advertising, together with the emergent culture of consumerism challenges the pharmacist's function as the custodian of readily available drugs and medicines. There is a danger of inappropriate need for a drug product being created via these trends. Pharmacy has to adapt to these trends to ensure its future as the guardian of the public's consumption of drugs.

FURTHER READING

Bradley, C. and Blenkinsopp, A. (1996) The future of self medication. *British Medical Journal*, **312**, 835–837.

Dyer, C. (1999) Incontinence campaign tests limits of advertising rules beneficence. *British Medical Journal*, **319**, 591.

Hoffman, J.R. and Wilkes, M. (1999) Direct to consumer advertising of prescription drugs. An idea whose time should not come. *British Medical Journal*, **318**, 1301.

Kennedy, J.G. (1996) Over the counter drugs. *British Medical Journal*, **312**, 593–594.

WEB SITE

Association of the European Self-Medication Industry (AESGP): *www.aesgp.be/index.html*

REFERENCES

Crown, J. (1999) *A Review of The Prescribing, Supply and Administration of Medicines*, Department of Health, London.

SELF-ASSESSMENT QUESTIONS

Question 1: Outline the principles of bioethics, and reflect on how traditional roles of drug retailing may conflict with these.

Question 2: What are the arguments put forward to support drug deregulation policies?

Question 3: How may drug advertising present ethical conflicts for pharmacists and consumers alike?

KEY POINTS FOR ANSWERS

Question 1: Autonomy, non-maleficence and beneficence may all be in conflict with retailing activities connected with drugs. As a pharmacist earning a living, one may be tempted to sell more expensive drugs or even non-proven remedies. The dilemma is between your ethical obligations and the need to support yourself and family in an essentially commercial market.

Question 2: Governments are keen to harmonise laws, whenever possible, and to reduce the public tax burden. A wider choice of publicly available drugs would, in theory, achieve this aim by reducing subsidised prescribing and physician consultations. Physicians see this as a benefit, allowing them to focus on more serious, acute illness in communities. The pharmaceutical industry claims that increased sales, and profits, will allow them to continue to invest in R&D. Pharmacists claim that a wider choice of supervised drug availability will increase their professional status and allow them to effectively treat a wider range of illness.

Question 3: The primary purpose of advertising is to increase sales. This may not always be a good thing where drugs are concerned (why?). A secondary purpose is to inform, and this is claimed by advertisers of drugs to be desirable, as it will increase autonomy with respect to self-medication. However, is it possible to persuade a person to purchase a (potentially unnecessary) drug? Are the current trends in consumerist advertising actually creating a need for a drug treatment where none previously existed? It is clearly a difficult balance between ethically informing the public and the commercial promotion of branded drug products, with the pharmacist in a pivotal position in this milieu.

10 **Promoting Health**

Alison Blenkinsopp, Claire Anderson and Rhona Panton

INTRODUCTION	152
WHAT IS HEALTH PROMOTION?	152
MYTH ONE: INDIVIDUALS EXERCISE CONTROL OVER THEIR HEALTH	154
The role of lifestyle	155
MYTH TWO: THE UNENLIGHTENED PUBLIC	155
MYTH THREE: INFORMATION ALONE CHANGES BEHAVIOUR	156
CAN BEHAVIOUR BE CHANGED?	157
HEALTH PROMOTION IN PHARMACY PRACTICE	159
THE EVIDENCE FOR PHARMACISTS' CONTRIBUTION TO HEALTH PROMOTION	160
CONCLUSION	162
FURTHER READING	162
REFERENCES	162
SELF-ASSESSMENT QUESTIONS	163
KEY POINTS FOR ANSWERS	163

INTRODUCTION

Community pharmacists are ideally placed to act as health promoters. Health promotion is commonly perceived as being about lifestyle change and personal choice and the pharmacist's role tends to be discussed in that context. However, health promotion has a wider meaning, incorporating a range of actions with the potential to improve health. This chapter will present health promotion and the pharmacist's role in its wider context. It will begin by presenting definitions and models for health promotion and will then go on to consider three myths: the myth of individual control over health, the myth of the unenlightened public and the myth that information alone changes behaviour. Finally we review health promotion in pharmacy practice and consider the evidence for pharmacists' contribution to health promotion.

WHAT IS HEALTH PROMOTION?

Health promotion aims to maintain and enhance good health and prevent ill-health. It has been argued that '*the overall goal of health promotion may be summed up as the balanced enhancement of physical, mental and social facets of positive health, coupled with the prevention of physical, mental and social ill-health*' (Downie *et al.* 1992). The term encompasses a range of activities and issues including both individual and societal aspects. At one end of this range are government policy and legislation affecting health. These include actions with a direct influence on health (for example, legislation to ban tobacco advertising) as well as those which affect the determinants of health (for example, social welfare and benefits policies).

Pharmacists' training largely takes place using a perspective where ill-health is considered a biomedical problem, wherein medicines and other technologies alone are regarded as curative, and health professionals assume the role of 'expert' regarding knowledge about illness and cure.

Thus, when pharmacists receive a health-related inquiry they are likely to translate it into a disease-oriented request and think first of a medical treatment or referral. This is not necessarily inappropriate professional practice, but it can lead to the bio-medicalisation of health – that is, health and illness are considered as exclusively biologically determined (see also Chapters 7 and 25). Pharmacists and other health professionals are beginning to provide information to promote and maintain good health, to support people's actions and behaviours related to health, and to contribute to improving quality of life. However, pharmacists are likely to continue to link the offering of such advice to the use of medicines and other health-related goods, as the provision of medicines is their core function.

The traditional view of the health professional as an expert instructing the public about what to do is, however, outmoded

Beattie's strategies of health promotion (Beattie 1990), is a useful way to explore the pharmacist's current and potential future contribution (Figure 10.1).

In Beattie's framework, pharmacists' involvement in health promotion to date has primarily fallen within quadrant 1 – providing expert information to individual clients. It is easy to see how health professionals, who know only too well the health consequences of certain behaviours, may be tempted to act in a '*telling*' rather than a '*discussing*' mode. However the evidence shows that people tend not to respond positively to such approaches.

Current thinking is that the pharmacist's most effective contribution would be through adopting a general style consistent with quadrant 3 – working with individuals to negotiate change.

Health professionals engage in '*people-centred health promotion*', which is:

'*An enterprise involving the development over time, in individuals and communities of basic and positive states of and conditions for physical, mental and social and spiritual health. The control of and resources for this enterprise need to be primarily in the hands of the people themselves, but with the back up and support of health professionals, policy makers and the overall political system. At the heart of this enterprise are two key concepts: one of development (personal and community) and the other of empowerment*' (Raeburn and Rootman 1998).

Thus, health promotion embraces the notions of community as well as individual development. Models for health promotion include health education, prevention and health protection. The pharmacist has an important role as an articulate and informed advocate for their

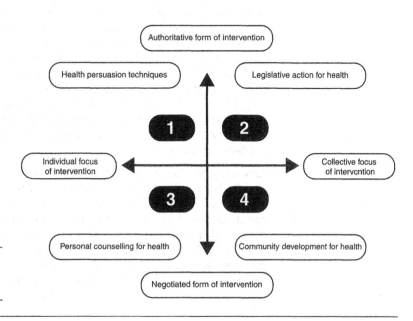

Figure 10.1 Strategies for health promotion (Beattie 1990)

community, in lobbying at local and national level, and supporting local community groups working for health improvement. However, in order to effectively engage with the health promotion agenda, pharmacists need to understand its relationship with the social and economic context. In the next section three myths which relate to health promotion are considered.

MYTH ONE: INDIVIDUALS EXERCISE CONTROL OVER THEIR HEALTH

Over the last two decades the evidence of inequalities in health has mounted (see Chapter 8 for a fuller discussion). In the UK, in the 1980s and early 1990s, Government policy on health focussed on individual behaviour rather than on the interaction between individuals and their environment. The 1998 Government Green Paper in England, *Our Healthier Nation*, was the first such document to acknowledge that health chances are determined by a more complex set of factors than simply peoples' lifestyle choices. Purchasing wholemeal bread or fresh fruit and vegetables is difficult if you live on a housing estate or housing project which is a '*food desert*', where most local shops have closed down, and those that remain do not sell healthy food choices, you do not have a car and the nearest supermarket is two bus rides away. Or, in relation to smoking, as Downie *et al.* (1992) put it:

'*Imagine a society in which there is no mythological imagery surrounding cigarette smoking: no spurious association with manliness, elegance, sophistication, achievement, "grown-upness", smartness, and so on; where there is open portrayal in tobacco advertising (if it exists at all) that cigarettes are dirty and smelly, and that smoking kills around one in seven of the population; where there are decent health education programmes from the cradle to the grave; where it is acknowledged that tobacco does not soothe the nerves until one is already "hooked" on it; where no other false values are attached to smoking; and where there are no social pressures to smoke. Suppose that in this environment an adult wakes up one day and announces that, having weighed up all the pros and cons, he or she has arrived at the unfettered decision to take up smoking 20 cigarettes daily for life, thereby running a one in four risk of dying prematurely. One might reasonably say that that person has freely chosen to smoke*'.

Emerging evidence continues to show how the effects of relative deprivation and affluence on future health are determined before birth. As a result, health professionals have revised their assumptions about the extent to which individuals can exercise real choices about their health, and previous '*victim blaming*' approaches have been recognised for what they were – inappropriate and unrealistic. The concepts of '*social exclusion*' and '*underclass*' are used worldwide to describe those in societies who are most in need of support, financial and otherwise. For pharmacists working in deprived areas and providing services for people whose health chances most need to be improved, the challenges have to be recognised. Pharmacists should reflect on:

- Their own socioeconomic status
- The gap between this and the socioeconomic circumstances of their customers
- The implications in terms of differences in educational level, vocabulary, culture
- The potential credibility of any advice they may offer

Pharmacists should work more closely with client groups within local communities, e.g. drug users, mothers and toddlers. Playing a more active part in determining the needs of their communities is the basis for pharmacists to consider how they, acting as facilitators, can help empower individuals to meet their needs.

The role of lifestyle

Pharmacists can offer information and advice about a range of issues including those highlighted in Box 10.1

Box 10.1 Issues about which pharmacists can offer information and advice

- Smoking cessation
- Baby and child health
- Healthy eating
- Physical activity
- Drug misuse
- Contraception and sexual health
- Stress
- Oral health
- Concordance in medicine-taking (e.g. for treatments to prevent heart disease and osteoporosis)
- Prevention of accidents
- Prevention and early diagnosis of cancer (e.g. skin cancer)
- Promotion of screening and vaccination programmes

However advice and information are not given in a vacuum and no individual is a '*blank sheet*'. People bring with them to the pharmacy their own beliefs and information system about health, and the pharmacist needs to be aware of the background against which further information might be offered (see also Chapter 7).

MYTH TWO: THE UNENLIGHTENED PUBLIC

Previously it was believed that lack of information was the reason why people made less healthy lifestyle choices. With the proliferation of information over the last decade, the public has become increasingly better informed about the factors that affect health. The lay media is full of stories and information on health, and the internet enables access to detailed technical information which would once have been the province of health professionals. For the time being, access to the internet is greater among the higher social classes, but this is changing and the next decade is likely to see a great expansion in its availability.

Research shows that the public is generally well aware of the health risks of smoking. Yet about one third of the population continues to smoke and far from declining, smoking amongst women and children is increasing. Why is this? People make their own risk-benefit calculations in relation to behaviour. Smoking might be seen as the only way of coping with an otherwise unbearable life, and living longer by giving up smoking may not be an attractive prospect. Thus 'concepts of future' play a key role. The underlying theme of many health promotion messages has focussed on extending life. As Pitts (1996) puts it, 'the aim of much preventive health therefore is to substitute an early death, say before the age of 60 years in the UK, for a later one'. Such an outcome may not be perceived as a benefit and thus an incentive to change by those who are poor. Consequently, pharmacists need to adapt the message to the circumstances of the recipient.

MYTH THREE: INFORMATION ALONE CHANGES BEHAVIOUR

It might be expected that the changes in the public's knowledge about health would lead to the adoption of healthier lifestyles. However, research shows that providing information does not in itself inevitably lead to the expected effect. In particular, providing negative information about the consequences of behaviours that are likely to be harmful to health (for example, government advertisements about drug misuse which were intended to frighten people into stopping) does not work. Pharmacists have an important role to play in interpreting health information and in clarifying areas where the messages seem to be in conflict or information has been misunderstood. An example of this may be media presentation of new research findings which contradict previous health messages. In 1998 and 1999 for example, large studies showed that eating a diet high in fibre did not reduce the incidence of bowel cancer, and that eating a diet low in fat did not reduce the incidence of breast cancer. Both of these studies produced results that contradicted hitherto accepted evidence. Some of the popular media portrayed these findings as showing that eating fibre in the diet, or trying to reduce fat intake, was not worthwhile. The fact that many previous studies had shown health benefits from eating more fibre or eating less fat was largely ignored or underplayed in the presentation of the 'story'. In cases such as these, pharmacists can interpret new findings and set them in the context of the bigger picture.

CAN BEHAVIOUR BE CHANGED?

Even though information in itself is unlikely to result in behaviour change, it is an important part of attempts to persuade people to adopt healthy choices. Research by behavioural psychologists resulted in the development and testing of a model to explain why individuals change and why they sometimes revert to previous behaviour. The Trans Theoretical Model (TTM) of behaviour change drew on theories from several disciplines to develop a model which is both explanatory and the basis for tailoring intervention (Prochaska and DiClemente 1992). The TTM is commonly referred to as the '*Stages of Change*' model and has been tested in a range of behaviours where change could enhance health. There are five stages: Pre-contemplation, Contemplation, Preparation, Action and Maintenance. Table 10.1 describes each stage and sets out the implications for pharmacists.

The stages are not linear and the TTM should be regarded as a cycle which people may enter at any stage, leave and re-join (Figure 10.2). People who want to stop smoking, or misusing drugs, for example, often make several attempts before they eventually quit. Failure at one

Table 10.1 Applying the Stages of Change model in pharmacy health promotion (From: Blenkinsopp, Panton and Anderson 1999; adapted from Berger 1997 which contains a more detailed version)

Stage	Behaviour	Implications for pharmacist intervention
Pre-contemplation	The individual is content with current behaviour and has no intention of changing; is not considering change	Listen and respond to questions. Attempts to persuade unlikely to be successful
Contemplation	The person is thinking about the possibility of changing, but has made no plans to change	Listen and respond to questions. Provide information
Preparation	The decision has been made to change and the person is getting ready to make the change	Help in planning and goal-setting
Action	The change is implemented	Encourage return to pharmacy to discuss progress. Supportive approach
Maintenance	The person works to prevent relapse to the previous behaviour	Continue supportive approach. Encourage discussion of possible problems that might lead to relapse. Give positive feedback

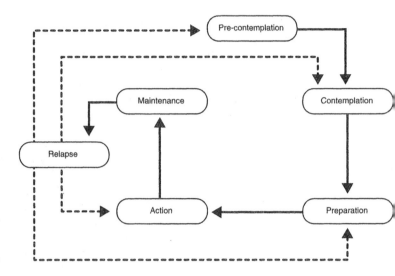

Figure 10.2 The stages of change cycle

attempt does not mean that a future attempt cannot be successful. An individual may re-enter the cycle at the planning or action stages, or may revert to pre-contemplation for a period.

Pharmacists can use the model in practice, by using careful questioning to assess which stage the person is currently at and tailoring information, advice and questions appropriately. Appropriate questions might include those in Box 10.2.

Box 10.2 Possible questions pharmacists might ask to establish the position of an individual in relation to the Stages of Change model of behaviour

- Have you ever thought about changing/stopping?
- Would you like to try to change?
- Would you like some information about…?
- If you could use some help, I'm available here, just ask to speak to me

One of the key elements of this approach is that when an individual is in the pre-contemplation stage, health professionals should not attempt to push them to the next stage. Information might be offered but the person is left to make their own decision. Pre-contemplation may continue for months or years. Support for allowing people the space and time to reach the next stage comes from research on their attitudes to smoking cessation advice from general practitioners. Smokers anticipated that they would be given anti-smoking advice by the doctor whenever they consulted about health. The respondents felt that they and most other smokers were well aware of the risks they were taking with their health and held a strong belief that the decision about quitting belonged to them, having taken into account their circumstances. Patients receiving doctors' repeated advice on smoking cessation showed that their responses ranged from anger, resentment and guilt to not seeking medical advice when it was needed because the anticipated '*ritualistic*' advice to stop smoking was a barrier (Butler *et al.* 1998).

The Stages of Change approach has been adopted by those working in health promotion worldwide. While there is good evidence from clinical trials that it produces change (for example, in smoking cessation, diet modification, drug misuse), studies have generally included counselling sessions that would be unfeasibly long in many pharmacy settings. Evidence for the effectiveness of TTM in brief interventions is less extensive to date, and concerns have been expressed at its widespread adoption by health professionals ahead of the evidence. Nevertheless TTM is valuable in that it appeals to health professionals, is easily remembered and provides a basis for response that recognises the need to tailor information and advice.

HEALTH PROMOTION IN PHARMACY PRACTICE

Pharmacists wishing to develop '*health promoting*' activities may adopt a style of consulting which involves listening and negotiating rather than telling, crucially taking into account the individual's social circumstances. For example, when discussing a person's drug therapy, the pharmacist can focus on the individual's needs in a holistic way, tailoring therapy to age-specific or culturally-specific needs. This may involve the role of family members, carers or friends in the management of therapy, while taking into consideration living conditions, health status and socioeconomic resources. Any pharmacist may participate in health promotion and those working in community and hospital practice are well placed to do so. Their level of input can be classified as:

Level 1: displaying leaflets on health topics and responding to requests for advice and information about health.
Level 2: in addition to level 1, offering information and advice opportunistically and pro-actively, working in a co-ordinated way with community-based health care workers.

The difference in these two levels is essentially that in the first the pharmacist is passive and working at an individual level, and in the second active and using community networks effectively.

The components of health promotion input from pharmacists are summarised in Box 10.3. Pharmacists should adopt a holistic approach and think creatively about the opportunities to promote health. By holistic we mean addressing issues not traditionally associated with pharmacy, but which may be linked to the sale or supply of medicines or health-related goods. Pharmacists may be uncomfortable when

Box 10.3 The components of pharmacists' health promotion activities

providing dietary advice, or recommending physical activity programmes. This initial discomfort may be alleviated by targeting advice to particular groups of people, for instance:

- Target information about effective physical activity to those receiving prescriptions for medicines to prevent or treat osteoporosis. This might be the availability and timing of local sessions to promote strength and balance as part of a *'falls reduction programme'*
- Ask patients presenting prescriptions for medicines for heart problems whether they would like further information about diet and physical exercise

Forward-looking health care organisations are experimenting with, for example, the prescription of exercise sessions by pharmacists, in which the patient receives vouchers for exercise sessions at local leisure facilities.

THE EVIDENCE FOR PHARMACISTS' CONTRIBUTION TO HEALTH PROMOTION

In medicine, the randomised controlled trial (RCT) is considered the gold standard for the generation of evidence (see also Chapter 25). However RCTs may not encompass the sorts of multi-component behavioural interventions that are utilised in health promotion programmes. There has been a vigorous debate about appropriate research methodologies to evaluate health promotion programmes. One of the major methodological difficulties is differentiating the effects of health promotion initiatives from other services and information which the public might obtain. Another issue is measuring the resultant health gain, since many health promotion initiatives are designed for long-term effects (for example, preventing heart disease). Educational gain, following a health promotion intervention, may be more readily measured. Two major RCTs of community pharmacists' provision of smoking cessation advice based on brief interventions using Stages of Change and the use of Nicotine Replacement Therapy (NRT) have been conducted in Scotland and Northern Ireland. Both have shown that pharmacists' intervention produces a significantly higher and more sustained rate of quitting when compared with no intervention.

Numerous pharmacy-based health promotion schemes have been developed but tend to be small scale, measuring processes rather than health outcomes. Many of these have demonstrated public acceptance of pharmacists' involvement in health promotion. In the UK, a major study in one area showed that pharmacy customers collecting prescriptions were the most likely to expect to receive general health information in the pharmacy and to value it (Anderson 1998).

The findings of a qualitative consumer study conducted in Austria in 1996 suggested that while pharmacists were perceived as close to everyday life, representing a trustworthy institution and a link to primary health care, they were perceived as primarily concerned with selling medicines. Only 10% of consumers perceived the pharmacy as a source of health/illness related information (compared with 50% for the family doctor).

There are few published studies of pharmacy health promotion in Europe, an exception being evaluations of campaigns on smoking, skin diseases and asthma based in Swedish pharmacies. All of these illustrated the contribution that pharmacists could make in these areas. In the Swedish Asthma Year the public were offered brochures and leaflets in pharmacies and information articles in the national pharmacy magazine. The evaluation estimated that the campaign impacted on 42% of the Swedish population with twice as many patients using adequate amounts of inhaled steroids for asthma following the campaign than previously (Lisper and Nilsson 1996). Throughout Europe, health promotion by community pharmacists has been linked to the wider concept of pharmaceutical care and forms part of a number of ongoing studies. Examples include training on inhaler technique for patients with asthma and promoting healthy lifestyles as part of overall management of hypertension by pharmacists.

Research suggests that while pharmacists themselves are committed to involvement in health promotion, the feasibility of spending time on a one to one basis, in patient-centred health promotion with their customers, depends on staff skill mix and working arrangements. In particular, personal involvement in the dispensing process acts as a barrier to spending more time at the *front of the shop* talking with customers.

Conclusion

Pharmacists have the potential to contribute to health promotion activ
ities in the community. To achieve this potential, pharmacists wil
need to develop working styles that embrace the notions of negotiatior
and partnership with the public. Changes in working arrangements
particularly reducing the amount of time spent on mechanica
and technical aspects of dispensing, will be a prerequisite to the
development of the health promotion role. As the public's access tc
information increases, the pharmacist's role in interpreting anc
contextualising information will become more important.

Further reading

Blenkinsopp, A., Panton, R.S. and Anderson, C. (1999) *Health Promotior
for Pharmacists* (2ⁿᵈ Edn.) Oxford University Press, Oxford.

Bury, M. (1997) *Health and Illness in a Changing Society*, Routledge
London.

Ley, P. (1997) *Communicating with Patients – Improving Communication
Satisfaction and Compliance*, Stanley Thorne, Cheltenham.

References

Anderson, C. (1998) Health promotion by community pharmacists
consumers' views. *International Journal of Pharmacy Practice*, **6**, 2–12

Ashworth, P. (1997) Breakthrough or bandwagon? Are intervention:
tailored to Stage of Change more effective than non-staged
interventions? *Health Education Journal*, **56**, 166–174.

Beattie, A. (1990) Knowledge and control in health promotion
In: J. Gabe, M. Calman and M. Bury (Eds.) *Sociology of the Healtl
Service*, Routledge, Kegan and Paul, London.

Berger, B. (1997) Readiness to change – implications for pharmac)
practice. *Journal of the American Pharmaceutical Association*, **NS37**
321–329.

Butler, C.C., Pill, R. and Stott, N.C.H. (1998) Qualitative study o
patients' perceptions of doctors' advice to quit smoking
Implications for opportunistic health promotion. *British Medica
Journal*, **316**, 1878–1881.

Downie, R.S., Fyfe, C. and Tannahill, A. (1992) *Health Promotion: Model.
and Values*, Oxford University Press, Oxford.

Johnson, S.S., Grimley, D.M. and Prochaska, J.O. (1998) Prediction o
adherence using the transtheoretical model: implications fo:

pharmacy care practice. *Journal of Social and Administrative Pharmacy*, **15**, 135–148.

Lisper, P. and Nilsson, J.L.G. (1996) The asthma year in Swedish pharmacies: a nationwide information and pharmaceutical care programme for patients with asthma. *Annals of Pharmacotherapy*, **30**, 255–460.

Pitts, M. (1996) *The Psychology of Preventive Health*, Routledge, London.

Prochaska, J.O. and DiClemente, C.C. (1992) Stages of change in the modification of problem behaviours. In: M. Hersen., R.M., Eisler and P.M. Miller (Eds.) *Progress in Behaviour Modification*, Sycamore Press, New York.

Raeburn, J. and Rootman, I. (1998) *People-Centred Health Promotion*, Wiley, Chichester.

SELF-ASSESSMENT QUESTIONS

Question 1: How might the Trans Theoretical Model (TTM) be applied in the pharmacy setting?

Question 2: In what ways might pharmacists be passive and active promoters of health?

Question 3: In what ways could pharmacists be advocates for health promotion at both a local and a national level?

KEY POINTS FOR ANSWERS

Question 1: The TTM (States of Change) model can be used as a means to assess and understand an individual's current behaviour, and as a basis for tailoring advice and information to that person. It can be applied to a range of health related behaviours including the use of medicines (adherence), as well as *'lifestyle'* aspects such as smoking, nutrition, contraception and alcohol.

Question 2: Passive promotion of health might include stocking information leaflets, policies on stockholding (e.g. not stocking and displaying confectionery; stocking sugar-free medicines). Active promotion of health might include opportunistically offering advice and information (e.g. discussing smoking cessation with someone requesting a cough remedy; discussing the use of folic acid with a woman purchasing an ovulation testing kit; raising the issue of physical activity with a person receiving treatment for osteoporosis). Establishing contact with other agencies in the community and working with them to support health promoting initiatives would be another type of active involvement (e.g. liaising with services for drug users; working with community psychiatric nurses to support people with mental health problems).

Question 3: Advocacy at local level might involve supporting the community by lobbying the local authority and/or health service providers or commissioners for improved services. Letter writing and participation in meetings and campaigns as an informed and concerned community member can make an important contribution. At national level, advocacy might involve liaison with, and lobbying of, government, professional bodies and patient groups.

Compliance, Adherence and Concordance

Robert Horne

INTRODUCTION	166
COMPLIANCE, ADHERENCE OR CONCORDANCE?	166
CONSEQUENCES OF NONADHERENCE	167
CAUSES OF NONADHERENCE	168
Characteristics of the disease	168
Characteristics of the treatment regimen	169
Socio-demographic characteristics: the search for the 'nonadherent patient'	170
Medication knowledge and adherence	171
Quality of interactions between patients and health care practitioners	171
PATIENTS' BELIEFS: THE PSYCHOLOGY OF ADHERENCE	173
Perceptions of illness	174
Adherence decisions and beliefs about medication: balancing necessity beliefs against concerns	175
Common sense origins of necessity beliefs and concerns	176
THE CONCORDANCE INITIATIVE	177
From concordance to compliance: the 'perceptions and practicalities' approach to facilitating adherence	178
CONCLUSION	179
FURTHER READING	181
REFERENCES	181
SELF-ASSESSMENT QUESTIONS	183
KEY POINTS FOR ANSWERS	183

INTRODUCTION

Pharmacy practice serves to facilitate the appropriate use of medicines. In traditional approaches to clinical pharmacy it was thought that this could be achieved by helping to ensure that individual patients received the *'correct medicine in the correct dose at the correct time'*. However, providing a patient with the appropriate medication is only the first stage in the therapeutic process. The patient then has to use the medicine in a way that ensures optimum benefit. If one assumes that the prescription was evidence-based and appropriate then presumably this will be achieved by following the prescriber's instructions. However it is thought that at least a third of all prescribed medication is not taken as directed.

The fact that many patients do not use medication as prescribed has generated much research and debate over the last three decades, and it has become a major issue in medical care. The topic identifies some of the limitations of modern medicine, and highlights the vital role of self-care in the treatment of illness. It shows that good prescribing requires an understanding and knowledge of psychology as well as pharmacology. Nonadherence to prescribed medication may be intentional as well as accidental. Many patients actively decide to take their medication in a way that differs from the instructions. At first glance it may seem odd that someone would go to the trouble of consulting a physician and then not follow the prescribed treatment. Understanding why patients might do this has been a key target for recent research into adherence.

This chapter will outline current knowledge about the causes of nonadherence and will identify some of the controversies surrounding the topic. It will pay particular attention to the psychology of adherence and will illustrate how understanding the causes of nonadherence has led to renewed interest in models of care which emphasise partnership between patients and clinicians, leading to the concept of concordance.

COMPLIANCE, ADHERENCE OR CONCORDANCE?

Although the term *compliance* is commonly used in the medical and pharmaceutical literature, it has been criticised because it has unfavourable connotations in terms of the clinician-patient relationship. It seems to denote a relationship in which the role of the clinician is to decide on the appropriate treatment and issue the relevant instructions, whilst the role of the patient is to comply with the *'doctor's orders'*. Within this model noncompliance may be interpreted as patient incompetence, in being unable to follow the instructions or worse, as deviant behaviour. The term *adherence* has been adopted by many as an alternative to compliance, in an attempt to emphasise that the patient is free to decide whether to adhere to the doctor's recommendations and that failure to do so should not be a reason to blame the patient. Recently, the term, *concordance*, has been used to denote the degree to which the patient and clinician agree about the nature of the illness and the need for treatment. Concordance is now often used in relation to adherence and the meaning of concordance will be considered in more detail later in this chapter. However, concordance is not another term for compliance/adherence. Concordance relates to the process and outcome of a medical consultation, whereas compliance/adherence describes the patient's behaviour. In this chapter the term '*adherence*' will be used in the sense of conceptualising medicine-taking as a partnership between a patient and a clinician.

CONSEQUENCES OF NONADHERENCE

Nonadherence is a difficult phenomenon to grasp. The definition and measurement of adherence are even more problematic. For example, when does nonadherence become clinically significant? How should we assess levels of nonadherence? A detailed discussion of definitions and measurement is beyond the scope of this chapter but is dealt with elsewhere (Horne 2000). Suffice it to say that although variations in the way in which adherence has been defined and measured hamper comparisons between studies, it is thought that at least 30% of prescribed medication is not taken as directed, and that nonadherence is an important barrier to achieving the best from medication. This is an important issue with ethical implications. Adherence research seems to be fuelled by an implicit assumption that high adherence is good for patients and low adherence is bad. This will only be true if the prescription represents the best treatment option for the individual patient.

Individualising the prescription to the needs of the patient is a complex process, wherein the clinician needs to apply principles of therapeutics, knowledge of current evidence (usually obtained from data of large scale clinical trials), and prescribing policies to the needs of the individual, whilst taking into account patient preferences. The practice of clinical pharmacy may have a useful input into this process, if accepting the assumption that the role of the health care professional is to help the patient make an informed decision about adherence rather than to '*improve compliance*' per se.

If we take a leap of faith and imagine that each prescription represents the best possible intervention for each particular patient, then nonadherence represents a significant loss to patients, the health care system and the pharmaceutical industry. For the patient it is a lost opportunity for health gain, for the health care system a potential waste of resources (medicines are purchased but not used) and there is a possible increase in future demands for health care related to the lack of treatment effect. The pharmaceutical industry also loses, as patients whose adherence is low may redeem their prescriptions less frequently. For many illnesses, and treatments, the relationship between adherence and outcome is unclear. However, there is some evidence that high rates of adherence to medication are associated with more favourable outcomes. The importance of adherence to health outcomes is illustrated by the study described in Box 11.1

Box 11.1 Example of the importance of adherence to health outcomes

The importance of adherence is illustrated by a retrospective review of the data from a large clinical trial of beta-blockers in myocardial infarction (Horwitz *et al.* 1990). Patients with high rates of adherence (>75%) were more than twice as likely to have survived after one year than matched patients with low adherence (<75%). A striking and unexpected result was that this was also found to be the case for patients in the placebo arm of the trial. That is, patients with high rates of adherence to placebo (>75%) were twice as likely to survive than those with low rates of adherence to placebo (<75%). The explanation for this result is unclear, but the authors postulate that high adherence may be a marker for effective coping strategies. This viewpoint is enhanced by recent work which shows that cognitive factors, such as patients' beliefs about the illness and treatment, influence their coping patterns, which in turn, influence psychosocial adjustment and outcome of the illness.

See Horwitz and Horwitz (1993) for a review of the literature linking medication adherence to health outcomes.

CAUSES OF NONADHERENCE

The issue of patient adherence came to prominence with the publication of the classic review by Haynes *et al.* (1979) which summarised the findings of more than 200 research papers. Since then, many more studies of adherence have been published and have provided an insight into the causes of nonadherence. The type of factors that have been investigated can be grouped under the headings shown in Box 11.2.

Box 11.2 Approaches to understanding adherence

- Characteristics of the disease and treatment regime
- Socio-demographic characteristics of the patient
- Patients' knowledge
- Quality of interactions between the patients and health care practitioner
- Patients' beliefs

Characteristics of the disease

There is circumstantial evidence that general levels of adherence may be higher in some conditions than others. For example, Horwitz and colleagues reported that only 10% of patients recovering from a myocardial infarction were classed as non-adherent, whereas studies involving patients with hypertension tend to report higher levels with nonadherence rates averaging around 50% (Meichenbaum and Turk 1987). Similarly, adherence rates in acute conditions are often higher than in chronic disease, especially where treatment of the latter seems to produce little symptomatic benefit. However, the fact that considerable variation in adherence is noted among patients with the same disease, suggests that variations in adherence arise from the effect of the disease *on the individual,* rather than from a property of the disease which has a generalisable effect on adherence in all patients. In order to understand nonadherence we should therefore focus on patients and how they interpret or manage the challenges imposed by the disease.

Characteristics of the treatment regimen

The formulation or packaging of the medication may act as a barrier to adherence. Some patients may have difficulty in swallowing large capsules or may lack the manual dexterity to use complex dosage forms such as metered dose inhalers, or to open blister packs or child-resistant containers. Patients with arthritic conditions may be particularly prone to these problems.

There is evidence to support the common sense notion that the more complex the treatment demands, the lower the adherence. There are several sources of complexity: the prescription of a large number of individual medications, the need to take medication at frequent intervals, or medications which are difficult to use, such as inhaler devices. Complex regimens carry the risk of information overload and related problems of poor understanding or poor recall of instructions. Additionally, a complex regimen may be so disruptive to the patient's daily routine that they become de-motivated and may avoid or delay doses. The observed relationship between regimen complexity and nonadherence seems to have led to the assumption in some quarters that simply reducing the frequency of dosing is enough to prevent nonadherence. This is evidenced by the marketing of '*once daily*' pharmaceuticals. However, there is little evidence to suggest that this strategy alone is sufficient to prevent nonadherence. Complexity *per se* is not the key issue, but how well the treatment fits in with the individual patient's routine, expectations and preferences.

Approximately half the UK population are exempt from prescription charges. For the other half, it is thought that some patients may fail to redeem prescriptions because they cannot afford to pay the prescription charge (co-payment). One study of primary nonadherence involving nearly 5,000 patients attending a large general practice in England, showed that nonexempt patients redeemed significantly fewer prescriptions than those who were exempt from charges (33% as opposed to 17%) (Beardon *et al.* 1993). This suggests that cost may be a barrier to adherence for certain patients/medications. Further research is needed to clarify the impact of prescription cost on adherence.

Socio-demographic characteristics: the search for the 'nonadherent patient'

No clear relationship has emerged between race, gender, educational experience, intelligence, marital status, occupational status income and ethnic or cultural background and adherence behaviours. Similarly the relationship between age and adherence appears to be complex and inconsistent. A number of studies which have compared adherence rates over a fairly wide range of ages, suggest that the commonly held view that elderly patients are less adherent than their younger counterparts is misguided. Indeed, there is evidence to suggest that adherence rates are often lower in younger than in older adults. Recent research suggests that the explanation for this finding may lie in age-related differences in attitudes to health maintenance and management of illness, with elderly patients being more cautious about their health (Leventhal and Crouch 1997).

There is little evidence that adherence behaviours can be explained in terms of trait personality characteristics. Even if stable associations existed, they would serve to identify certain 'at risk' groups to facilitate targeting of interventions, but could do little to inform the type or content of interventions. Furthermore, socio-demographic characteristics and personality traits are not generally amenable to change and therefore present few opportunities for interventions. Establishing a link between socio-demographic or personality variables does little to explain *why* such factors are associated with high or low adherence. We are therefore none the wiser about what to do to facilitate adherence, since we cannot influence a person's age, gender or personality. Moreover, the idea that stable socio-demographic factors (e.g. age, gender or intelligence) or dispositional characteristics (i.e. personality) are the main determinants of adherence is discredited by evidence that adherence rates do not just vary between patients, but within the same patient over time and between different aspects of the treatment. This is not to say that socio-demographic or dispositional characteristics are irrelevant. Rather, it would seem that associations with adherence may be indirect and best explained by the influence of socio-demographic and dispositional characterises on other relevant parameters, such as motivation or ability.

In summary then, the typical *'nonadherent patient'* is something of a myth: most patients are nonadherent some of the time. Stable characteristics such as the nature of the disease and treatment, or socio-demographic variables influence the adherence behaviour of some patients more than others. This has led to a greater emphasis on understanding the interaction of the individual with the disease and treatment, rather than identifying the characteristics of the *'nonadherent patient'*. An early example of a more patient-focused approach is research linking patients' knowledge to adherence.

Medication knowledge and adherence

Patients do not always understand prescription instructions and may forget considerable portions of what clinicians tell them. It is well recognised that many patients have a poor understanding of the terminology that is often used by doctors in communicating details about their illness, and many patients have little or no understanding of the details of their medication regimen. However, the relationship between a patient's knowledge of their medication regimen and their adherence to it, is by no means simple or clear-cut. The associations between knowledge and adherence are at best small and inconsistent, and enhancing knowledge does not necessarily improve adherence. Another reason for inconsistencies in the association between knowledge and adherence is that medication knowledge is not a unitary concept, but rather comprises different knowledge components. This is illustrated by the early work of Ascione and colleagues (1986) who found wide intra- and inter-patient variations in the level of knowledge about three aspects of medication among 187 cardiovascular patients. Patients knew most about the purpose of the medication and how to take it. Fewer patients knew what to do if they missed a dose and only a small minority could identify the common side effects associated with their treatment. Thus the observed inconsistencies in relations between medication knowledge and adherence may be partially explained by variations in the way in which medication knowledge is conceptualised and measured.

Why do many patients have such poor knowledge about their medication? At least part of the answer to this question lies with patients' understanding and recall of information provided by health care professionals. Addressing these issues extends the scope of adherence research to include the role of the doctor and patient-health professional interactions.

Quality of interactions between patients and health care practitioners

There is increasing interest in the role of patient satisfaction as a mediator between information provision, recall and adherence. Surveys conducted over the past two decades indicate that many patients are dissatisfied with aspects of consultations with health care professionals and the amount of information offered to them about their illness and treatment. In a national UK survey of patients' satisfaction with medicines information received, an average of more than 70% of subjects wanted more information than they were given (Gibbs *et al.* 1990). Dissatisfaction with attributes of the practitioner or the amount of information and explanation provided may act as a barrier to adherence by making the patient less motivated towards the treatment. Ley and Llewellyn (1995) have summarised the findings of

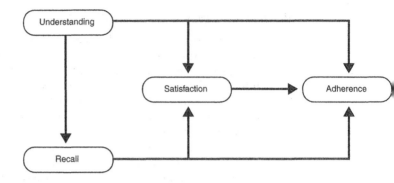

studies exploring links between understanding, recall, satisfaction
and adherence in the form of a correlational diagram reproduced in
Figure 11.1.

More recent studies have attempted to relate patient satisfaction to
the degree to which patient expectations about specific aspects of the
consultation were fulfilled as shown in Box 11. 3. A further aspect of
patient satisfaction in relation to medication use is the extent to which
their desire to be involved in the decision to prescribe is fulfilled. More
studies are needed to establish whether patients' degree of perceived
empowerment within the prescribing decision is correlated with
adherence.

In a study involving 504 patients of 25 general practitioners in 10 London
practices, patient expectations – defined in terms of needs, requests and
desires, prior to seeing the doctor – and their fulfilment were assessed using
validated questionnaires. Patients were generally much more eager to obtain
an *'explanation of their problem'* than they were to obtain *'support'* or *'tests and
diagnosis'* and the degree to which their expectations were met was predictive
of satisfaction with the encounter (Williams *et al.* 1995).

Further insight into the importance of addressing patients' needs for clear
explanations of their illness and treatment is provided by the Medical
Outcomes Study – a large study of how patients fare with health care in the
USA (DiMatteo *et al.* 1993). One aim of this study was to examine the influence
of physicians' characteristics on patient adherence to a range of treatments. In a
cohort of over 8,000 patients, reported medication adherence at 2 years was
related to reported medication adherence at baseline and to the tendency of
the physician to report that they saw a greater number of patients per week,
and arranged a specific follow-up appointment. It is interesting that the
socio-demographic characterises of patients and doctors had no influence on
adherence and that adherence to one aspect of the treatment (e.g. medication)
did not predict adherence to any other (e.g. diet, exercise). The authors
hypothesised that adherence was stimulated by scheduling frequent follow up
visits in which patients' experience with medication could be monitored.

Box 11.3 Recent studies
of patients' satisfaction
with medical
consultations

Most interventions to improve adherence are targeted towards improving patients' ability to take their medication as instructed (e.g. by providing clear instructions or simplifying the regimen or by issuing reminders). These interventions are often very useful. Unfortunately, they only address part of the problem. There is an implicit assumption that nonadherence is fundamentally caused by a lack of competence on the part of the patient. However, nonadherence may be deliberate as well as unintentional. Unintentional non-adherence occurs when the patient's intentions to take the medication are thwarted by barriers such as forgetfulness, and inability to follow treatment instructions because of poor understanding or physical problems such as poor eyesight or impaired manual dexterity. Deliberate or intentional non-adherence, arises when the patient *decides* not to take the treatment as instructed.

Thus, two issues should be considered when trying to understand adherence: *ability* and *motivation*. Unintentional nonadherence is linked to problems of ability. To understand deliberate nonadherence the patient's motivation to take or not to take the medication as prescribed should be considered (see Figure 11.2). The discipline of health psychology is particularly helpful for this. Health psychology is concerned with the study of psychological and behavioural processes in health and health care. The health psychology approach to adherence begins by focusing on motivation and starts with the assumption that *'what people do is influenced by what they think'*. Thus, if we want to understand why people respond to their illness by not following treatment advice we should look at what they think about the illness and treatment.

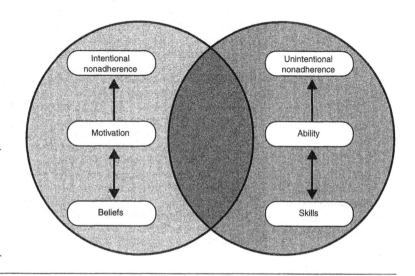

Figure 11.2
Unintentional and intentional aspects of nonadherence (Reproduced from Horne 2000, with permission)

Perceptions of illness

Health psychology theories suggest that the personal beliefs a patient forms about their illness can have a profound influence on their willingness to follow the advice of health care practitioners. This approach is exemplified by the *self-regulatory theory* or *common sense model* developed by Leventhal *et al.* (1992). This conceptualises the patient as an *'active problem solver'* whose behaviour in response to an illness (e.g. taking or not taking prescribed medication) reflects an attempt to manage the illness in a way which makes sense to them. The model suggests that people are rarely inclined to *'blindly'* follow health advice, even if it is provided by clinicians whom they respect. Rather people tend to interpret the advice and make a decision about whether they should follow it.

This model suggests that when we are faced with a *'health threat'* (e.g. experiencing symptoms or being told by a physician that we have a particular disease) our first response is to form a *'mental-map'* or *'model'* of the condition. This helps us to *'make sense'* of the condition and guides the action we take to remedy the perceived problem. Patients' models of illness are referred to using several terms: illness beliefs, illness perceptions and illness representations. For the purposes of this discussion these terms are considered interchangeable as they essentially mean the same thing: the patient's personal ideas about their illness. Leventhal suggests that illness perceptions have several important attributes shown in Box 11.4.

- Patients' personal ideas about their illness are often organised around five components: identity, timeline, cause, consequences and control/cure. These can be thought of as the answers to five basic questions about the illness or health threat: What is it? How long will it last? What caused it? How will it/has it affected me? Can it be controlled or cured? People form a mental model or representation of the illness, which is made up of their answers to these questions
- Perception of symptoms has a strong influence on patients' ideas about their illness and upon subsequent behaviour. Patients are more likely to perceive their condition as a problem, and try to rectify it, if they associate it with unpleasant symptoms. This is illustrated by the example of hypertension in Box 11.5. In other words the experience of symptoms is fundamental to our thinking about illness. Taking a treatment for a condition which does not appear to have any symptoms may appear to go against *'common sense'* unless the patient is provided with a clear rationale for why the treatment is being recommended (e.g. for prophylaxis)
- Illness perceptions influence behaviour and outcomes.
- Patients' own ideas about the illness may have a stronger influence on their behaviour than the advice of health care practitioners. This is illustrated by the example in Box 11.6

Box 11.4 Important attributes of illness perceptions (Leventhal *et al.* 1992)

Box 11.5 Illustrating the importance of symptoms of common sense models of illness: the case of hypertension

Adherence decisions and beliefs about medication: balancing necessity beliefs against concerns

Once patients are perceived as active problem solvers, it follows that in deciding whether to adhere to a treatment schedule, the patient has to think not only about whether the illness warrants treatment, but also whether the treatment is appropriate for the illness. When patients are

Study 1: Researchers from New Zealand and the UK assessed whether illness perceptions influenced adherence to recommendations (attending rehabilitation sessions) and recovery (return to work and everyday functioning) after a heart attack. They found that patients' models of the MI (beliefs about the symptoms associated with the condition, its causes, likely duration, personal consequences and potential for control or cure), elicited during convalescence in hospital shortly after the acute event, were stronger predictors of attendance at rehabilitation classes and return to work, than were clinical factors such as the severity of the MI. Those who saw their heart condition as an acute problem were less likely to turn up for rehabilitation classes (Petrie et al. 1996).

Study 2: The finding that initial illness perceptions predicted attendance at rehabilitation classes was replicated by a recent study involving MI patients in London (Cooper et al. 1999).

Study 3: Illness perceptions have also been shown to influence how patients respond to the acute event. A recent study showed that patients' interpretation of their symptoms was a key predictor of delay to seek help and reach hospital. Many patients experienced their heart attack as a gradual onset with a complex array of symptoms including nausea and feeling feverish. For many, this contrasted with their 'prototypic' view of a heart attack as a dramatic event characterised by crushing chest pain and collapse. The degree of mismatch between symptom experience and expectation was significant predictor of delay to seek help (Horne et al. 2000).

Box 11.6 Illness perceptions influence behaviour and outcomes: evidence from three studies involving patients with myocardial infarction (MI)

faced with taking prescribed medication, two types of belief seem to be particularly influential in determining levels of adherence. These are: the degree to which the patient believes in the *necessity* of the prescribed medicine and their *concerns* about taking it. Patients' concerns are often linked to commonly held beliefs that taking regular medication would result in harmful long-term effects or cause dependence and that having to take medication is disruptive.

Studies involving patients from several illness groups (including asthma, diabetes, kidney disease, heart disease and cancer) have shown that necessity beliefs and concerns are related to reported adherence. Patients with stronger beliefs in the necessity of their medication were more adherent: those with stronger concerns were less adherent (Horne and Weinman 1999).

The negative correlation between concerns and reported adherence suggests that patients may respond to fears about potential adverse effects by trying to minimise the *perceived* risks of medication by taking less. This is after all a logical response if the patient believes that the medication is necessary to control the illness, yet is simultaneously concerned about potential adverse effects of taking it. This can result in the patient taking part of, rather than the total recommended dose.

Studies also suggest that adherence to medication is influenced by a cost-benefit analysis in which beliefs about the necessity of their medication are weighed against concerns about the potential adverse effects of taking it. However, this does not imply that each time the patient is required to take a dose of medication, they sit down and think through the pros and cons of doing so! The cost-benefit analysis may be implicit rather than explicit. For example, in some situations, non-adherence could be the result of a deliberate strategy to minimise harm by taking less medication. Alternatively, it might simply be a reflection of the fact that patients who do not perceive their medication to be important may be more likely to forget to take.

Common sense origins of necessity beliefs and concerns

Patients' ideas about their illness and treatment are usually related to one another in a logically consistent way. This is illustrated by considering some of the correlates of necessity beliefs and concerns. For example, studies of patients' beliefs about medicines show that some people have more negative attitudes towards medicines than others. These patients may be more reluctant to accept that the prescribed medication offers the best treatment for their illness and are likely to have stronger concerns about the potential adverse effects of medicines prescribed for them (Horne, 1997).

Two factors appear to have a particularly strong link to patients' perceptions of the necessity of prescribed medication: their beliefs about the illness and their experience of symptoms. Patients will be more likely to agree with the necessity for prescribed medication if this accords with their perception of the illness. For example, an asthma patient who perceives their asthma to be a fairly short-lived problem with few personal consequences (i.e. *'I am ill when I suffer from an asthma attack but otherwise feel normal'*), may not have strong beliefs in the necessity of regular prophylactic medication and may be more inclined to manage their condition using medication for symptomatic relief alone. The effect of symptom experiences on views about medication-necessity may be complex. At one level, symptoms may stimulate medication use by acting as a reminder or by reinforcing beliefs about its necessity. However, patients' *expectations* of symptom relief are also likely to have an important effect. This could be problematic if the expectations are unrealistic. For example, a patient who expects their newly prescribed antidepressant medication to relieve their symptoms of depression after a few doses is likely to be disappointed when they find that the medication takes several days or weeks to have any effect. This might cause them to believe that the medicine is ineffective and that continued use is not worthwhile. Symptom experience may also influence medication concerns if they are interpreted by the patient as medication side-effects. Research into patient beliefs about their illness and treatment illustrates the key principles about the psychology of adherence shown in Box 11.7.

Box 11.7 Key principles of the psychology of adherence

Eliciting patients' own beliefs about the necessity of prescribed medication and their concerns about potential adverse effects offers a basis for concordance. Addressing potentially misplaced beliefs offers a route to helping patients make informed decisions about their medication.

THE CONCORDANCE INITIATIVE

The importance of patients' perceptions of their illness and treatment was acknowledged in a report on adherence commissioned by the Royal Pharmaceutical Society of Great Britain in 1997. The report concluded that patients would be more likely to adhere to their medication if patient and practitioner were in agreement about the nature of the illness, and the relative risks and benefits of the proposed treatment. The term *concordance* describes this *'agreement'* or *'shared understanding'*. It is important to recognise that concordance is not the same as adherence or compliance. Concordance describes the outcome of an interaction between patient and clinician (e.g. doctor, nurse or pharmacist). Adherence (compliance) describes the patients' behaviour. Concordance does not necessarily guarantee adherence (concordance may be attained but the patient may still fail to take their medication because they forget or because the regimen is too complex). The concordance initiative makes an important contribution to the adherence debate by highlighting the fact that good prescribing is a process of negotiation between patient and practitioner in which the patient's views are taken into account. However, the concept of concordance is in an early stage of development, with many outstanding questions about its development and how it might be translated into practice.

From concordance to compliance: the 'perceptions and practicalities' approach to facilitating adherence

How can insights from research into the psychology of adherence and philosophies of practice, such as concordance, inform the practice of pharmacy? I would suggest a *'perceptions and practicalities'* approach as a possible model for practice (Horne 2000). Pharmacists are in a good position to help patients get the best from medication by adopting a *'partnership model'* which takes account of patients' perceptions of their medication. The decision to take or not to take a medicine should, in almost all cases, be taken by the patient. However, this is problematic if the decision is based on mistaken perceptions about the relative benefits and risks of treatment. Clinicians could help patients by ensuring that their decision is informed by fact, rather than by mistaken beliefs about the necessity of the medication, or misplaced concerns about adverse effects. This entails eliciting patients' views about their medication and addressing concerns about adverse effects in a frank and open discussion. Thus, interventions to facilitate adherence should be based on a *'perceptions and practicalities'* approach. This follows a model of adherence shown in Figure 11.3, which recognises that nonadherence may be intentional or unintentional. It shows that patients make decisions about taking medication based on whether this makes sense in the light of their beliefs about the illness and treatment, and their expectations of outcome. If using the medicine as prescribed does not make sense to the patient (e.g. taking regular inhaled steroids, in the absence of symptomatic benefit), they are unlikely to follow it, even if the regimen is convenient and easy to use. Thus, interventions which only focus on the practicalities of using the medication (e.g. easy to read labels, clear instructions, convenient

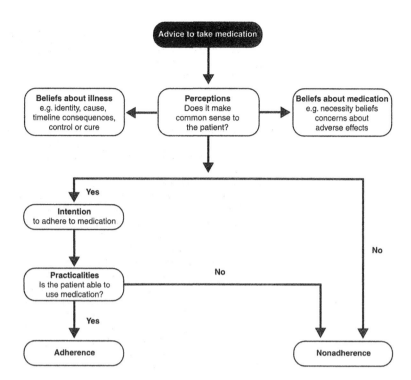

Figure 11.3 The perceptions and practicalities model of adherence (Reproduced from Horne 2000, with permission)

packaging) will be much more effective if patients' beliefs about their illness and treatment are first addressed.

Over the course of a chronic illness, patients may need more than one opportunity to discuss their treatment with a health care practitioner. A single discussion at the start of treatment may be insufficient. Patients should also be able to feedback their experiences of their medication and raise any concerns or questions which arise over the course of their treatment. In collaboration with other health care professionals, pharmacists may have an important role in this. Box 11.8 identifies a number of opportunities for pharmaceutical care, which focus on adherence issues.

CONCLUSION

Nonadherence to medication is perceived to be a significant barrier to treatment efficacy and is detrimental to patients and the health care system. Research shows that nonadherence may have many causes but these may be simplified into perceptions and practicalities. Nonadherence may be linked to beliefs about the illness and the *necessity* of medication as well as to *concerns* about potential adverse effects. When viewed from the patient's perspective nonadherence is often seen to be a common sense response to the illness and treatment. For

Box 11.8 Some examples of how pharmacists might implement a perceptions and practicalities approach to facilitating adherence

example, it may be a logical, albeit mistaken attempt to moderate the perceived risk of treatment by taking less medication.

Future interventions to help patients manage their medication require a patient–centred approach which takes account of the patients' perceptions of their illness and treatment, and the degree to which they wish to be involved in treatment decisions. To help patients get the most from prescribed medicines, pharmacists and other health care professionals should address patients' beliefs about the treatment as well as their ability to use it. Patients frequently want to know 'why' as well as 'how'. Patients should be provided with a rationale for *why* their medication is necessary, and be given an opportunity to discuss their concerns about its use. These approaches should be coupled with initiatives addressing the practicalities of using the medication for example by making the regimen as convenient to use as possible and by tailoring it to fit the patient's capabilities and lifestyle. These approaches should occur over the course of a chronic illness providing patients with an opportunity for feedback. This may be a method for moving towards an ideal: a concordant partnership between patient and clinician.

FURTHER READING

Myers, L. and Midence, K. (1998) *Adherence to Medical Conditions*, Harwood Academic Publishers, Amsterdam.

Ogden, J. (1997) *Health Psychology*, Open University Press, Buckingham.

Petrie, K. and Weinman, J. (1997) *Perceptions of Health and Illness*. Harwood Academic Publishers, Amsterdam.

REFERENCES

Ascione, F.J., Kirscht, J.P. and Shimp, L.A. (1986) An assessment of different components of patient medication knowledge. *Medical Care*, **24**, 1018–1028.

Baumann, L.J., Cameron, L.D., Zimmerman, R.S. and Leventhal, H. (1989) Illness representations and matching labels with symptoms. *Health Psychology*, **8**, 449–470.

Beardon, P.H.G., McGilchrist, M.M., McKendrick, A.D. and MacDonald, T.M. (1993) Primary non-compliance with prescribed medication in primary care. *British Medical Journal*, **307**, 846–848.

Cooper, A., Lloyd, G., Weinman, J. and Jackson, G.(1999) Why patients do not attend cardiac rehabilitation: role of intentions and illness beliefs. *Heart*, **82**, 234–236.

DiMatteo, M.R., Sherbourne, C.D., Hays, R.D., Ordway, L., Kravitz, R.L., McGlynn, E.A., Kaplan, S. and Rogers, W.H. (1993) Physicians' characteristics influence patients' adherence to medical treatment: results from the Medical Outcomes Study. *Health Psychology*, **12**, 93–102.

Gibbs, S., Waters, W.E. and George, C.F. (1990) Prescription information leaflets: a national survey. *Journal of the Royal Society of Medicine*, **83**, 292–297.

Haynes, R.B., Taylor, D.W., and Sackett, D.L. (1979) *Compliance in Health Care*, Johns Hopkins University Press, Baltimore.

Horne, R. (1993) One to be taken daily: reflections on non-adherence (non-compliance). *Journal of Social and Administrative Pharmacy*, **10**, 150–156.

Horne, R. (1997) Representations of medication and treatment: advances in theory and measurement. In: K.J. Petrie and J. Weinman (Eds.) *Perceptions of Health and Illness*. Harwood Academic Publishers, Amsterdam, pp 155–188.

Horne, R. (2000) Nonadherence to medication: causes and implications for care. In: P. Gard (Ed.) *A Behavioural Approach to Pharmacy Practice*, Blackwell Science, Oxford, pp 111–130.

Horne, R. and Weinman, J. (1999) Patients' beliefs about prescribed medicines and their role in adherence to treatment in chronic physical illness. *Journal of Psychosomatic Research*, **47**, 555–567.

Horne, R., Weinman, J. and Hankins, M. (1999) The Beliefs about Medicines Questionnaire (BMQ): the development and evaluation of a new method for assessing cognitive representations of medication. *Psychology and Health*, **14**, 1–24.

Horne, R., James, D., Petrie, K., Weinman, J. and Vincent, R. (2000) Patients' interpretation of symptoms as a cause of delay in reaching hospital during acute myocardial infarction. *Heart*, **83**, 1–5.

Horwitz, R.I. and Horwitz, S.M. (1993) Adherence treatment and health outcomes. *Archives of Internal Medicine*, **153**, 1863–1868.

Horwitz, R.I., Viscoli, C.M., Berkman, L., Donaldson, R.M., Horwitz S.M., Murray, C.J., Ranshoff, D.F. and Sindelar, J. (1990) Treatment adherence and risk of death after a myocardial infarction. *Lancet* **336**, 542–545.

Leake, H. and Horne, R. (1998) Optimising adherence to combination therapy. *Journal of HIV Therapy*, **3**, 67–71.

Leventhal, E.A. and Crouch, M. (1997) Are there differentials in perceptions of illness across the life-span? In: K.J. Petrie and J. Weinman (Eds.) *Perceptions of Health and Illness*. Harwood Academic Publishers, Amsterdam, pp. 77–102.

Leventhal, H., Diefenbach, M. and Leventhal, E. (1992) Illness cognition: using common sense to understand treatment adherence and affect cognition interactions. *Cognitive Therapy and Research*, **16**, 143–163.

Ley, P. and Llewellyn, S. (1995). Improving patients' understanding, recall, satisfaction and compliance. In: A. Broome and S. Llewellyn (Eds.) *Health Psychology: Processes and Applications* (2nd Edn.) Chapman and Hall, London, pp. 75–98.

Meichenbaum, D. and Turk, D.C. (1987), *Facilitating Treatment Adherence: A Practitioner's Handbook*, Plenum Press, New York.

Petrie, K.J., Weinman, J., Sharpe, N. and Buckley, J. (1996) Predicting return to work and functioning following myocardial infarction: the role of the patient's view of their illness. *British Medical Journal* **312**, 1191–1194.

Royal Pharmaceutical Society of Great Britain. (1997) From Compliance to Concordance; Achieving Shared Goals in Medicine Taking, Pharmaceutical Press, London.

Williams, S., Weinman, J., Dale, J. and Newman, S. (1995) Patient expectations; what do primary care patients want from the GP and how far does meeting expectations affect patient satisfaction. *Family Practice*, **12**, 193–201.

SELF-ASSESSMENT QUESTIONS

Question 1: List the elements of self-regulatory theory

Question 2: How could self-regulatory theory be extended when applied to medication adherence?

Question 3: What is concordance and how does it relate to compliance/adherence?

Question 4: Outline the *'perceptions and practicalities'* approach to facilitating treatment adherence

KEY POINTS FOR ANSWERS

Question 1:

- Patients are active problem solvers whose decisions about whether to follow health care advice are influenced by their own *'common sense'* ideas about the illness
- Patients ideas about illness (*'common sense models'*) are structured around five components or themes which can be thought of the answers to five basic questions about the symptoms or diagnosis: 'What is it? (Illness Identity), What caused it? (Causal Attributions), How long will it last? (Illness Timeline), How will it affect me and those close to me? (Illness Consequences), Is it amenable to control or cure? (Cure/Control Beliefs)
- A person's common sense model of a health threat (e.g. experiencing symptoms or being presented with a medical diagnosis) helps them to *'make sense'* of their condition and guides their decision about how to deal with it (e.g. whether to take prescribed medication)
- Patients' common sense models of illness often differ from the medical yet can have a greater influence on illness–related behaviour (e.g. taking or not taking medication) than medical advice
- The model also highlights the importance of patients' emotional reactions to illness as determinants of behaviour
- Common sense models of illness are strongly influenced by symptoms
- Patients evaluate the outcome of their decisions (Appraisal) and may change their coping procedure or model of the illness accordingly

Question 2:   The ability of self-regulatory theory to explain variations in adherence to treatment may be enhanced by including beliefs about medication. Research has shown that patients' personal beliefs about the *necessity* of their medication for maintaining present and future health and their *concerns* about the potential adverse effects of taking it influence adherence. Thus, including beliefs about their medicines as well as their perceptions of illness may enhance the theory. There is preliminary evidence that perceptions of medicine may have a stronger effect on medication adherence than illness beliefs, but that common sense models of illness influence perceptions of medication necessity.

Question 3:   Concordance relates to the process and outcome of medical consultations. It is an idea in development but includes the notion that clinicians need to understand how their patients perceive their illness and treatment. It is **not** a synonym for adherence or compliance and does not replace these terms. (The terms *'adherence'* and *'compliance'* reflect different perspectives of the same phenomenon: the degree to which the patients' behaviour matches medical advice: for many purposes the terms are interchangeable). We do not yet know if concordance influences compliance/adherence. Research in this area requires an operational definition of concordance and a valid method for measuring it.

Question 4:   Helping patients to get the best from their medicines requires a dual approach that takes account of the *perceptions* that inform decision making as well as the *practicalities* of medication taking. The *'Necessity-Concerns Model'* offers pharmacists and other clinicians a means of addressing relevant perceptions. To facilitate the appropriate use of medication, clinicians should first help the patient to make an informed decision about their treatment by providing a clear *'common sense'* rationale for the *necessity* of the treatment and then elicit and address any *concerns* they might have about it. This should be combined with more traditional approaches to facilitating adherence (such as making the regimen convenient and providing clear instructions) which address the practicalities of using it.

PART FOUR

Professional Practice

12 Pharmacy as a Profession

Geoffrey Harding and Kevin Taylor

INTRODUCTION	188
PROFESSIONS AND PROFESSIONALISATION	188
Defining professional status	188
Core features of a profession	189
A functionalist analysis of professions	190
Professional judgements	190
The process of professionalisation	191
The professional project	192
Mystification and social distance	192
THE OCCUPATIONAL STATUS OF PHARMACY	192
Applying the criteria of the *Trait Theory* to pharmacy	193
Constraints to pharmacy's occupational development	193
Social closure	193
Controlling the use of medicines	194
Drug information	195
Commodification of medicines	195
Mercantilism	195
Pharmacy ownership	196
Technology	196
Potential opportunities for occupational development	197
Promotion of pharmacists as first port of call for health issues	197
Devolution of dispensing duties	197
Pharmacists as health care advisors	198
Pharmaceutical care	198
The symbolic transformation of drugs into medicines	198
CONCLUSION	199
RECOMMENDED FURTHER READING	200
REFERENCES	200
SELF-ASSESSMENT QUESTIONS	201
KEY POINTS FOR ANSWERS	201

INTRODUCTION

Before addressing the occupational status of pharmacists as professionals, we shall first consider what is meant by the term '*profession*' Opinions vary as to what distinguishes an occupation as a profession Some occupations, such as law and medicine, have acquired a preeminent status in society and have historically been endowed with power and prestige, commensurately attracting social and economic rewards. For these occupations, the term profession has a specific meaning distinct from its more colloquial sense, i.e. the opposite of amateur. Thus, '*professional*' sports persons, though skilled and paid to play their chosen sport, do not possess the key characteristics of a profession. Occupations aspiring to professional status do so in order to gain and protect certain privileges such as a monopoly of practice, autonomy of action and enhanced remuneration. This chapter is divided into two sections in which we shall deal firstly with definitional issues of professions and professionalism, and secondly, with an analysis of pharmacy as a profession.

PROFESSIONS AND PROFESSIONALISATION

Defining professional status

There has been much debate over what defines a profession. The development of this debate is summarised in Box 12.1.

- Professions are essential to the maintenance of the social order; an important stabilising force (Parsons 1939)
- Professions possess a statutory licence to perform certain actions (Hughes 1953)
- Professions possess characteristic traits (Goode 1960)
- Professions are self-regulating (Friedson 1970a)
- Professions need to promote an esoteric or indeterminate knowledge in order to attract social and economic rewards within a free market (Jamous and Peloille 1970; Johnson 1972; Larson 1977)
- Professions have particular relations with both the state and the public (Ritzer 1975; Weber 1978)
- Occupations aspiring to be a profession undergo a 'professional project' (MacDonald 1995)

Box 12.1 Landmarks in theoretical analysis of professions

Until the 1970s, professions were conceptualised as privileged occupations within capitalist societies, uniquely characterised by a commitment to a universal standard of service which was delivered in a neutral and non-profit motivated way. At this time analyses of professions centred on identifying and listing attributes specific to professions (Goode 1960). This has been referred to as the '*attribute*' or the '*trait*' theory of professions. The most frequently cited traits of a profession are outlined in Box 12.2.

Box 12.2 Attributes of professions

Core features of a profession

The traits identified by Goode and others can be further distilled down to what might be considered the core features of professions. These are summarised in Figure 12.1.

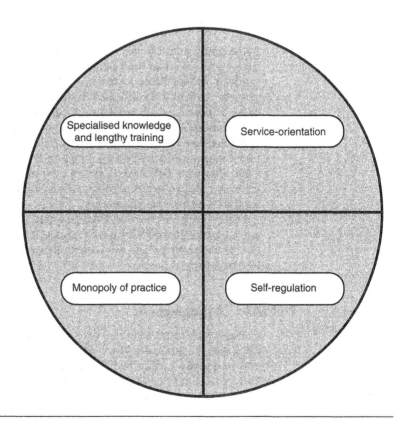

Figure 12.1 Core features of a profession

To be granted entry into a profession an individual must acquire *specialised knowledge* and undergo *lengthy training*. Extensive training is necessary, because the professional must possess a specialised knowledge, unavailable to the public, which in turn ensures the public's reliance on their service. During training, aspiring professionals also acquire the attitudes, values and belief systems specific to that profession, i.e. they undergo professional socialisation. Another characteristic of a profession is that of *service-orientation* i.e. a professional acts in the public's best interests, rather than pursuing their own self-interest. This is very important because professions have a *monopoly of practice* granted and secured by the State, which also sanctions their right to monitor and control their activities. For example, in most countries, pharmacists have an exclusive legal right to sell certain categories of medicines, but are bound by their own code of professional practice not to exploit this monopoly for personal financial gain. Professions also determine the content and scope of training, arbitrate over eligibility of membership and assess competency to practice, i.e. they *'self-regulate'*. This is necessary, it is argued, because the specialised skill and knowledge of the professional precludes non-professionals from evaluating or regulating their activities.

A functionalist analysis of professions

Some commentators have suggested that professions achieve their high status because they perform functions vital to the workings of modern industrialised society, rather than simply because they possess particular attributes. Within sociology, this has been referred to as a *'functionalist'* analysis. A functionalist perspective regards society as analogous to a living organism. All social institutions function to ensure the cohesion of the social order, rather like the various physiological systems which function to ensure our body's healthy state. Complex industrial societies depend on expert knowledge and informed judgement, and the function of professions is to supply this for the benefit of the community.

Whilst both the trait and the functionalist approaches have been supplemented by more critical analyses, it is apparent that professions do (a) possess certain important characteristics, and (b) fulfil an important social function.

Professional judgements

Professionals claim to make *'professional judgements'* (see also Chapter 13) based on particular forms of knowledge and skill that are esoteric and frequently cannot be fully articulated in written form (codified). Jamous and Peloille (1970) have described how a professional judgement is informed by a greater proportion of indeterminate knowledge

(I) than technical knowledge (T), i.e. professional judgements are characterised by a high I/T ratio. Indeterminate knowledge is personal knowledge acquired through professional experience, whilst technical knowledge is rational and codified i.e. available from texts. The centrality of a professional judgement for professions has been identified in the case of medicine by Elliot Freidson (1970b), who describes the *'clinical mentality'*. The professional, Freidson argues, *'believes what he is doing'*, i.e. is likely to display personal commitment to a chosen course of action, and is essentially pragmatic, relying on results rather than theory, and trusting personal, rather than book knowledge. Similarly, pharmacists might be argued to exercise their professional judgements when deciding on the appropriate response to patients' symptoms.

Professional judgements do not in themselves demarcate a professional. To obtain, sustain and justify its status, it is not sufficient for an occupation to claim its judgements to be *'professional'*. The State and public must also place sufficient value on an occupation's knowledge (esoteric or otherwise) for professional status to be conferred.

The process of professionalisation

So far it has been assumed that what constitutes a profession is dependent on something special or exceptional about a particular occupation. However, whilst the length of training, service-orientation, ethical practice and expertise are all significant in convincing the State and the public of its importance, they are not *'causes'* of an occupation achieving professional status. The success of medicine, for instance, in establishing and promoting itself as a profession has been argued not to be attributable to the quality of medical knowledge or doctors' expertise (Wright 1979). When doctors first organised themselves as an occupational group, there was no evidence that they were any more effective than astrologers in influencing health. Historically doctors, rather than astrologers, were successful in establishing their claim to professional status because of the high social standing of doctors and their patrons.

How an occupation both achieves and maintains professional status is termed the process of *'professionalisation'*. This process involves the profession in successfully controlling its relationship with those who fund and use its services. Professionalisation is a dynamic process founded on complex social relations between the public, the occupational group, and the State. In this sense, it may be considered an accomplishment achieved through negotiation: it is not given by right but is subject to continual validation by the State and public. Thus the professions must be sensitive to social, political and technological change which may undermine their claims to privileged status. For example, the emergence of a consumer culture has led to more open accountability in professional practice and challenges to the traditional basis of professional authority and self-regulation.

The professional project

What can an occupational group do to legitimise its claim to professional status? The professionalisation process involves the deployment of a strategy which has been termed a *'professional project'* (MacDonald 1995). The success of this project does not rely on attaining a list of attributes, but rather on an occupational group (a) persuading the State that its work is reliable and valuable, and (b) the public's willingness to accept, or their inability to successfully challenge, the group's area of expertise.

Mystification and social distance

A *'professional project'* depends in part on the power relationship between the occupation's members and the public. An important element of this relationship is that of *'mystification'* (Johnson 1972). An occupation that aspires to professional status may only achieve this objective if it succeeds in promoting its knowledge and services as mystical or esoteric. By creating a dependence on their knowledge and skills, members of such occupations effectively reduce the areas of knowledge and experience they share with those they serve. This increase in the *'social distance'* between themselves and their clients provides professionals with an opportunity for autonomous control over their practices by warding off potential challenges to their status from the lay public.

A successful claim to professional status is an outcome of on-going political struggles and power conflicts, not just with the public and the State, but also rival occupational groups. An occupation becomes a profession not so much because of improvements in its skills and knowledge, but rather because the profession's leaders are successful in convincing the State and public that autonomy and self-regulation best serve the interests of all concerned. Thus, it may not be the characteristics of professionals *per se* that determine their status so much as their relationships with the public, the State, and other occupations. Instead of pondering the question of whether or not an occupation is a profession, it may therefore be more appropriate to consider the circumstances in which occupations attempt to establish and maintain themselves as professions.

THE OCCUPATIONAL STATUS OF PHARMACY

Pharmacy's status as a profession has been the subject of numerous analyses summarised in Box 12.3.

Box 12.3 Key analyses of pharmacy's occupational status

Applying the criteria of the *'Trait Theory'* to pharmacy

Pharmacists exhibit a number of professional *'traits'*. They have a virtual *monopoly of practice* in dispensing prescribed medication and in the sale of certain over the counter medicines; they possess *specialised knowledge* and undergo *lengthy training*; pharmacy is *service-oriented*, and is *self-regulating* with its own regulatory and disciplinary bodies. Therefore application of the *'trait'* approach would indicate that pharmacy is indeed a profession.

However, pharmacy has been described by Denzin and Mettlin (1968) as an example of *'incomplete professionalisation'*. This, they claim, is due to pharmacy's failure to recruit altruistic people; to exercise control of the supply and manufacture of drugs; to develop a unique body of scientific knowledge and to maintain occupational unity. This analysis has however been challenged by Dingwall and Wilson (1995) who argue that when these features are considered in the context of the professions of medicine and the law, doctors and lawyers are no more *'professional'* than pharmacists.

Notwithstanding this, we have seen that professionalisation is a dynamic process. If pharmacy is to establish and sustain its status as a profession, the concept of a professional project has to be embraced. However, several factors, outlined in Table 12.1, might hinder its future claim to privileged occupational status.

Constraints to pharmacy's occupational development

Social closure

For an occupation to aspire to professional status, its members must be licenced for practice by the State (Hughes 1953). In the case of community pharmacy this correlates with their legal entitlement to dispense prescribed drugs and medical appliances. Clearly, some form of formal qualification to practise is required to protect the public from unlicensed practitioners, but the credentials required to practise the core function of pharmacy – dispensing or supplying prescribed medication – are not exclusive to pharmacy. Currently, in the United Kingdom at least, physicians, dentists and nurses may all, in certain limited circumstances, supply medication to patients. Thus credentialism as a means of excluding competitors from supplying prescribed

Consumerism:	Public's willingness to challenge professional knowledge and authority
Technology:	Automation, routinisation and loss of mystique
Mercantilism:	Juxtaposition of market forces and service-orientation
Corporatisation of pharmacy:	Bureaucracy in pharmacy diminishes professional autonomy
Failure to achieve social closure:	Non-exclusivity of pharmacists' functions
Incomplete control over medicines:	Dependence on physicians and diminishing responsibility for OTC medicines

Table 12.1 Factors undermining pharmacy's professional status

medication, or '*social closure*' is not effective in distinguishing the occupation of pharmacy as a profession. Pharmacists however, do have an exclusive legal entitlement to sell certain categories of medicines establishing an element of '*social closure*'. This may become key to pharmacy's future professional project as prescribed medicines are increasingly de-regulated.

Controlling the use of medicines

Denzin and Mettlin (1968) claim that while possessing a licence and mandate to supply prescribed drugs, pharmacists have:

'... failed to engage in long term activities which ensure their control over the social object around which their activities are organised ... the drug. ... The major problem which prevents pharmacy from stepping across the line of marginality is its failure to gain control over the social object which justifies existence of its professional qualities in the first place'.

i.e. pharmacists cannot legally prescribe potent medications, but instead are required to supply them in accordance with prescribers' instructions. Thus, decisions about who uses which prescribed drug for which ailment, and how, are beyond the controlling power of pharmacists.

The prescribing and dispensing functions of physicians and pharmacists emphasise the differences in control each has over medications. However, it is overly simplistic to argue that doctors alone control the public's access to prescribable drugs as they themselves may be constrained by legislation and formularies. Pharmacists, on the other hand, may have '*control*' in terms of their contribution to formularies, input on ward rounds, the choice of product for a generically prescribed drug, refusal to dispense prescriptions on legal or therapeutic grounds, and simply through pharmacy opening hours and stock holding.

Drug information

An occupation's professional status is founded on the promotion of its advice and services as indispensable and esoteric in nature. Claims to the indispensable nature of pharmacists' advice and information are undermined by the fact that pre-packaged medicines contain written inserts giving detailed instructions for their use. Moreover pharmacists compete with other sources of advice and information such as doctors, the media and the lay community (see also Chapters 7 and 9). The open and wide availability of alternative sources of advice and information on minor illnesses and medication thus challenges pharmacy's claim to privileged occupational status on the basis of the esoteric, indeterminate and indispensable nature of its knowledge base. However, professional judgement can be argued to be necessary when pharmacists ensure the individual patient's informational requirements are met, tailoring written information and, in so doing, drawing on their indeterminate knowledge and professional experience.

Commodification of medicines

The wide availability of medicines from non-pharmacy outlets, together with the increasing deregulation of medicines, once obtained exclusively from pharmacies, means that medicines are increasingly perceived by the public, and promoted by the manufacturers and suppliers as commodities, qualitatively indistinguishable from other retail goods. If medicines can be purchased from supermarkets, petrol filling stations etc, it follows that no accompanying *'expert'* supervision or advice is necessary when they are purchased, essentially making the pharmacist's contribution in this area redundant.

Mercantilism

Community pharmacists practice in an economic environment where commercial viability is of primary importance. Commercial interests would appear to be at odds with the ethos of impartial service orientation and professional altruism (see also Chapter 9). Consequently pharmacists may experience *'role strain'* or *'role ambiguity'*, as they balance the conflicting demands of professional and retail practice. For instance, evidence suggests that pharmacy proprietors are more likely than employee pharmacists to recommend customers to purchase a product. Even when the provision of goods or services would be beneficial to customers, these may only be offered when pharmacists perceive there is sufficient demand and it is commercially advantageous to do so. That said, there is also evidence suggesting that conflict between professional altruism and commercial interests is not inevitable.

Pharmacy ownership

In recent years there has been an increasing proliferation of multiple and supermarket-based pharmacies (see also Chapter 2). Successful large organisations such as these require complex bureaucratic procedures for maximising their efficiency and profitability. This results in rationalised, standardised pharmaceutical services as dictated by corporate policies. This has implications for the professionalisation of pharmacy since it has been claimed that the intrinsic knowledge and skill of an occupation claiming professional status:

'... is asserted to be so esoteric as to warrant no interference by laymen, and so complex, requiring so much judgment, from case to case as to preclude governing it by an elaborate system of detailed work rules or by supervision exercised by a superior official' (Friedson 1994).

The increasing corporatisation of community pharmacy thus raises questions as to whether the professional autonomy of pharmacists is susceptible to compromise by commercial interests, with their activities constrained, controlled and regulated by routinised bureaucratic procedures.

Technology

The increased availability of pre-formulated medicines and the emergence of original-pack and patient-pack dispensing clearly diminishes the utilisation of pharmacists' compounding and formulating skills, and the time taken to dispense medicines is less than in the past. Consequently, the 'mystique' traditionally associated with the compounding aspects of their role has largely disappeared. Likewise, pharmacists' intellectual input into the dispensing process has been largely usurped and rationalised by computer software which identifies potential drug interactions and inappropriately prescribed doses, and produces medicine labels with appropriate directions and warnings. Pharmacy's exposure to such occupational and technological change has been described as an example of 'deprofessionalisation', wherein the increasing automation of tasks has undermined the traditional basis for its claim to professional status (Birenbaum 1982 Holloway et al. 1986). Thus pharmacists' expertise and practice becomes routinised and the public may perceive them as merely suppliers of pre-packaged medicines. Correspondingly, there is limited scope for pharmacists to bring their own unique knowledge and skills to their day-to-day tasks. That is to say, they are too highly trained for the jobs they do.

When a profession's specialised knowledge becomes codified and rationalised its very existence is threatened. As Turner (1989) suggests 'objective changes in tasks, brought about for example, by technological advance, inevitably threaten to transform or possibly obliterate, a particular profession'.

Potential opportunities for occupational development

Health care is continually developing. As pharmacists take on new responsibilities this will necessarily impact on their occupational status. Table 12.2 illustrates the impact that developmental changes may have on their claims to professional status based on the application of theoretical analyses of professionalisation.

Promotion of pharmacists as first port of call for health issues

Pharmacists have promoted themselves as '*first port of call*' health professionals, available to the public without appointments, providing advisory and health care services. The rationale for their acting as 'gatekeepers' to primary health care rests on their ability to make a professional judgement regarding the appropriate action in response to patients' symptoms, including self treatment or referral to other services. However in adopting such a strategy, it is important to recognise the symbolic importance of rationing the public's claims on professionals' time. This demarcates a social distance between professional and public by reinforcing the concept that because a professional's time is highly valued it must be rationed.

Devolution of dispensing duties

In recent years the de-skilling associated with dispensing prescribed medication has reduced pharmacists' input in the dispensing process. This has provided an opportunity to increase their activities in, for example, the provision of health care advice and diagnostic testing. To take on such activities the manipulative aspects of dispensing have been largely devolved to pharmacy technicians with pharmacists'

Strategy	Pros	Cons
Promoting open access	Platform for indeterminate knowledge	Diminishes value of 'experts' time
Devolving dispensing duties	Reduction in time spent on technical activities	Distances pharmacists from their traditional role
Promoting advisory function	Opportunities for professional judgement	May eclipse 'core dispensing functions'
Pharmaceutical Care	Defines boundaries of pharmaceutical responsibility	Possible boundary encroachment
Enhancing service delivery	Delivers best practice	Constrains professional autonomy
Promoting a symbolic function	Exclusive function of pharmacy	Ethereal and unevaluated

Table 12.2 Evaluation of pharmacy's professionalising strategies

involvement restricted to checks for accuracy. These developments form part of a professionalising strategy, as pharmacists take on new roles and responsibilities in health care.

Pharmacists as health care advisors

Assuming an advisory role on medication and other health issues and offering diagnostic tests such as blood cholesterol and blood pressure measurement provides pharmacists with an opportunity to shed their image of over-educated and under-utilised health workers. This in turn would appear to have the effect of increasing pharmacists' I/T ratio, i.e. as pharmacists become increasingly involved in providing health care advice and education, and interpreting test results there is a commensurate rise in the use and promotion of their indeterminate knowledge, enhancing claims to professional status.

Pharmaceutical care

The various activities pharmacists currently perform have, in recent years, been encompassed by the concept of *'pharmaceutical care'* defined as *'the responsible provision of drug therapy for the purpose of achieving definite outcomes that improve a patients quality of life'* (Hepler and Strand 1990). What actually comprises pharmaceutical care is currently poorly defined. To some people, it is indistinguishable from clinical pharmacy, whilst in the community it might be argued to encompass pharmaceutical services additional to dispensing, such as the provision of advice to patients, residential homes and other primary care workers. The practice of pharmaceutical care, with its emphasis on the patient, and in particular, its outcome-orientation will, it has been argued, serve as a professionalising strategy by imparting to pharmacy the key elements of other health care professionals, namely a practice philosophy, a process of care and a practice management system (Cipolle *et al.* 1998). Pharmaceutical care requires pharmacists to be directly responsible and accountable to patients for the outcomes of drug therapy and as such represents an opportunity for pharmacists to exercise control over medicines use. Putting pharmaceutical care into practice however, will necessarily involve pharmacists in negotiating with other health professionals where this impinges on their areas of professional responsibilities. This has been referred to, in the context of the development of clinical pharmacy, as *'boundary encroachment'* (Eaton and Webb 1979).

The symbolic transformation of drugs into medicines

Historically, the physical transformation from drug to medicine was almost the sole province of pharmacists as they compounded medicines from their constituent ingredients. While this physical transformation function is now undertaken predominantly within the pharmaceutical industry, the symbolic meaning and value attributed to a medicine is still acquired within the pharmacy.

Pharmacists are authorised by the State and the public to transform potent pharmacological entities into medicines, i.e. they inscribe prescribed, or purchased drugs with a particular meaning for the user (e.g. to alleviate or control a biological dysfunction). For example, warfarin, a rodenticide, is transformed into a medicine with specific meaning for a patient when supplied by a pharmacist for a specific medical purpose. Similarly, aspirin can be considered a drug because of its ability to inhibit a particular enzyme. However, aspirin can also be considered a commodity, widely available to the public to relieve mild to moderate pain. In such circumstances, aspirin is loaded with no more symbolic significance than any other product available from retail outlets, because it is supplied beyond the surveillance of drug *'experts'*. However, when aspirin is selected (from a range of alternative drugs) by a pharmacist, sanctioned to interpret its appropriateness for a specific individual, this commonly available drug has the potential to be symbolically transformed into a medicine.

This benefits the public by investing a prescribed or purchased product with *'added value'*, in that a drug becomes a medicine for an individual's specific condition. Moreover, opportunities for pharmacists' input into such transformations may increase in the future due to the accelerating rate of reclassification of prescription to OTC medicines. This important social function is taken for granted by both pharmacists and the public and has not been exploited, yet it is a function which pharmacists alone are able to perform.

CONCLUSION

Increasingly, questions are being raised as to whether the privileged status of professions can be justified. Professions have historically wielded disproportionate power and influence, with minimal accountability for their activities. Increasingly the State and public are questioning professional practice and traditional *'restrictive practices'* are being eroded. Pharmacy is no exception. Currently there are important questions concerning pharmacists' activities and their contribution to the provision of health care. This will have implications for their relationships with other health professionals as well as their relationships with the public. If pharmacy is to maintain and sustain a privileged occupational status in the future, with its effective monopoly of practice, it must respond strategically to social, political and technological change. This response should be in the form of a *'professional project'* which capitalises on pharmacists' unique knowledge and skill. Privileged occupational status is not bestowed. It is an outcome of continual negotiation of social relationships between the public, the State and the occupation.

Recommended further reading

Cipolle, R.J., Strand, L.M. and Morley, P.C. (1998) *Pharmaceutical Care Practice*, McGraw-Hill, New York.

MacDonald, K.M. (1995) *The Sociology of the Professions*, Sage Publications, London.

Turner, B.S. (1995) *Medical Power and Social Knowledge* (2nd Edn.) Sage Publications, London, Chapter Seven.

References

Birenbaum, A. (1982) Reprofessionalisation in pharmacy. *Social Science and Medicine*, **16**, 871–878.

Cipolle, R.J., Strand, L.M. and Morley, P.C. (1998) *Pharmaceutical Care Practice*, McGraw-Hill, New York.

Denzin, N.K. and Mettlin, C.J. (1968) Incomplete professionalisation: the case of pharmacy. *Social Forces*, **46**, 375–381.

Dingwall, R. and Wilson, E. (1995) Is pharmacy really an 'incomplete profession'? *Perspectives on Social Problems*, **7**, 111–128.

Eaton, G. and Webb, B. (1979) Boundary encroachment: pharmacists in the clinical setting. *Sociology of Health and Illness*, **1**, 69–89.

Freidson, E. (1970a) *Profession of Medicine; A Study in the Sociology of Applied Knowledge*, Dodd, Mead and Co, New York.

Freidson, E. (1970b) *Professional Dominance*, Atherton Press, Chicago.

Friedson, E. (1994) *Professionalism Reborn*, Polity Press, Cambridge.

Goode, W.J. (1960) Encroachment, charlatanism and the emerging professions: psychiatry, sociology and medicine. *American Sociological Review*, **25**, 902–914.

Harding, G. and Taylor, K.M.G. (1997) Responding to change: the case of community pharmacy in Great Britain. *Sociology of Health and Illness*, **19**, 547–560.

Hepler, C.D. and Strand, L.M. (1990) Opportunities and responsibilities in pharmaceutical care. *American Journal of Hospital Pharmacy*, **47**, 533–543.

Holloway, S.W.F., Jewson, N.D. and Mason, D.J. (1986) 'Reprofessionalisation' or 'occupational imperialism'?: some reflections of pharmacy in Britain. *Social Science and Medicine*, **23**, 323–332.

Hughes, E.C. (1953) *Men and Their Work*, The Free Press, Glencoe.

Jamous, H. and Peloille, B. (1970) Changes in the French university hospital system. In: J.A. Jackson. (Ed.) *Professions and Professionalisation*, Cambridge University Press, Cambridge.

Johnson, T. (1972) *Professions and Power*, Macmillian Education Ltd, London.

Larson, M.S. (1977) *The Rise of Professionalism: A Sociological Analysis*, University of California Press, London.

MacDonald, K.M. (1995) *The Sociology of the Professions*, Sage Publications, London.

Messier, M.A. (1991) Boundary encroachment and task delegation: clinical pharmacists on the medical team. *Sociology of Health and Illness*, **12**, 310–331.

Parsons, T. (1939) The professions and the social structure. *Social Forces*, **17**, 457–467.

Ritzer, G. (1975) Professionalisation, bureaucratization and rationality: The views of Max Weber. *Social Forces*, **53**, 627–634.

Turner, B. (1987) *Medical Power and Social Knowledge*, Sage Publications, London.

Turner, B. (1989) Review of Abbott, A. *Sociology*, **23**, 472–473.

Weber, M. (1978) *Economy and Society*, University of California Press, Berkeley.

Wright, P. (1979) A study of the legitimisation of knowledge: the success of medicine, the failure of astrology. In: R. Walls. (Ed.) *On the Margins of Science*, Sociological Review Monograph **17**, Keele.

SELF-ASSESSMENT QUESTIONS

Question 1: List the elements of the trait theory.

Question 2: By what criteria may pharmacy be considered an incomplete profession?

Question 3: How might the increased use of technology in pharmacy, for example the use of Information Technology and pre-packaged medicines, be argued to (a) enhance and (b) compromise its claims to professional status?

Question 4: What impact has technology had on the occupational status of pharmacy?

KEY POINTS FOR ANSWERS

Question 1:

- A profession determines its own standards of education and training
- Requires extensive training
- Operates within a particular belief system
- Is legally recognised by some form of licensure

- Is regulated by its members
- Influences legislation affecting its members
- Attracts higher income, power and status
- Attracts high calibre applicants
- Is relatively free from lay evaluation
- Enforces standards of practice higher than those required by legislation
- Is likely to be a life-time occupation

Question 2:

- Lack of autonomy and control over the drug/medicine
- Mercantilism
- Unregulated and open access by the public – could be argued to diminish social distance and mystique

Question 3:

a) Enhances claims to professional status by:

- Liberating pharmacists from mechanistic and routine processes and procedures, permitting them to concentrate on the provision of expert knowledge and advice

b) Compromises claims to professionals' status by:

- Removing the traditional mystique surrounding their compounding and dispensing activities
- Judgmental skills replaced by computer software

Question 4:

a) *Positive* impact of technology includes:

- Freeing pharmacists from technical activities to exercise professional judgements
- Patient information leaflets may be a useful focus for pharmacists advice giving

b) *Negative* impact includes:

- Negating pharmacists' traditional technical functions
- Technology constrains professional judgement, promotes routinisation and removes mystique
- Patient information leaflets and package inserts undermines pharmacists' claims to unique knowledge base

Professional Judgement and Ethical Dilemmas

Richard O'Neill

INTRODUCTION	204
THE REGULATION OF PHARMACY	204
LEGAL DIMENSION	206
Negligence	206
Standard of care	207
Pharmacists' civil liability	208
ETHICAL DIMENSION	209
Morality and ethics	209
Deontological theory	210
Utilitarian theory	210
Ethical Principles	210
Non-maleficence	211
Beneficence	211
Autonomy	211
Justice	211
Ethics and pharmacy	212
Ethical dilemmas	213
PROFESSIONAL DIMENSION	214
Personal professional development	214
Professional audit and guidelines for practice	215
Risk management	215
DECISION-MAKING AND PROFESSIONAL JUDGEMENT	216
The dispensing process	217
Prescription errors	218
Errors arising during dispensing or issuing dispensed medicines	219
Non-prescription medicines	220
CONCLUSION	221
FURTHER READING	221
GUIDELINES	222
WEBSITE	222
REFERENCES	222
SELF-ASSESSMENT QUESTIONS	224
KEY POINTS FOR ANSWERS	224
DILEMMAS FOR DEBATE	226

INTRODUCTION

Pharmacy education has traditionally emphasised the acquisition of specialised knowledge and the development of selected skills required in the preparation and distribution of medicines. Over recent years, a far greater range of activities has been envisaged for pharmacists, including a greater involvement in the prescribing and supply of medicines, necessitating a much wider range of skills in which competence must be achieved. Central to these changes is a greater emphasis on the provision of advice and information to patients.

The aim of pharmacists' early education is to provide a durable foundation for a lifetime of practice. As well as an understanding of theory and its application to practice, the development of personal effectiveness, together with a sense of appropriate attitudes and values, within a framework of professional behaviour, is a necessary requirement of preparation for practice. This is addressed and developed during the period of supervised experience in practice and, thereafter, by ongoing, self-development and learning. Competence in problem-solving and communication are essential elements in pharmacy practice. As problem-solvers, pharmacists need to be able to think clearly and logically and to make, and take responsibility for, decisions based on sound analysis and appropriate evidence. This requires a recognition of personal limitations, an ability to self-appraise, a commitment to continuing competence, and due regard to the legal, professional and ethical implications that accompany every decision and action taken.

THE REGULATION OF PHARMACY

Pharmacists are expected to provide a wide range of services, although the work of community pharmacists is still mainly centred on the dispensing of prescriptions and the supply of non-prescription medicines. Dispensing incorporates a range of activities from the receipt of the prescription in the pharmacy to delivery of the medicine to the patient. As part of the dispensing process, for example, the pharmacist must ensure that patients are adequately and appropriately informed about medicines to enable patients to gain maximum benefit from their medication. Pharmacists' contribution to consumers' health is shown in Box 13.1.

Box 13.1 Pharmacists' contribution to consumers' better health (Royal Pharmaceutical Society of Great Britain 1996)	• Management of prescribed medicines • Management of chronic ailments • Development of advisory role in health care • Management of common ailments • Promoting and supporting healthy lifestyle

Advising on the management of minor ailments and ensuring patients can make informed choices about over the counter (OTC) medicines, requires competence in symptom recognition and a detailed knowledge of non-prescription medicines. These are areas of everyday practice where pharmacists are expected to take decisions and make professional judgements.

Increased responsibility implies a potential for increased liability, and an increased basis for misconduct or malpractice. Health care and health care professionals are regulated, not by a single body or group, but in a number of ways. The most direct form of regulation involves legislation and judicial precedents, concerned with the standard and delivery of health care, and enforced through the courts. Another form of regulation is entrusted to supervisory bodies, established by law and given jurisdiction to enforce standards of conduct by controlling entry to the profession and through disciplinary powers (see Chapter 12). Pharmacists work in an environment governed by ethics, their primary focus being to serve the interests of the patient and the community. It is fundamental that both the legal controls on pharmacy and the ethical framework within which pharmacists operate, allow them to exercise their professional discretion as independent health care professionals. The three dimensions of pharmacy regulation are shown in Figure 13.1.

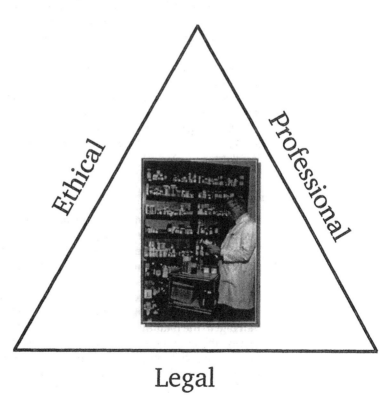

Figure 13.1 The three dimensions of pharmacy regulation

LEGAL DIMENSION

Pharmacy is perhaps the most regulated of all health care professions. There is a plethora of laws, regulations and standards with which the pharmacist is expected to comply, and liability may arise from a variety of different situations. The law may operate in a number of ways to maintain standards of pharmacists' practice (Box 13.2).

Box 13.2 The ways in which the law operates to maintain standards

Liabilities that derive from the professional practice of pharmacy typically concern one of the following categories:

- Pharmacy and medicinal laws (criminal liability)
- Standards of care (civil and criminal liability)
- Ethical considerations (professional misconduct/malpractice)

Pharmacists are expected to be familiar with the responsibilities and duties imposed upon them, and this necessitates a thorough knowledge and understanding of the law as it relates to pharmacy practice. Statutory obligations are, of course, wider than pharmacy legislation itself; they include many other areas such as health and safety, consumer and environmental protection, and employment legislation.

Negligence

In civil law, an individual who fails to take the care a reasonable person would exercise in any given situation is described as negligent. Clearly there are degrees of negligence. Negligence which is so severe as to warrant punishment under the criminal law is described as gross negligence.

Liability in negligence arises when the breach of a duty owed by the defendant to the plaintiff (the person bringing the action) results in damage to the plaintiff: damage that should have been foreseeable and reasonably avoidable (Box 13.3). It follows that the first step in establishing such liability is to show that such a duty exists. It is well established in law that pharmacists, in common with other health care professionals, owe a duty of care to their patients to act with a reason

Box 13.3 Elements of the tort of negligence

able level of skill and care. Patients depend upon health care professionals and their standards of professional conduct, and rely on the special skill and knowledge of the pharmacist when she or he sells, dispenses, or counter-prescribes medicines. If a pharmacist makes a mistake, or falls below the proper level of care, then harm may be caused to patients and to the public reputation of pharmacy. With regard to the dispensing process, a pharmacist's duty of care will relate to all aspects of checking the prescription, dispensing the medicine, and providing advice and counselling. A cause of action may, therefore, relate to incorrect interpretation, failure to supply the correct medicine, mislabeling or from inappropriate counter-prescribing (Kayne 1996a; 1996b; 1996c). A person has a duty of care to all those people whom he or she can reasonably foresee might be harmed by their actions or inactions. While it is reasonably foreseeable that forgetting or failing to check the correct dosage of a drug could cause harm, this may also apply to such actions as giving advice or failing to pass on critical information to patients or other health care professionals.

Standard of care

To be liable for negligence there must also have been a breach of the duty of care by failing to provide the required standard of care. A pharmacist is not negligent when he acts in the way that reasonably competent members of the profession would act. The question is: what is the appropriate standard of care? Pharmacists are required to practice to a minimum common standard that takes into account evolving standards. This necessitates that pharmacists keep up to date and give due consideration to professional guidelines. The degree of skill demonstrated by pharmacists should be appropriate to the task undertaken and the standard of care should be related not to the individual but to the position they hold. Otherwise, a subjective standard of care would mean that a patient's expectations would depend upon the experience of the particular professional. A single standard of care for patients can only be achieved by relating the reasonableness of a professional's conduct to the task that is undertaken and, therefore, what is objectively reasonable does not change with the experience of the professional. Thus, the minimum standard of care to be expected from a newly qualified pharmacist is no lower than that to be expected from an experienced one.

The law courts have accepted that responsible practitioners recognise their own limitations. One way of meeting the appropriate standard of care is to seek help and advice when appropriate. As a matter of practice and common sense, inexperienced practitioners will normally undertake fewer complex tasks than their experienced colleagues and seek their assistance to check their work. Importantly, a pharmacist's responsibility for the dispensing of medicines cannot be delegated, so even if the functions are performed by a dispensing assistant, the pharmacist is ultimately responsible for them.

When a judge decides a case, details describing the rationale under which the case was decided (the *ratio decidendi*) are published and may act as a precedent for subsequent cases. A body of law is thereby created which supplements statutes and regulations. The normal outcome of a successful action in negligence is damages, the amount being based upon the principle that the plaintiff should, as far as possible, be put into a position he would have been in but for the injury to him. The primary purpose of law of negligence is to compensate the injured party and, as a secondary purpose, to deter negligent conduct. Professional indemnity insurance is a professional requirement for pharmacists.

Negligence involves some form of careless conduct and is usually the result of some inadvertence. Errors of judgement may not themselves amount to negligence; some errors may be consistent with the due exercise of professional skills, while others are so glaringly below proper standards as to make a finding of negligence inevitable. A single dispensing error can, if sufficiently serious, constitute misconduct on the part of the pharmacist. Several errors may indicate a failure to take due care. A pharmacist's prime duty is to see that the public is protected: '*This is an important duty, for one can hardly imagine anybody who could be more dangerous to the public than a pharmacist who is liable to make errors in dispensing what may be dangerous drugs*' (Sir Gordon Willmer, Chairman of the Statutory Committee, reported in Pharmaceutical Journal 1974).

Pharmacists' civil liability

In the past, pharmacists have enjoyed virtual immunity from liability in exchange for accuracy in dispensing of prescriptions. Provided the prescription was dispensed correctly, the pharmacist was not liable for subsequent problems caused by the drug itself. A '*no-mistakes allowed*' legal approach to pharmacy reflected the technical nature of the pharmacist's traditional role of prescription processing (compounding and dispensing), '*... and recognition that an honest error in judgement cannot occur when judgement has not been used*' (Brushwood 1995). Pharmacists have always accepted responsibility for accurate processing of prescriptions - the correct drug product, strength and directions to the correct patient - which was seen very much as a technical process. As such, a pharmacist could be held to be negligent as a matter of law for a dispensing mistake no matter how careful they might have been – (*res ipsa loquitur*) the fact of the error speaks for itself (Brushwood 1995). Today, arguably, the pharmacist's duty of care to a patient has expanded in conjunction with the expanded professional roles that have been adopted, and a pharmacist might be expected, amongst other things, to prevent unwanted or negative outcomes from drug therapy. Pharmaceutical care, first defined by Hepler and Strand (1990) covers all the services that pharmacists provide and can be thought of as '*a practice in which the practitioner takes responsibility for a patient's drug related needs and holds him or herself accountable for meeting these needs*' (Simpson 1997).

A pharmacist cannot act as a mere conduit in the supply of medicines. A pharmacist who knows (or should reasonably have known) of a potential problem with drug therapy, who can foresee (or should reasonably have foreseen) harm to the patient, may be held accountable for failing to protect the patient's interests. While there remains the requirement to be error-free in the technical act of prescription processing, pharmacists are also required to recognise potential problems in a prescription and to take corrective action if a potential problem exists.

ETHICAL DIMENSION

Health care law governs professional practice and is an important regulator of professional standards and conduct. However, the law does not, and cannot, answer all questions about what constitutes morally correct behaviour. There are many instances when professionals are confronted with choices that are significantly different in moral terms, but on which the law is uncommitted. Moral obligations are normally seen as going beyond the legal obligations. The law, by its nature, cannot enforce an ideal standard of care, but aims to prevent care falling below an acceptable minimum standard. Hence the law of negligence is concerned with guaranteeing that a minimum level of competence is achieved. Unlike simple, reactive decisions made rapidly, professional judgements are complex and often demand unravelling of moral and ethical issues. They are questions of value beliefs and assumptions at personal and professional levels.

Morality and ethics

Morality concerns itself with relations between people and is made up of values and duties based on beliefs shared by society or a section of society; they tell those who share them what is right and wrong. Ethics is the application of values and moral rules to human activities; it centres around interpersonal relationships and how best to manage them. It is also concerned with the process of making moral judgements. There are two main approaches to resolving moral issues and health care dilemmas: deontological (rule-based approach) and utilitarian (a form of consequentialism).

Deontological theory

Deontologists contend that morality is grounded in pure reason and objectivity. Decisions are ethically valid if they conform with a proper moral rule, and wrong if they violate such a rule. The person most closely associated with the deontological approach was Emmanuel Kant (1724–1804), who held that every person has an inherent dignity and as such is entitled to respect. This respect is shown by never using people to achieve goals or consequences; people are ends in themselves. The morally correct thing is always to be guided by moral duties, rights and responsibilities, and some actions are intrinsically immoral, irrespective of how positive or beneficial the consequences might be, whilst others are intrinsically moral, irrespective of how negative the consequences. Amongst the commonly accepted types of rules are: telling the truth, keeping promises, respecting privacy, helping others and protecting the right to life. However, deontologists do not always agree on the same precepts, or the importance they ascribe to different rules, or how flexible they are in making exceptions to the rules. Adherence to moral rules, whatever the consequences, governs the deontologist's approach to ethical dilemmas. However, such a process is not self-evident. There is no obvious way to give order, or varying weight, to various duties, rights and responsibilities when the moral rules they have adopted come into conflict.

Utilitarian theory

Utilitarianism places the focus on the consequences of actions. This approach was developed by Jeremy Bentham (1748–1832) and John Stuart Mill (1806–1873). The attraction of the utilitarian theory is that it offers a simple explanation of what makes actions right or wrong, the right act being that which results in the best available outcome. A utilitarian approach to a dilemma would be to consider alternative courses of action, then predict the probable consequences of each of them, and then evaluate the likely implications for everyone affected. Having weighed each value factor, the action that produces the best balance of benefits over burdens is the one that must be implemented. Conflicting moral rules can be disregarded: the best solution is that which leads to the best consequences overall. Duties, rights and responsibilities can be ignored with such an approach; people may be used as '*means to an end*'.

Ethical principles

Utilitarian and deontological philosophies suffer when it comes to applying them to everyday ethical decision-making, due to their innate generality. With regard to health care ethics, various norms or guiding principles have emerged from further development of the basic obligation-based (deontological) and consequence-based (utilitarian

Principle	Application
Non-maleficence	Avoid harm
Beneficence	Act to benefit
Respect for autonomy	Respect choice
Justice	Treat fairly

Table 13.1 Ethical Principles (Beauchamp and Childress 1994)

ethical theories. Such principles enable varying weight to be given to various duties, rights and responsibilities and so help to guide action. The four principles proposed by Beauchamp and Childress (1994) have been widely accepted in the biomedical field and are increasingly apparent in professional codes of ethics (Table 13.1).

Non-maleficence

This is considered to be at the confluence of medical ethics and pharmacy, and is the most compelling moral element driving decision-making. Harm may be caused in many ways: by some deliberate action; by incorrect action perhaps through neglect or ignorance; or through omission such as by failing to prevent others doing harm.

Beneficence

This is closely allied with non-maleficence, in that it also concerns preventing harm or removing harm as well as bringing about positive good. According to Beauchamp and Childress (1994), a health professional would have a positive duty of beneficence towards a person when that professional has the capacity to promote the person's well-being.

Autonomy

This involves individuals being able to formulate and carry out their own plans, desires, wishes and policies, thereby determining the course of their own life. Paternalism is often used to legitimise infringements of another's autonomy, supported as it is by the principle of beneficence. Paternalistic behaviour usually means acting on behalf of another person in that person's best interest. Competence in decision-making is closely related to autonomous decision-making and to questions about the validity of consent. The increasing emphasis on a more patient-centred approach to health care and patient involvement in decision-making, necessitates that patients receive adequate information in order to make informed choices about their health care. Patient preferences and values need to guide decisions about choices of treatment in addition to professional knowledge.

Justice

This requires that the interests of all those concerned are considered, and they are given that to which they are entitled. People should be treated fairly (or equally) and not differentiated on grounds such as gender, race or creed. Different types of justice are relevant in professional ethics situations: *distributive*, *compensatory* and *procedural* (Purtilo 1999). The principle of distributive justice, for example, requires that benefits and burdens be distributed equitably, in accordance with the level of need or merit. Many codes of ethics contain other principles such as fidelity (faithfulness) and veracity (truthfulness) and other personal virtues, although some may be considered to be covered under the umbrella of the four outlined by Beauchamp and Childress.

Ethics seeks to answer the questions: *what should we do*? and *what should we not do*? Ethics is concerned not only with making the right decision but also with justifying those decisions. When there are conflicting moral responsibilities, when in following one guiding principle we desert another, the situation becomes an ethical dilemma. Situations which involve some ethical decision include those where there is more than one solution, no obvious correct solution, and where ethical principles such as beneficence, non-maleficence, autonomy and justice conflict. In deciding how to act, health care professionals ought to consider certain principles for ethical decision making (Box 13.4).

Box 13.4 Principles for ethical decision-making

- Avoid harm
- Where possible achieve benefit
- Respect the autonomy of the individual
- Consider, fairly, the interests of all those affected

These principles may act as guides in ethical decision-making: a broad framework for organising deliberations and debate. They should not be considered as a simple formula or easy method for solving ethical dilemmas, but rather, a reminder of the key elements of ethical thinking. Ethical judgement depends crucially on questions of fact as well as questions of principles.

Ethics and pharmacy

All rules, whether legal, moral or customary, lay down standards of behaviour. They specify what ought to be done and aim to mark the boundaries between acceptable and unacceptable conduct. While the law requires that a basic standard of practice is maintained, codes of professional practice express a higher expectation and ethics requires that this standard be at the highest possible level.

A common feature of all professions is an ethical code which encompasses those beliefs and behaviours to which members of the profession subscribe. It embodies ideals, or guiding principles by which a member can judge their own conduct and by which this conduct can be viewed by others. Codes may range from those which are extremely detailed, covering a wide spectrum of activities, to those which are shorter and more idealistic.

Detailed codes typically comprise principles and standards. *Principles* are rules that should always be obeyed unless an exception is available, and statements of principle can be made relatively precisely; *standards*, by comparison, should always be under review and changing. These emphasise pharmacists' duties to their patients. A code, however detailed, cannot hope to cover every situation, and a short aspirational code, consisting only of ethical principles, may provide professionals with a clearer understanding of where their obligations originate when dealing with conflicts, as well as greater freedom in professional judgement (Barber and O'Neill 1999).

Ethical dilemmas

Pharmacy ethics involves the application of ethical rules and principles to the practice of pharmacy. When faced with an ethical dilemma, a pharmacist is expected to use his, or her, professional judgement in deciding on the most appropriate course of action. An expanded professional role and a closer involvement with the patient will increase the opportunities for ethical problems to arise. Every encounter with a patient raises ethical issues, although such issues do not necessarily present ethical dilemmas. Many issues confronting the pharmacist are unambiguous and straightforward to resolve. Ethical dilemmas arise from fundamental conflicts among beliefs, duties and principles. Pharmacists can be faced with an ethical dilemma in diverse areas. For instance:

- When asked by a patient or carer what a medicine is used for
- When asked to dispense or sell a medicine that contravenes one's religious or moral beliefs
- When involved in questions concerning the behaviour or competency of a colleague

The application of ethical principles and decision-making is needed to solve such dilemmas, and this requires pharmacists to develop a working knowledge of formal and systematic ethical analysis, as well as learning to distinguish ethical issues from, for example, social or legal issues. Ethical decision-making is a multi-step process (Box 13.5), requiring judgement, reasoning and analysis. It involves evaluating facts and values, as well as duties, in order to arrive at a reasoned and justifiable solution to resolve the conflict. It is a process of problem-solving which requires critical thinking, in which the cause, alternative actions and potential effects of each action must be considered (Justice 1990; Weinstein 1993).

The question of what is right is not just decided within an ethical framework, but also within legal and professional obligations. The law establishes the ultimate standard for evaluating conduct and the phar-

Box 13.5 Steps in the process of ethical decision-making

macy profession sets out those things that a pharmacist is obliged to do. Ethical analysis therefore requires that all of these elements are considered.

PROFESSIONAL DIMENSION

The role of a professional body is to set standards of professional practice, to safeguard the best interests of the public and the profession. Self-regulation is an important element of a profession and in contemporary society, with rising expectations of the professions, this cannot be taken for granted (see Chapter 12). The stringent level of professional care to be exercised by, and expected of, a pharmacist is evidenced, among other things, by the onerous obligations placed on them by their professional codes of practice. Pharmacists have a responsibility to remain up-to-date and to maintain competence and effectiveness as a practitioner, and to base their practice on a 'best evidence' approach. In order to fulfil this responsibility, it is necessary for them to participate in continuing professional development which includes continuing education and professional audit.

Personal professional development

Pharmacists need to perfect a process of continual learning in order to cope with the constant change with which they are confronted, and will continue to be confronted. Continual learning can be depicted as a cycle, the components of which have been identified as *learn, analyse, question* and *act* (Woodward 1998). Participation in structured continuing education programmes is one approach but, importantly, pharmacists need to be effective self-learners. Sources of drug information are numerous; ranging from the World Wide Web, computer databases, drug information centres, reference books, textbooks, professional journals, distance learning material, local formularies and bulletins. It is essential to appreciate the nature and source of material, whether it is independent or noncommercial, and whether it has been subject to external validation/peer review, in order to determine the reliance that can be placed upon it. Pharmacists must decide how best to keep their knowledge and skills up-to-date and have access to the best evidence on which to base their practice. In the future, this will undoubtably result in professional bodies placing increasing emphasis on standards of knowledge and professional performance as well as on professional misconduct.

Professional audit and guidelines for practice

Audit is the process by which standards of practice may be improved. Individual performance standards concerning some part of the structure, process or outcome of pharmacy practice (such as dispensing procedures, health promotion, and response to symptoms) are measured against some model standards that are consistent throughout the profession (Hayes *et al.* 1992). Standards in professional practice should be continually improving (See also Chapter 32).

There is a danger that over-regulation of a profession can result in diminution of its professionalism. Guidelines, or rules of procedure, by their very nature, set out to influence both the way in which pharmacists practise and their accountability. However, detailed guidelines can run the risk of dictating how pharmacists are to perform their duties, thereby diminishing professional judgement and the provision of true pharmaceutical care. Certainly, following guidelines slavishly is to invite problems as it implies a lack of thought and a failure to check whether these guidelines are up-to-date. It could be negligent not to be up-to-date with current literature on a subject. Guidelines do not, and cannot, remove the need for professional judgement. They must be interpreted sensibly, and appropriate interpretation and application is likely to result in better patient care than either disregard or unthinking compliance.

Risk management

Awareness of the law of negligence is a valuable tool for analysing whether a proposed risk is sensible or not, i.e. in '*risk management*'. Pharmacy in not a profession associated with risk-taking. The pharmacist's relationship with a patient primarily involves the prevention, or minimisation, of the risks of drug therapy. The checking of a prescription for errors, ensuring that the correct medicine is supplied with appropriate directions and that the patient is warned of potential dangers or unwanted effects, are all intended to minimise risk to the patient. In order to minimise the risk of dispensing errors, for example, safety procedures need to be adopted in which checks can be made at various stages of the process. A risk-management system needs to be developed (Box 13.6) beginning with the identification and analysis of potential problems and the implementation and monitoring of suitable risk-minimisation techniques (Baker and Mondt 1994).

- Address the various activities taking place
- Identify the risks
- Analyse the risks
- Identify solutions towards reducing or eliminating the risk
- Evaluate the risk management strategy

DECISION-MAKING AND PROFESSIONAL JUDGEMENT

Pharmaceutical care requires pharmacists to make decisions. Decision-making can be considered a manifestation of professional knowledge and is essential to the authority and mission of a profession.

Decision-making has been described as a series of steps, each building upon the other, finally culminating in the actual decision. A hierarchy of levels may be involved (Box 13.7).

Box 13.7 Hierarchy of
decision-making
(Campagna 1995)

- *Recognition* of the problem
- *Formulation* or exploration of the problem
- Identification or generation of *possible solutions*
- *Information searching; judgement* against a normative standard
- *Choice* of solution
- *Action*

Other elements such as *clarification* and *feedback* also play a part in the process

The types of decision a pharmacist is required to make clearly depends upon the practice setting, but have been classified by Brodie *et al.* (1980) as:

- Managerial decisions
- Non-clinical decisions
- Clinical decisions

Some practical aspects of pharmacy practice are largely technical or routine, and can often be broken down into their component parts. These are regarded as '*skills*' and, as such are capable of being mastered. They may involve little in the way of reasoning and lend themselves to routine and simple application of knowledge. However, there is a limit to how far a professional role can be codified in terms of activities and skills. Professional practice is not merely a matter of delivering a service to clients through a predetermined set of clear-cut routines. Far from being simple and predictable, professional practice is more complex and less certain. The pharmacist is involved in making many complex decisions which rely on a combination of knowledge, professional judgement and common sense which cannot be set into absolute routines (see Chapter 12).

Practitioners should be alert to the complex nature of practice, treating the knowledge they have as adaptable, and be conscious of the principles upon which practice is based. Knowledge is not permanent nor totally mastered. Rather, it is, temporary, dynamic and problematic. A health care professional must be a *lifelong learner* rather than a mere *knower*. Where undergraduate education emphasises factual information and certainty, and looks at the theory (the basics), professional knowledge emerges from critical reflection on, enquiry into and deliberation about experience. Formal knowledge (i.e. knowledge formulated outside practice) is transformed in practice to become personal professional knowledge. Theory underpins practice, but practice is the starting point for understanding theory (Fish and Coles 1998).

The dispensing process

Dispensing of prescriptions remains the core activity of community pharmacists and provides an example of pharmacist decision-making with varying degrees of professional judgement involved. The dispensing process involves all of the activities which take place from the receipt of the prescription in the pharmacy until the collection of the medicine by the patient or their representative. Every prescription for a medicine must be seen by the pharmacist, who bears the legal and professional responsibility, and a judgement is made as to the appropriate action(s) required. Dispensing includes a number of stages: the initial screening of the prescription; any actions necessary to remedy omissions, errors or ambiguities; the correct assembly or preparation of the medicine with a suitable label; and the provision of advice and information as appropriate (Table 13.2). Each stage involves a number of steps each requiring specific knowledge, skills and competencies.

Pharmacists undertake a considerable responsibility when dispensing prescriptions – a responsibility that is not offset or undermined by the fact that the prescriber may have made an error. They have a duty to make an independent assessment of a prescription, requiring the ability to accurately interpret and evaluate the prescription and to make a professional judgment whether or not it should be dispensed,

Requirement	Application of knowledge on
Verification of the authenticity, completeness and legality of the prescription	Legislation controlling medicines, the practice of pharmacy and requirements for the supply of dispensed medicines
Appropriateness of the dose, frequency, duration, dosage form and route of administration	Pharmacology, therapeutics and pharmaceutics
Appropriateness of prescribed medication with existing medication (if any) and evaluation of possible contra-indications	Therapeutics, drug interactions and clinical pharmacy

Table 13.2 Initial screening and dispensing of prescriptions

and to determine what action is necessary to rectify any problems or ambiguities. A pharmacist's primary concern must be the welfare of the patient. If the pharmacist, having contacted the prescriber about a prescription and been told to dispense, still has reservations, it is doubtful whether they would avoid all liability should she or he proceed with the dispensing and the patient subsequently suffers harm. It would not be seen as a proper exercise of professional judgement, although it could perhaps be argued that any initial negligence on the part of the prescriber was exacerbated by his or her response to the query (McKevitt 1988).

Pharmacists have a legal duty to verify the legitimacy of a prescription. To be valid, a prescription must comply with certain legal requirements, and a supply made in the absence of these can constitute a criminal offence. Similarly, since the dispensing of a forged prescription for a prescription-only medicine can also constitute a criminal offence, if the prescriber's signature is unknown, there is a requirement that the pharmacist takes sufficient steps to satisfy him or herself that it, and the prescription, is genuine. While the law itself may provide little in the way of constructive direction when dealing with some prescription problems such as a prescription from an unknown prescriber, professional guidelines do offer advice. Situations arise when the law and professional/ethical requirements conflict, for example an incorrectly written, but genuine, controlled drug prescription for which there is an immediate clinical need. The pharmacist is then confronted with the need to exercise a professional judgement as to whether or not to make an illegal supply, a judgement which cannot be delegated.

Prescription errors

The types of errors associated with prescriptions may be those associated with incomplete details (omission) or those associated with incorrect details (commission) (Table 13.3).

Errors of omission	Errors of commission
Absence of legal requirements	Incorrect drug or indication for use
Absence of dosage form or strength	Incorrect dosage form or strength
Absence of dose or dosage regimen	Incorrect dose or dosage regimen
Absence of quantity or duration of treatment	Incorrect quantity or duration of treatment
	Duplicate therapy
	Drug interactions
	Contraindicated or inappropriate therapy

Table 13.3 Examples of prescription errors

Procedures, or professional guidelines, are typically available for dealing with omissions from prescriptions. Such omissions may, however, present the pharmacist with a legal or ethical dilemma. Errors of commission represent a far greater threat to the safety of the patient if not identified and corrected, but are less easy to identify than omissions.

In reality, since a pharmacist is not usually privy to the diagnosis, ascertaining the appropriateness of a prescribed item might be difficult in some circumstances. However, whether or not the prescribed dose or dosage regimen lies within the usual range for the patient and, where appropriate, the condition being treated, can be checked and information sought from appropriate texts or references for particular situations such as drug interactions, contraindications, incompatibilities, and adverse effects. Pharmacists are increasingly using information technology as an aid in identifying problems such as drug interactions and inappropriate dosing regimens. However, it is important to recognise that the role of computer systems is to support or supplement the pharmacist's input, not to supplant it. The pharmacist must evaluate each situation and make a professional decision.

Errors arising during dispensing or issuing dispensed medicines

Dispensing errors frequently fall into one of two categories (Baker and Mondt 1994):

1. Mechanical errors which are technical in nature
2. Intellectual or cognitive errors which typically involve professional judgement

Possible mechanical and intellectual errors are indicated in Box 13.8. An organised and systematic method of dispensing and an effective checking system at various stages throughout the dispensing process are essential.

Additionally, techniques that might be employed in dispensing prescriptions to lessen the possibility of mechanical errors, include the use

---

Mechanical errors:

- Incorrect dosage form or strength supplied
- Incorrect quantity supplied
- Incorrect medication supplied
- Labelling errors/omissions

Intellectual errors:

- Absence of counselling/advice/information
- Improper counselling/advice/information

Box 13.8 Errors in the dispensing process

---

of dispensing baskets/trays as a receptacle for each prescription and a separate area for dispensing and checking. The public expectation of pharmacists is one of absolute accuracy, and being busy is no excuse for a dispensing mistake. The pressures of time must be managed effectively.

Errors may also occur in the issuing of medication to a client. To minimise such errors, medication items should not be delivered in a sealed bag, whilst a docket system may act as additional positive identification of patients. The pharmacist should check through each item with the patient against the prescription, which can be attached to the bag on completion of the final check, having first used the prescription to make an absolute check of names and address.

Pharmacists have a responsibility to ensure the safe and effective utilisation of medicines, by providing comprehensible information in the form of labels and information leaflets, as well as verbal advice. Patients need to be adequately and appropriately informed about their medication and advice should be consistent with, and reinforce that provided by the prescriber, so as to ensure patients receive maximum benefit.

Finally, a written record should be kept of all interventions made, and action taken, by the pharmacist. Similarly, records should be kept of any mistakes made, whether they reached the patient or not, so that actions may be taken to correct the process and learn from the mistakes.

Non-prescription medicines

Self-medication is an integral part of health care. A key activity of pharmacists is in advising patients on dealing with minor ailments. This requires the pharmacist to maintain a competence in symptom recognition, maintain sufficient knowledge to make the appropriate choices about non-prescription medicines, and the ability to judge when to refer a patient on to a medical practitioner. Pharmacists are expected to meet the standard of professional conduct set by professional bodies regarding health care advice. A safe and structured approach is needed when responding to symptoms in order to elicit the necessary information on which to make a professional judgement. A number of questioning approaches have been advocated, such as *WWHAM* (Box 13.9) and *ENCORE* (Figure 13.2).

Box 13.9 WWHAM Questions (National Pharmaceutical Association)

- W – Who is it for?
- W – What are the symptoms?
- H – How long have the symptoms been present?
- A – Action already taken?
- M – Medicines they are taking for other problems?

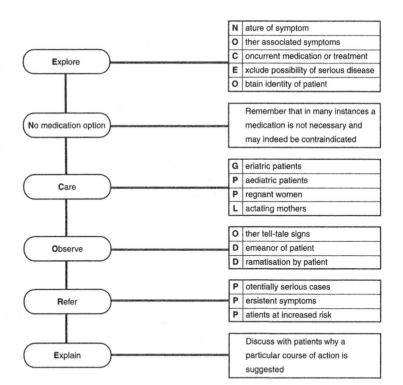

N	ature of symptom
O	ther associated symptoms
C	oncurrent medication or treatment
E	xclude possibility of serious disease
O	btain identity of patient

Explore

No medication option — Remember that in many instances a medication is not necessary and may indeed be contraindicated

G	eriatric patients
P	aediatric patients
P	regnant women
L	actating mothers

Care

O	ther tell-tale signs
D	emeanor of patient
D	ramatisation by patient

Observe

P	otentially serious cases
P	ersistent symptoms
P	atients at increased risk

Refer

Explain — Discuss with patients why a particular course of action is suggested

Figure 13.2 ENCORE, a mnemonic for a structured approach to responding to symptoms (Li Wan Po 1992)

CONCLUSION

One of the principal concepts of a profession is the ability to make personal professional decisions. Decision-making is an expression of professional knowledge and responsibility. Pharmacists work to help patients gain maximum benefit from their medication, in so doing they need to make decisions and judgements. Like other health care professionals, pharmacists are under a duty to exercise reasonable care and skill in all the disparate tasks they undertake, requiring a commitment to maintaining good standards of conduct, up-to-date knowledge and continuing competence. Pharmacists must be adept at making sound decisions and judgements; patients, society and the pharmacy profession expect nothing less.

FURTHER READING

Abood, R.R. and Brushwood, D.B. (1997) *Pharmacy Practice and the Law* (2nd Edn.) Aspen Publishers Inc, Gaithersburg, Maryland.

Appelbe, G.E. and Wingfield, J. (1997) *Dale and Appelbe's Pharmacy Law and Ethics* (6th Edn.) The Pharmaceutical Press, London.

Appelbe, G.E., Wingfield, J. and Taylor, L.M. (1997), *Practical Exercises in Pharmacy Law and Ethics*, The Pharmaceutical Press, London.

Beauchamp, T.L. and Childress, J.F. (1994) *Principles of Biomedical Ethics* (4th Edn.) Oxford University Press, Oxford.

Mullen, K. (2000) *Blackstone's Pharmacy Law and Practice*, Blackstone Press, London.

Purtilo, R. (1999) *Ethical Dimensions in the Health Professions* (3rd Edn.) W.B. Saunders Company, Philadelphia.

GUIDELINES

Medicines, Ethics and Practice. A Guide for Pharmacists No. 22 (1999) Royal Pharmaceutical Society of Great Britain, London.

Royal Pharmaceutical Society of Great Britain *(1996) Pharmacy in a New Age: the New Horizon*, The Royal Pharmaceutical Society of Great Britain, London.

WEBSITE

Pharmweb: Pharmacy in Practice; *Ethics in Pharmacy Practice* http:// www.pharmweb.net/pwmirror/uk/stjames/ethics

REFERENCES

Baker, K.R. and Mondt, D. (1994) Risk management in pharmacy *American Pharmacy*, **NS34**, 60–61.

Barber, N. and O'Neill, R. (1999) Suggestions for a new code of ethics *Pharmaceutical Journal*, **262**, 923–925.

Beauchamp, T.L. and Childress, J.F. (1994) *Principles of Biomedical Ethics* (4th Edn.) Oxford University Press, Oxford.

Brodie, D.D., Parish, P.A. and Poston, J.W. (1980) The decisions pharmacists make. *American Journal of Pharmacy Education*, **44**, 40–43.

Brushwood, D.B. (1995) The pharmacist's expanding legal responsibility for patient care. *Journal of Social and Administrative Pharmacy*, **12**, 53–62.

Campagna, K.D. (1995) Pharmacists' levels of performance in making drug therapy decisions. *American Journal of Health-Systems Pharmacy*, **52**, 640–645.

Fish, D. and Coles, C. (1998) *Developing Professional Judgement in Health Care. Learning Through the Critical Appreciation of Practice*, Butterworth Heinemann, Oxford and Boston.

Hayes, P., Kayne, S., Martin, T. and McMurdo, A. (1992) Use of professional self audit in pharmacy practice. *Pharmaceutical Journal*, **249**, 650–652.

Hepler, C.D. and Strand, L.M. (1990) Opportunities and responsibilities in pharmaceutical care. *American Journal of Hospital Pharmacy*, **47**, 533–543.

Justice, J. (1990) Objectivity and critical thinking to resolve ethical dilemmas in pharmacy practice. *Journal of Social and Administrative Pharmacy*, **7**, 93–98.

Kayne, S. (1996a) Negligence and the pharmacist: Part (1) aspects of the law and duty of care. *Pharmaceutical Journal*, **256**, 654–656.

Kayne, S. (1996b) Negligence and the pharmacist: Part (2) areas of liability. *Pharmaceutical Journal*, **257**, 31–32

Kayne, S. (1996c) Negligence and the pharmacist: Part (3) dispensing and prescribing errors. *Pharmaceutical Journal*, **257**, 32–33.

Li Wan Po, A. (1992) ENCORE. A structured approach to responding to symptoms. *Pharmaceutical Journal*, **248**, 158–161.

McKevitt, T. (1988) Doctors, pharmacists and prescriptions. The standard of care owed to the patient. *Professional Negligence*, **December**, 185–188.

Pharmaceutical Journal (1974) Pharmacist to be struck off register for dispensing errors. *Pharmaceutical Journal*, **212**, 11.

Purtilo, R. (1999) *Ethical Dimensions in the Health Professions* (3rd Edn.) W.B. Saunders Company, Philadelphia.

Royal Pharmaceutical Society of Great Britain (1996), *Pharmacy in a New Age: the New Horizon*, The Royal Pharmaceutical Society of Great Britain, London.

Simpson, D. (1997) Pharmaceutical care: the Minnesota model. *Pharmaceutical Journal*, **258**, 654–656.

Weinstein, B.D. (1993) Ethical decision making in pharmacy. *American Pharmacy*, **NS33**, 48–50.

Woodward, B.W. (1998) The journey to professional excellence: a matter of priorities. *America Journal of Health-Systems Pharmacy*, **55**, 782–789.

Question 1: To whom does a pharmacist have a responsibility?

Question 2: To which persons/bodies might a pharmacist be held accountable for his/her actions?

Question 3: List some mechanical and intellectual dispensing errors that might occur

Question 4: What do you consider to be the relative merits and criticisms of the utilitarian and deontological approaches to resolving moral issues?

Question 5: Indicate the steps of decision-making

KEY POINTS FOR ANSWERS

Question 1:

- patient
- public
- pharmacy profession
- professional colleagues
- other health care professions
- employer
- oneself

(You may wish to debate the order)

Question 2:

- **Patient** → negligence claim → civil action → damages
- **Society** → criminal offence → criminal prosecution → conviction/penalty
- **Employer/Health Contractor** → breach of contract → disciplinary action → termination of employment/contract
- **Profession** → professional misconduct/malpractice claim → disciplinary body hearing → removal from the professional register

Question 3:

a) **Mechanical** – problems in the way the drug product is dispensed, including:
- wrong product
- wrong strength
- wrong formulation
- wrong labelling

b) **Intellectual** – decision-making or discretionary matters
- failure to warn, counsel or advise the patient

Question 4:

Note how the strengths of one system relate to the weaknesses of the other:

Utilitarian	**Deontologist**
Merits	**Merits**
• Actions not intrinsically right or wrong – best result is that which leads to greatest happiness (best consequences) for those affected	• Morality found in pure reason
	• Moral rules, duties and values
	• No emotion/subjectivity involved
	• Rational/objective criteria used
• Clear way of determining what is the right thing to do – consider all parties involved; weighs factors	• People as ends in themselves
• Flexibility in dealing with moral dilemmas	**Criticisms**
• Avoids conflict between moral rules	• Too rigid
Criticisms	• Less clear argument concerning the importance of morality; morality important *per se*
• Lacks justice/morality	• Problem of conflicting moral rules
• Fails to consider individual rights	
• Subjective criteria included	• Ends cannot justify means even if outcome is good
• The ends can justify the means	• Insufficient weight to intuition or feelings
• *Slippery slope* objection	

Question 5:

Action

↑

Choice of Solution

↑

Judgement

↑

Information Search

↑

Identification of Possible Solution

↑

Formulation/Exploration of the Problem

↑

Recognition and Clarification of the Problem

DILEMMAS FOR DEBATE

Consider how the pharmacist might deal with:

1. An incorrectly written controlled drug prescription issued for a regular patient with terminal illness
2. A request from a mother for information about some tablets she has found in her teenage daughter's bedroom
3. A request from a young woman for an emergency, post-coital contraceptive
4. A concern regarding the professional competence of a colleague

You may wish to consider these under the headings of *legal, ethical* and *professional* aspects. Also, whilst it is often said that moral dilemmas have no *right answer*, there are undoubtably some options which are much more appropriate than others, and all solutions have to be justified.

14 Effective Communication

Norman Morrow and Owen Hargie

INTRODUCTION	228
THE NEED FOR GOOD COMMUNICATION	229
Patients often do not understand, or forget, information they are given	230
Patients are often dissatisfied with the advice and information they are given	230
Lack of patient-practitioner concordance	231
Patient satisfaction and concordance are related	231
Inattentiveness to patients' psychosocial needs	231
KEY COMMUNICATION SKILLS	232
Building rapport	234
Explaining	235
Questioning	235
Listening	237
Nonverbal communication	238
Suggesting and advising	238
Opening	239
Closing	240
Assertiveness	240
Disclosing personal information	241
Persuading	242
COMMUNICATION AND DISABILITY	243
CONCLUSION	245
FURTHER READING	245
REFERENCES	245
SELF-ASSESSMENT QUESTIONS	247
KEY POINTS FOR ANSWERS	247

INTRODUCTION

Communication in the context of pharmacy practice is concerned primarily with health and illness. The concept of *'health'* can be viewed in six different dimensions (Box 14.1).

Box 14.1 Six dimensions of health (Ewles and Simnett 1992)

In an interview we conducted, an elderly woman with longstanding rheumatoid arthritis demonstrated the importance of a wide perspective of health when describing what being healthy meant to her:

'Well, I think that a day that I would be free enough of pain to enjoy reading. Now my neck is so bad that I cannot keep it at an angle and the day that I would be able to read in comfort would be a really good day; or a day that I would have somebody coming to visit that I would really enjoy their conversation, for instance my own children and some members of the family and a lot of friends that we have. I have my Christian faith. I think psychologically it is the mainstay of how I feel. Then, of course, I have a wonderful husband and I just don't know how I could cope without him. I know that is something not everybody who has this pain and disease enjoys, so it's a great blessing to me.'

The relational dimension of care has grown in importance in recent years, with a remarkable change in the nature of practitioner-patient relationships. One dimension of this was the introduction of the Patient's Charter in the UK (Department of Health 1992), which highlighted the health care provisions to which members of the public were entitled. From a Government viewpoint, it sought to stimulate greater efficiency and effectiveness within the National Health Service (NHS). From a professional practice standpoint, it has instilled a greater consciousness of service quality, whilst from a consumer perspective, it articulated standards whereby services could be judged for overall quality and satisfaction. One effect of this has been to raise the expectations of patients about what they are entitled to as consumers of health care services. The production and display of a practice leaflet in each community pharmacy, detailing the pharmaceutical services available, is but one example of this consumer-oriented approach.

In their book on pharmaceutical care practice, Cipolle *et al.* (1998) made the important observation that: *'Care means communication. Quality care means quality communication'*. Indeed, communication is now widely recognised as central to effective health care, and, *'Patients rate communication skills as the most sought after quality of the primary health care provider'* (Ross *et al.* 1994). In confirming its importance, the Audit Commission (1993) in their report of communication in NHS hospitals concluded that: *'there is increasing evidence of a positive relationship between communication and clinical outcomes across a range of clinical conditions and types of treatment'*.

Against such a background, this chapter will examine the role of communication in pharmacy practice. It will highlight the need for, and benefits of, effective communication, and the negative consequences of poor or inappropriate communication. The key interpersonal skills required by pharmacists will be elaborated upon. Further, the problems posed by patients with special communication needs will be examined, together with ways in which these needs can best be met.

THE NEED FOR GOOD COMMUNICATION

Interpersonal communication is a two-way, transactional, process. As we send messages to others, at the same time we receive verbal and nonverbal signals from them. Our interactive style is to a large extent shaped, and even determined, by the other person. For instance, a pharmacist who is dealing with a happy, young mother showing off her newborn infant will behave very differently compared to when dealing with a recently bereaved 80 year old widow. Pharmacists must be cognisant of the goals, nature and expectations of each individual patient.

In relation to communication with patients, a distinction has been made between *'blunters'* who deliberately avoid information about their condition, particularly if it may have negative implications, and *'monitors'* who actively search for, and request such detail (Miller *et al.* 1988). In their study of information-giving in community pharmacies, Blenkinsopp *et al.* (1994) described patients as *'active'* or *'passive'* depending upon the extent to which they introduced new topics into the consultation. Active patients received almost twice as much information as passive ones, although in a follow-up one day after their visit, it was found that both groups had forgotten two-thirds of the information they had been given. Interestingly, those patients who complain most about the amount of information or explanation they have been given may paradoxically be better informed than those who do not complain (Armstrong 1991).

The need for good communication is demonstrated by research evidence, which indicates a range of problems with both the content of the communication and the process by which information is conveyed.

Dickson *et al.* (1997) summarised the results of this research at the practitioner-patient interface under the headings shown in Box 14.2 and discussed below.

Box 14.2 Key issues of practitioner–patient interaction (Dickson *et al.* 1997)

- Patients often do not understand, or forget, information they are given
- Patients are often dissatisfied with the advice and information they are given
- Lack of patient-practitioner concordance
- Patient satisfaction and concordance are related
- Inattentiveness to the patient's psychosocial needs

Patients often do not understand, or forget, information they are given

The main findings here are:

- The more information given the more is forgotten. In general patients forget approximately half the information they are given by practitioners
- Patients remember best what they hear first, as well as what they consider to be most important
- Patients often have minimal biological knowledge, such as the location of vital organs
- Patients with a higher level of medical knowledge recall more of what they are told
- A patient's age is not necessarily an indicator of retentive ability
- Patients who are highly anxious at one extreme, or not at all anxious at the other, remember less than those with a moderate level of anxiety
- Many patients, even if they do not understand, do not like to ask questions
- Complicated oral or written instructions compromise understanding

Patients are often dissatisfied with the advice and information they are given

Dissatisfaction with advice is usually linked to the following factors:

- Poor practitioner rapport-building skills, e.g. poor level of eye contact, little empathy, and lack of encouragement
- Patients not receiving the amount of information they require
- Limited time available for the consultation
- Lack of specificity and precision in the information given
- The way in which information is provided
- Being unable to access the right person to deal with their problem

Lack of patient-practitioner concordance

In all practitioner-patient exchanges there is an imbalance, or asymmetry in the perspectives and roles of the individuals concerned (Pilnick 1998). For example, the practitioner has the knowledge base and the status that the patient does not usually have, while the latter has the condition that the former does not have. This can lead to discordance in the relationship. The concept of concordance has been advocated to empower patients to meet their specific needs. Concordance is based on the notion that the consultation is a negotiation between practitioner and patient acting as equals, with the aim of achieving a therapeutic alliance (see also Chapter 11). The importance of achieving this alliance is underscored by the research literature, which abounds with evidence of therapeutic failure. For example, the Royal Pharmaceutical Society of Great Britain (1997) report indicated that approximately 50 per cent of patients who suffer from chronic conditions are not fully compliant with their medication regime and consequently do not derive optimal therapeutic benefit.

Patient satisfaction and concordance are related

Lack of adherence with clinical advice has been shown to be directly related to the following factors:

- Level of satisfaction with the consultation
- The persuasiveness and credibility of the practitioner, and of the information provided
- Patients' perceptions of the severity of their condition and their vulnerability to it
- The duration and complexity of the treatment regime
- Treatment effectiveness
- Patients' expectations, outlook and attitude
- Influence of family and friends
- The level of supervision provided

Inattentiveness to patients' psychosocial needs

Research demonstrates a reluctance by practitioners to discuss the psychosocial dimensions of a patient's wellbeing. Patients react negatively to this, particularly as they deem their emotional needs to be as important, if not more important, than their physical needs. Dissatisfaction is, therefore, often attributed to:

- Overly directive practitioners
- Practitioner insensitivity to the patient's feelings, concerns and opinions

- A concentration purely on the patient's medical condition to the exclusion of accompanying worries – listening only to facts and ignoring feelings
- Failure to tune in to the patient's nonverbal cues which signal other needs
- Lack of support to manage a condition where coping rather than a cure is the only realistic option

Given all of the above issues, the necessity for the pharmacist to become a skilled communicator is apparent. The key benefits which will ensue are shown in Box 14.3.

Box 14.3 Consequences of the pharmacist as a skilled communicator

- Improved patient outcomes
- Improved patient satisfaction with services
- More patient-friendly pharmacy practice
- Reduction in patient anxiety
- Increased pharmacist status
- Enhanced pharmacist satisfaction and self-esteem
- Increased patronage of pharmacy and subsequent business advantage
- Decrease in complaints and litigation

By contrast when pharmacists' communication is ineffective the consequences are equal and opposite to the above. The likely outcomes are shown in Box 14.4.

Box 14.4 Consequences of the pharmacist as an unskilled communicator

- Reduced adherence to therapeutic regimes
- Decreased satisfaction with the content and process of the communication
- Insensitivity to the needs of customers
- Increased worry and concern amongst patients
- Decreased pharmacist status
- Job dissatisfaction
- Loss of business and reduced client base
- Increases in formal complaints and legal action

KEY COMMUNICATION SKILLS

A study of communication among pharmacists identified eleven key skill areas, together with relevant sub-skills, through analysis of video recordings of actual practice (Hargie *et al.* 2000). These are presented in Table 14.1 in rank order of perceived importance. Knowledge and application of these skills are fundamental to effective practice and they are summarised below.

1. **Building rapport**
   i   Preserving confidentiality
   ii   Being helpful
   iii Being available/accessible
   iv   Showing genuine concern
   v   Offering reassurance
   vi   Politeness in manner
   vii Showing interest in the patient
   viii Showing warmth
   ix   Engaging
   x   Showing pleasure
   xi   Accommodating patient's needs
   xii Use of humour
   xiii Greeting by name

2. **Explaining**
   i   Reasoned instructions
   ii   Explaining for reassurance
   iii Informing
   iv   Repetition
   v   Reinforcing/emphasising
   vi   Directing

3. **Questioning**
   i   Other medication taken
   ii   Symptoms-related
   iii Exploring situation
   iv   Patient details
   v   Showing interest

4. **Listening**
   i   Showing sympathy/empathy
   ii   Encouraging patient to provide information
   iii Showing interest (beyond the problem)

5. **Nonverbal communication**
   i   Eye contact
   ii   Tone of voice
   iii Examining patient
   iv   Proximity
   v   Positioning
   vi   Using hand gestures
   vii Smiling and nodding
   viii Standing still
   ix   Touch
   x   Illustration/demonstration

6. **Suggesting/Advising**

7. **Opening**
   i   Identifying patient by name (prescription check)
   ii   Greeting, general
   iii Greeting by name

8. **Closing**
   i   Polite closing
   ii   Thanking patient
   iii Initiating ending of interaction

Table 14.1 Rank-order of effective communication skills and sub-skills

	9.	**Assertiveness**
		i Pharmacist politely standing ground
		ii Enhancing credibility by referring to view of other health professionals
Table 14.1 *(Continued)*	10.	**Disclosing personal information**
	11.	**Persuading**

Building rapport

There are two motivations for pharmacists to maintain rapport with patients. First, presentation of themselves as health care practitioners and second, the development and preservation of patient loyalty necessary to sustain business success.

Building rapport was the skill most frequently employed by community pharmacists, indicating that the relationship element of practice was particularly important. In addition, patients were more influenced by, and followed the advice of, practitioners with whom they formed a good relationship. Indeed, there is clear evidence that we require fewer reasons for accepting recommendations from friends than from strangers. The existence of a good relationship also allows for the expression of negative emotions by the practitioner (e.g. anger, anxiety, frustration), and this is related to greater patient adherence to the advice and direction offered. Genuine concern communicated by the pharmacist is reciprocated by a desire in the patient to please the practitioner by following treatment directives.

Many strategies contribute to the initiation, maintenance and enhancement of relationships. Among the most important are demonstrating friendliness and warmth, using the patient's name, expressing genuine interest and concern for patients and their needs, discussing shared interests, demonstrating appropriate sympathy and empathy, referring to previous encounters, being readily available, employing appropriate humour, and preserving confidentiality. Another crucial dimension of rapport building is that of offering reassurance. Negative media publicity about medicines has increased patients' need for reassurance concerning their therapy. In anticipation of questions such as *'is it safe to continue taking this?'*, pharmacists need firstly to deal with the factual aspect of the fear. Box 14.5 represents a four-step model of reassurance.

In parallel, pharmacists should use a range of reassurance strategies in order to address related emotional concerns (Box 14.6).

Box 14.5 A four step model of reassurance	1. Provision of general background information
	2. Review of scientific/clinical evidence
	3. A summary of the balance of risk:benefits
	4. Recommended action

Box 14.6 Reassurance strategies

Explaining

Client satisfaction occurs across three domains:

- *Affective satisfaction* is a product of factors such as empathy, friendliness and trust
- *Behavioural satisfaction* is determined by factors such as how the client's needs/problems are ascertained, length of waiting time and the pace of the interaction. The establishment of good rapport contributes to both of these dimensions
- *Cognitive satisfaction* relates to the explanations given by the pharmacist to the patient. Here the emphasis is on providing advice, information and instruction in sufficient detail and using language which can be readily understood (Hargie *et al.* 1994). The understanding, retention and utilisation of advice and information can be effected by pharmacists using the techniques shown in Box 14.7.

- Place the most important points at the beginning and at the end of any interaction
- Emphasise key points
- Give specific instructions
- Provide only essential information in order to prevent overload
- Simplify complicated messages
- Use examples and analogies relevant to the patient's experience
- Have a logical structure that patients can follow
- Present the oral message fluently
- Converse at the patient's pace
- Repeat instructions
- Accompany the oral message with a written or visual aid
- Address the needs of special patient groups (e.g. braille labels for the visually impaired; instruction leaflets in ethnic minority languages)
- Provide a demonstration
- Encourage the patient to repeat the demonstration
- Monitor feedback to check the extent of patient understanding
- End the consultation with a summary of key points

Box 14.7 Strategies used by pharmacists to ensure patients understand, retain and use advice and information

Questioning

The traditional medical model of health care has been that while patients might know what they *want*, health professionals, through their superior knowledge, believe they know what patients actually *need*. More recently, this imbalance between patient and practitioner goals has been strongly questioned. The predominant view now is that patients should be empowered, insofar as possible, to negotiate their own needs and be involved in the decisions involving all aspects of their care. This means that pharmacists in partnership with patients must agree the needs to be met. The acronym *FUN* (First Uncover Needs) is useful, in that it is only when the needs of patients have been fully established that the interaction can progress satisfactorily and messages be specifically tailored to address them. While there are recurring patient questions (see Box 14.8), it is important to respect the individuality of each patient and find out exactly what their specific needs and circumstances are. This means that pharmacists must pay careful attention to their questioning style.

- 'Why me?'
- 'Why now?'
- 'Why this particular illness?'
- 'What is this medicine for?'
- 'How do I take it?'
- 'Are there any side-effects?'
- 'How long do I need to take it for?'
- 'What will happen if I don't take it?'
- 'What is going to happen to me?'

Box 14.8 Questions commonly asked by patients

The research evidence consistently points to a predominantly closed style of questioning by pharmacists and an interviewing style in which the pharmacist controls and directs the consultation (Morrow *et al.* 1993; Tully *et al.* 1997). Closed and leading questions restrict the scope of responses, often requiring only a '*Yes*' or '*No*' answer, and assume prior knowledge on the part of the questioner, such that the information gathered maybe incomplete or inaccurate potentially resulting in compromised action. For this reason pharmacists need to develop effective interviewing techniques which will be objective in the collection of data and open to the needs of patients.

A distinction can be made between facilitative and restrictive questioning styles (Morrow and Hargie 1988). As shown in Table 14.2,

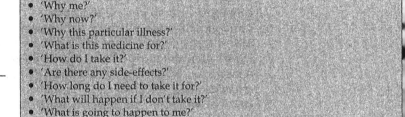

Facilitative style		Restrictive style
Open ←	Question Scope →	Closed
Psychosocial ←	Question Content →	Factual
Low ←	Question Bias →	High
Slow ←	Questioning Pace →	Fast
Indirect ←	Question Method →	Direct
Deep ←	Question Level →	Shallow
Patient ←	Main Questioner →	Pharmacist
Accepting ←	Receptivity to Patient Answers →	Ignoring

Table 14.2 Facilitative and restrictive questioning continua

the facilitative style allows patients to be centrally involved in the consultation, whereas the restrictive style largely ignores the needs of the patient. In the former, the style of the questions tends to be open, their content includes psychosocial dimensions, there is a low level of bias in terms of fewer leading questions, the pace is appropriate to the patient, and the health professional encourages patient questions and is accepting of responses.

In order to use questions effectively pharmacists should employ the strategies outlined in Box 14.9.

Box 14.9 Effective questioning

- Reduce the number of closed questions and use more open questions
- Ask only one question at a time
- Structure the sequence of questions to follow a logical pattern
- Use probing questions to follow up on patients' responses
- Increase participation by pausing both after asking a question and after the patient's initial response
- Encourage patients to ask questions
- Avoid questions that will bias responses
- Show concerted attention in delivering the question

Listening

As well as asking appropriate questions, pharmacists should listen carefully to what the patient has to say. Evidence from public surveys consistently demonstrates a very strong desire for community pharmacists to spend more time listening fully to patient concerns. Good listening behaviour demands concentrated effort and is indicated both verbally and nonverbally. As Davis and Fallowfield (1991) pointed out: *'Active listening is very hard work initially and demands considerable attention and practise but the advantages in terms of eliciting information and developing a good therapeutic relationship with a patient are worth the investment of time'*.

To optimise effective listening the points in Box 14.10 should be borne in mind:

Box 14.10 Optimising effective listening

- Do not stereotype the patient
- Be objective
- Show nonverbal indicators of interest and attention (eye contact, head nods, etc.)
- Arrange a conducive environment, avoiding distractions
- Be prepared to listen
- Keep an open, analytical mind, searching for the central thrust of the message
- Identify supporting arguments and facts
- Do not dwell on one or two aspects at the expense of others
- Delay judgement, or refutation, until you have heard the entire message
- Verbally follow up on what the patient has said (questions, reference to previous statements, summaries, etc.)

Nonverbal communication

There are two core purposes of nonverbal behaviour. First, *messag* *comprehension and recall* is facilitated by the use of nonverbal behaviours, such as communicative gestures (e.g. raising three fingers to signal 'three' of something). Second, *relational communication*, such as the expression of liking and friendship, is conveyed by a range of behaviours including: direct body and facial orientation, a close conversational distance, consistent eye contact, head nods, a forward leaning and open posture, smiles and pleasant facial expressions, frequent gestures, and appropriate touch.

Nonverbal communication is especially important in pharmacy for the four main reasons shown in Box 14.11.

Box 14.11 Four reasons for the particular importance of nonverbal communication in pharmacy

1. The role of patients as consumers of health care gives them the time and opportunity to monitor closely the nonverbal behaviour of the pharmacist
2. Fear and uncertainty about their illness increases the attention they pay to the pharmacist's often subtle nonverbal cues that indicate how and what they should be feeling
3. Patients often do not fully understand the verbal message, or believe it not to be wholly truthful, and so they analyse nonverbal cues for information on which to base their judgements about their condition
4. The patient's treatment or condition may interfere with their ability to communicate verbally. Nonverbal signals then become the prime channel for communication

While the pharmacist must be skilled in the use of nonverbal behaviour, the interpretation and assessment of the patient's nonverbal messages is also very important. For example, a patient showing nonverbal signs of embarrassment should be taken to a more private area of the pharmacy for the consultation. In addition, pharmacists also need to make important decisions about the truthfulness of what the patient is saying, especially if drug abuse or misuse is suspected. A range of research studies on deception indicators (e.g. Buller and Burgoon 1996; Vrij 1999) has revealed commonly recurring verbal and nonverbal behaviours (see Box 14.12).

Suggesting and advising

A comparison of consultations in the study by Hargie *et al.* (2000) revealed one skill that was commonly employed when dealing with over the counter (OTC) items but not used by pharmacists when handling prescription-related encounters. This skill, termed suggesting/advising, was defined as the offer of a personal/professional opinion about a particular course of action, while simultaneously allowing the final decision to lie with the patient. Examples of this skill included *'Have you tried an inhalation at all? Sometimes it can help ...'. 'I think you'd be better taking the adult cough mixture because it just thins the phlegm and*

Box 14.12 Indicators of deception

then you cough it up yourself ...' It may be that in the OTC context, patients have to fully negotiate their own needs (and pay directly for the service), and this in turn demands a more comprehensive response from the pharmacist. This is in contrast to the situation where the '*written order*' from the doctor (the prescription) following a medical consultation may already have dealt with many of the patient's needs, and the pharmacist does not wish to appear to '*intervene*'. At the same time, there are degrees of suggestion by the pharmacist, with some more forcefully expressed than others, to emphasise their importance. These were prefaced by expressions such as: '*I would strongly recommend you ...*'. '*You would be well advised to ...*'.

Opening

As the saying goes, '*You don't get a second chance to make a first impression*', and indeed the manner in which the pharmacist meets and greets the patient will influence how the former is perceived. The main steps involved in effective openings are shown in Box 14.13.

- Greet the patient using their name if possible ('*Good morning, Mrs Iverson. How are you today?*')
- Use appropriate nonverbals (move towards the patient, smile, engage in eye contact, etc.)
- Carefully observe the patient's nonverbal communication to determine the degree of privacy required
- Take up a suitable location for the consultation and give the patient undivided attention
- Use an approach which underlines to the patient that their involvement is both expected and desired
- Establish fully what the patient's needs and concerns are and convey to the patient your acceptance of these
- Check out '*what has gone before*', as appropriate
- Reward the patient for seeking advice ('*It's wise to ask about this*')

Box 14.13 Main steps in effective openings

Closing

It is important to terminate the consultation smoothly and satisfactorily, so that it comes to a natural end with both parties having achieved their goals. To achieve an effective closure, the checklist in Box 14.14 should be borne in mind.

Box 14.14 Achieving effective closure of communication

Assertiveness

The ability to assert oneself confidently is essential for effective social functioning. This involves standing up for personal rights and expressing personal thoughts and feelings openly, while at the same time respecting the rights of others. An assertive approach is particularly important when:

- Making reasonable requests of others
- Refusing to comply with unreasonable requests
- Handling unreasonable refusals

However, within the health setting it would seem that certain groups, including pharmacists, find this skill quite difficult to implement, especially when dealing with other professionals and with ancillary health care workers (Dickson *et al.* 1997). At the same time, it is now well established that *'assertion is a learned skill, not a "trait" that a person "has" or "lacks"'* (Rakos 1997). This means that pharmacists who have difficulty in being assertive can learn to overcome such inhibition. In fact there are three main behavioural styles of relevance here:

1. *Nonassertive style.* This style involves being subservient, self-effacing and apologetic, using hesitant speech with low voice

volume, avoiding eye contact, fidgeting frequently, not expressing opinions, and forgoing personal rights rather than becoming involved in any possibility of *'unpleasantness'*.

2. *Assertive style*. This involves the person seeking equality with others, readily expressing opinions and feelings, addressing contentious issues, speaking in a firm yet conversational tone, engaging in eye contact, and protecting the rights of themselves and others.

3. *Aggressive style*. This style involves vehemently expressing opinions, being self-opinionated and overbearing, revelling in contentious issues, speaking loudly and abusively, interrupting others and glaring at them, and taking no cognisance of their rights.

Of these styles, assertiveness has been clearly shown to be the most effective. Submissive people are not well respected, while aggressive individuals are actively disliked. When assertion is used skilfully, with due recognition given to the rights of others, then the most positive outcomes are obtained. The use of assertiveness often involves three elements, which may be illustrated in a situation where the pharmacist is confronted with a dubious prescription (Hargie and Morrow 1988):

- Description of the situation – *'This prescription has been altered'*
- Description, plus indication of noncompliance – *'This prescription has been altered and therefore I can't dispense it'*
- Description, noncompliance, plus request for the situation to be changed – *'This prescription has been altered and therefore I can't dispense it. Can you get your doctor to confirm this alteration?'*

Disclosing personal information

Self-disclosure is the act of verbally and/or nonverbally com-municating to others personal information (Tardy and Dindia 1997). It can be nonverbal, in that we can either hide feelings such as worry, happiness etc., or openly express them in our facial expressions, posture, and so on. However, most research on self-disclosure focuses upon the verbal component, and here the key defining feature is the use of a personal self-reference pronoun such as *'I'*, *'me'*, *'mine'* etc. (Hargie *et al.* 1994). Thus, the difference between the statements *'diabetes is very worrying'* and *'I am very worried about diabetes'* is that the former may or may not be a self-disclosure, whereas the latter definitely is.

A knowledge and skilled use of self-disclosure is important in pharmacy for two main reasons (Hargie and Morrow 1991). First, to effect an accurate diagnosis, patients must openly and honestly disclose personal details about their condition. Pharmacists therefore must use tactics that encourage patients to fully explain their situation. They can increase the level of self-disclosure from patients by:

- Establishing a relationship of trust, confidence, acceptance and empathy
- Having a professional personal appearance
- Providing a private environment in which personal matters can be discussed freely
- Dealing with patients in a receptive, caring, and unhurried style

Second, pharmacists have to decide what, and when, it is appropriate to self-disclose to patients. Here, self-disclosure can be divided into two main types – the pharmacist's own personal experiences, and the pharmacist's personal reactions to the patient's disclosures. Both are appropriate, but must be used judiciously. The first type can help to reassure patients that what they are experiencing is not unusual (a technique known as *'normalising'*), and also help to develop rapport by demonstrating shared experiences (e.g. *'I know what you're going through. When we had our first child, she kept us awake …'*). However patients do not expect a great deal of disclosure from pharmacists and so the second type is more common. Here, the focus of attention stays firmly upon the patient, and the pharmacist shows a willingness to become involved in their *'world'* (*'I really am determined to help you stop smoking …'*).

Persuading

Given the wealth of evidence indicating that patients often fail to follow advice about treatment regimes, a knowledge of the influencing tactics that can serve to increase patient compliance is important. A range of effective persuading strategies has been identified (Allen and Preiss 1998). To influence patients the pharmacist should:

Capitalise on their professional relationship with patients: we are more likely to be influenced by people we like, and for whom we have high regard. A positive pharmacist-patient relationship is the key to successful persuasion. In fact, the forceful delivery of negative messages within a positive relationship often leads to increased acceptance by a patient of the health threatening nature of their condition.

Engage feelings of threat and fear: this is an important influencing tactic in encouraging people to change their behaviour. In the health context the success of this approach depends upon four factors:

1. The magnitude and severity of the negative outcome
2. Its probability of occurring if nothing is done to avoid it
3. The effectiveness of the recommended response to remove the threat
4. The patient's belief in being able to adhere to the recommended treatment

Invoke moral appeals to promote positive health behaviour: this is an effective tactic since breaches of the moral code usually produce feelings of guilt. For example, a pregnant woman could be encouraged to give up smoking by telling her: '*You have a duty to your unborn child to give it the healthiest possible start in life, so you really must stop smoking*'.

Include logical arguments delivered with few hesitations or expressed doubts: a 'powerful' authoritative speech style (few hesitations or expressed doubts, coupled with the use of intensifiers such as '*definitely*', '*absolutely*' etc.) increase the influencing power of an argument.

Underline the power of the message: This is enhanced when the pharmacist projects a professional image in terms of personal appearance and bearing, and when the pharmacy, in its design, layout, product range and display, portrays a professional image.

These, then are the key communication skills central to effective pharmacy practice. There are no hard and fast rules about when, with which patients, or under what conditions, they should be used. Rather, the pharmacist must decide which combination of skills best meets the needs and requirements of each individual patient. However, for some patients, special communication efforts need to be made, owing to the nature of their conditions.

COMMUNICATION AND DISABILITY

Overcoming patients' communication difficulties is a major hurdle to effective patient counselling. This is especially the case when counselling patients who:

- Are confused about their medication
- Have age-related medication problems
- Are anxious about treatment

The groups of patients who may have particular communication difficulties are shown in Box 14.15.

The area of learning disabilities was explored in the Report on Mental Health Foundation Committee of Inquiry (1996) which pro-

Box 14.15 Patients who may have communication difficulties

- Disabled patients using wheelchairs
- The visually impaired
- The deaf or hard of hearing
- Those who do not speak English
- The elderly who are mentally ill
- Those with learning disabilities

vided a salutary insight into the range of communication problems faced by this group of people. The following quotation is indicative of the type of problem such individuals experience:

'The doctor gave me some tablets, but I had no idea what they were. He explained to me, but I didn't understand. It was Latin. People with learning disabilities find it hard to take tablets. They don't know what they are. They're afraid they will take the wrong kind of tablets and die.'

More recently, in an evaluation of 611 patients admitted to a University Hospital general medical service, 15.9% were found to have one or more disabilities affecting communication (Ebert 1998). Nine percent had altered mental states, 4.7% vision impairments, 2.8% speech impairments and 0.5% hearing impairments. Disability was more apparent in older age groups.

Clearly where communication difficulties exist and where they are not effectively managed, patient care is compromised and levels of patient dissatisfaction rise. There is, therefore, a crucial need for practitioners to be sensitive to the communication needs of such patients and to have developed strategies to facilitate effective dialogue between both parties.

The approach must operate at two levels: at the strategic or institutional level and at the personal level. At the strategic level clients' needs should be identified and defined, services should then be planned on the basis of need, implemented on a managed basis and monitored for effectiveness and quality. At the personal level, it will be concerned with the particular *'accommodations'* that need to be in place to facilitate communication. Some examples are given in Table 14.3.

A particular case in point is the inability of some patients to speak the language of the country in which they are resident. This is especially the case among ethnic minorities. Much has been done in respect of information produced in the ethnic minority languages and the importance of producing medicines-related information in such formats cannot be overemphasised (see also Chapter 16).

Disability	Accommodation
Visually impaired	Large print
	Braille
	Audiotape materials
Hearing impaired	Assistive listening devices
	Sign language and interpretation
Speech impairment	Tracheotomy speech adapters
	Communication boards
Impaired mental states	Compliance aids
	Surrogate sources of information e.g. carers

Table 14.3 Facilitating effective communication in disability

CONCLUSION

It is clear that communication plays a crucial role in the day-to-day working life of the pharmacist. As members of the public are being encouraged to have ever higher expectations of the care and treatment to which they are entitled, the communicative ability of the pharmacist will become crucial. While the pharmacist's technical expertise will continue to require updating and expansion, this needs to be matched by the development of the communicative aspects of practice. The old days when the '*hidden*' pharmacist could spend most of his/her time in the dispensary and use assistants as a shield to fend off patients are long gone. The Patient's Charter, changes such as POM to P Medicines and campaigns like '*Ask Your Pharmacist You'll Be Taking Good Advice*', have all contributed to a change in pharmacists' work patterns and led to an increase in the time they spend with patients. This increased contact, coupled with growing expectations of services by patients, means that high levels of communication skills will have to be the norm for members of the pharmacy profession.

Communication skills are particularly important in developing and maintaining good rapport with patients, uncovering their needs, providing clear advice and direction, and influencing them towards more healthy lifestyles. Given the incontrovertible evidence regarding the importance of communication to effective health care, it is clear that pharmacists will need to possess knowledge and ability in key skill areas. In this chapter we have highlighted the most important of these as being: rapport-building, explaining, questioning, listening, nonverbal behaviour, suggesting/advising, opening, closing, assertiveness, self-disclosure, and persuading.

FURTHER READING

Dickson, D., Hargie, O. and Morrow, N. (1997) *Communication Skills Training for Health Professionals* (2nd Edn.) Chapman and Hall, London.

REFERENCES

Allen, M. and Preiss, R. (Eds.) (1998) *Persuasion: Advances Through Meta-Analyses*, Hampton Press, New Jersey.

Armstrong, D. (1991) What do patients want? Someone who will answer their questions. *British Medical Journal*, **303**, 261–262.

Audit Commission (1993) *What Seems to be the Matter: Communication Between Hospitals and Patients*, HMSO, London.

Blenkinsopp, A., Robinson, E. and Panton, R. (1994) Do pharmacy customers remember the information given to them by the community pharmacist? In: G. Harding, S. Nettleton and K. Taylor (Eds.), *Social Pharmacy: Innovation and Change*, Pharmaceutical Press, London, pp. 84–94.

Buller, D. and Burgoon, J. (1996) Interpersonal deception theory. *Communication Theory*, **6**, 203–242.

Cipolle R.J., Strand L.M. and Morley P.C. (1998) *Pharmaceutical Care Practice*, McGraw-Hill, New York.

Davis, H. and Fallowfield, L. (1991) *Counselling and Communication in Health Care*, John Wiley, Chichester.

Department of Health (1992) *The Patient's Charter*, HMSO London.

Dickson, D., Hargie, O. and Morrow, N. (1997) *Communication Skills Training for Health Professionals* (2nd Edn.) Chapman and Hall, London.

Ebert, D.A. (1998) Communication disabilities among medical inpatients. *New England Journal of Medicine*, **339**, 272–273.

Ewles, L. and Simnett, I. (1992) *Promoting Health: A Practical Guide* (2nd Edn.) Scutari Press, London.

Hargie, O. and Morrow, N. (1988) Interpersonal communication 3 Assertiveness skills. *Pharmacy Update*, **4**, 243–247.

Hargie, O. and Morrow, N. (1991) The skill of self disclosure, parts 1 and 2. *Chemist and Druggist*, **235**, 343–344 and 769–770.

Hargie, O., Morrow, N. and Woodman, C. (2000) Pharmacists' evaluation of key communication skills in practice. *Patient Education and Counselling*, **39**, 61–70.

Hargie, O., Saunders, C. and Dickson, D. (1994) *Social Skills in Interpersonal Communication*. Routledge, London.

Miller, S.M., Brody, D.S. and Summerton, J. (1988) Styles of coping with threat: implications for health. *Journal of Personality and Social Psychology*, **54**, 142–148.

Morrow, N. and Hargie, O. (1988) Effective questioning skills in pharmacy practice. In: A. Balon (Ed.) *The Proprietary Articles Trade Association Official Reference Book*, Sterling Publications, London, pp. 37–40.

Morrow, N., Hargie, O., Donnelly, H. and Woodman, C. (1993) 'Why do you ask?' A study of questioning behaviour in community pharmacy-client consultations. *International Journal of Pharmacy Practice*, **2**, 90–94.

Pilnick, A. (1998) 'Why didn't you say just that?' Dealing with issues of asymmetry, knowledge and competence in the pharmacist/client encounter. *Sociology of Health and Illness*, **20**, 29–51.

Rakos, R. (1997) Asserting and confronting. In: O. Hargie (Ed.) *The Handbook of Communication Skills*, Routledge, London, pp. 289–319.

Report of Mental Health Foundation Committee of Inquiry (1996) *Building Expectations: Opportunities and Services for People with a Learning Disability*, The Mental Health Foundation, London.

Ross, F.M., Bower, P.J. and Sibbald, B.S. (1994) Practice nurses: characteristics, workload and training needs. *British Journal of General Practice*, **44**, 15–18.

Royal Pharmaceutical Society of Great Britain (1997) *From Compliance to Concordance. Achieving Shared Goals in Medicine Taking*. Royal Pharmaceutical Society of Great Britain and Merck Sharp & Dohme, London.

Tardy, C. and Dindia, K. (1997) Self-disclosure. In: O. Hargie (Ed.), *The Handbook of Communication Skills*, Routledge, London, pp. 213–235.

Tully, M.P., Hassell, K. and Noyce, P.R. (1997) Advice-giving in community pharmacies in the UK. *Journal of Health Service Research and Policy*, **2**, 38–50.

Vrij, A. (1999) Interviewing to detect deception. In: A. Memon and R. Bull (Eds.) *Handbook of the Psychology of Interviewing*, Wiley, Chichester, pp. 317–326.

SELF-ASSESSMENT QUESTIONS

Question 1: Why should pharmacists employ a facilitative questioning style when interviewing patients, rather than a restrictive style employing closed or leading questions?

Question 2: What are the two core purposes of nonverbal communication?

Question 3: How can pharmacists encourage patients to communicate personal information about themselves (self-disclosure)?

Question 4: What strategies might be employed by pharmacists in order to persuade patients to follow their advice?

KEY POINTS FOR ANSWERS

Question 1: A facilitative style, using open and non-leading questions, ensures that the patient remains central to the consultation. A restrictive style is not sensitive to the needs of the patient and by employing closed or leading questions limits the information that may be obtained.

Question 2:

- Communicative nonverbal gestures can enhance verbal messages
- Relational nonverbal communication, such as facial expressions, expresses how individuals feel about each other

Question 3:

- Establish an appropriate relationship with the patient
- Have a professional appearance
- Provide a private environment for the consultation
- Adopt an appropriate, unhurried, caring approach

Question 4:

- Capitalise on their professional status and relationship with the patient
- Encourage the patient to feel threatened by or to fear an event
- Use moral appeals
- Employ logical, authoritative arguments

Pharmacists and the Multidisciplinary Health Care Team

Christine Bond

INTRODUCTION	250
PHARMACISTS' CURRENT AND FUTURE ROLE	250
POWER AND STATUS IN INTER-PROFESSIONAL RELATIONSHIPS	251
Medicine, pharmacy and other health care professions	251
Separation of hospital and community pharmacy	254
The primary health care team and pharmacy	254
CHANNELS AND BARRIERS TO EFFECTIVE COMMUNICATION	254
Principles of team working	254
Inter-professional communication	255
The current position	255
Examples of good practice	256
PRESCRIBING AND MEDICINES MANAGEMENT	257
Pharmacists' influence on general practitioners' prescribing	257
Primary care pharmacists	260
Influences on changes in OTC prescribing	260
Information technology	263
CONCLUSION	263
FURTHER READING	264
REFERENCES	266
SELF-ASSESSMENT QUESTIONS	268
KEY POINTS FOR ANSWERS	268

INTRODUCTION

This chapter will consider the common background of pharmacy and medicine, and its impact on the development of pharmacy as it is practised today. Links with other professions in the health care team will also be discussed.

In the UK, general medical practitioners and pharmacists have a common ancestor in the mediaeval spicers who formed themselves into the Society of Apothecaries in 1617. They competed with the physicians, who by royal decree were the only group licensed to give and charge for, medical advice. The apothecaries dispensed medicines for physicians and recommended medicines for those members of the public unable to afford physicians' fees. However, they were not themselves permitted to charge for this advice.

In 1815 the Apothecaries Act allowed a charge to be made specifically for the provision of advice, as well as for the medicine which was dispensed. As a result of this legislation, the two distinct professions of general practice medicine and pharmacy emerged. A further bill before parliament, which sought to reform the law and prevent the Chemists and Druggists giving advice and recommending treatments for purchase, posed a threat to the future pharmacy profession. A leading group of Chemists and Druggists came together and argued that this would not be in the public's best interest. Parliament was convinced and the bill was defeated.

In 1840 the Society of Apothecaries and College of Surgeons agreed on a joint curriculum of study for general practitioners, and proposed that likewise the Chemists and Druggists should be compelled to undergo an examination in order to receive a licence to carry out their business. In 1841 Jacob Bell, son of a leading Chemist, formed the Pharmaceutical Society of Great Britain. The medical profession itself became united slightly later when the Medical Act of 1858 established the Medical Register which included the names of surgeons and apothecaries alongside those of physicians. A fuller exposition of the historical development of pharmacy is given in Chapter 1.

PHARMACISTS' CURRENT AND FUTURE ROLE

Recognition that the profession of pharmacy, within the UK, was not realising its full potential, was first officially identified in 1979 (Merrison 1979) and described in official reports, such as the Nuffield Report (1986) and subsequent Government White Papers. Extensive consultation both within and outwith the profession resulted in a definitive description of the future role of community pharmacy *Pharmaceutical Care: the Future for Community Pharmacy*, produced jointly by the Department of Health and the Royal Pharmaceutical Society of Great Britain (1992). This document considered various aspects of the community pharmacist's working practice under nine broad headings including services to general practitioners, the over the counter (OTC) advisory role, health promotion, and services to special needs groups such as the housebound. Thirty specific tasks were recommended to be either introduced nationally or on a pilot basis. Whilst some of these tasks merely formalised ongoing practice and were generally welcomed, others were innovative, covering areas as diverse as simple health care advice, therapeutic drug monitoring, and prescribing following agreed protocols. The report was received with some reservations by medical bodies and welcomed as *'pragmatic, prosaic, and progressive'* by the pharmaceutical profession.

The reality of the pharmacist's *'extended role'*, i.e. those activities additional to traditional dispensing activities, has been aided by an overall review of health care by central Government, culminating in a reconfigured service in Great Britain from April 1st 1999. This has provided a new opportunity for the professional base of pharmacy to expand, and for pharmacists to take their place in the multidisciplinary health care team.

Most new roles are concerned directly or indirectly with medicines management, and the optimisation of prescribed and non-prescribed medication. Thus, there are interfaces with general medical practitioners, and other health care professionals, and with the public. The needs of the patient will be central to all such interactions, which may cause problems when the patient's needs appear to conflict with the general medical practitioner's instructions. This two faceted role for the pharmacist has been contrasted with that of other health care professionals. Many of the new roles may not be new, but merely new to pharmacy, with resultant perceptions of boundary encroachment by the existing suppliers of the service. For example a wider role in the treatment of symptoms of minor ailments will inevitably result in an element of diagnosis. Diagnosis is often considered to be an activity solely for the medical profession, and any attempt by community pharmacists to participate in this is regarded as encroaching on medical territory. Thus, objective evaluation of pharmacists' new roles is very important and the relatively new academic discipline of *Pharmacy Practice Research*, a branch of *Health Services Research*, has a central part to play in the development of the profession (see also the chapters in Part 7 of this book).

This chapter will look at the effects of three key issues in influencing the above developments, namely, the influence of power and status in inter-professional relationships, channels and barriers to effective communication, and pharmacists' input into prescribing.

POWER AND STATUS IN INTER-PROFESSIONAL RELATIONSHIPS

Medicine, pharmacy and other health care professions

The main argument for maintaining the two professions of medicine and pharmacy, and thereby separating the prescribing and dispensing functions has been the acknowledged conflict which would otherwise exist when income is related to the quantity and cost of a medicine prescribed. For example, in Japan, where doctors are commonly responsible for both prescribing and dispensing, drug costs are higher than anywhere else in the world. Published figures for England and Wales indicate that the costs of drugs dispensed by dispensing doctors is higher than for doctors who only prescribe.

However, unlike the rest of Europe, pharmacists in the UK never quite achieved a monopoly over dispensing. There is a historical precedent allowing general medical practitioners to dispense, a right to which they still cling, which has resulted in repeated bitter controversy between the two professions. This reality is expressed graphically by Kronus (1976) as:

'Given a common origin, how did physicians come to dominate one set of work tasks (prescribing and diagnosis) and retain the right to engage in drug dispensing activity, whilst pharmacists lost any claim to medical practice as well as a monopoly over their own task territory?'

Once the professions of medicine and pharmacy had emerged in the mid-nineteenth century, the main role of the community pharmacist increasingly became that of dispenser. This change underwent a further acceleration after the National Health Service (NHS) Act in 1948. Once there was free public access to medical advice, there was a reduced advisory role for the community pharmacist whose task became more and more technical (see also Chapter 1).

A reversal of this trend depends on the public's perception of the pharmacist, and it has been suggested that the mission of all pharmacists should be to 'move the boundary of responsibility from the practice of a technique (the dispensing of medicines) to the patient' (Brodie 1981). This can be achieved by direct patient counselling alongside OTC medicine sales and by the increasing and accepted use of Patient Medication Records (PMRs), for both prescribed and non-prescribed medicines. PMRs create a direct link between the patient and the pharmacist and have been shown to be supported by the large majority of the public in the UK.

New pharmacy roles may encroach on the boundaries of other health care professions, particularly medicine. In the past the medical profession has refused to allow boundary encroachment by groups seeking to establish new roles for themselves. This is exemplified by the development of the sub-profession of medical pharmacology, by the medical profession, in response to the challenge from pharmacy. Another example is the establishment of the obstetricians and gynaecologists in response to the developing role of midwives. There have however, been some exceptions, such as the successful emergence of the dental profession, and the partial success of clinical psychologists. In other settings, for instance in third world countries, on ships, expeditions, and oil rigs, medical care has been successfully devolved to paramedics (for example allowing the treatment of minor symptoms following agreed protocols), and this has gradually been introduced into UK medical practice with nurse-led specialist clinics (e.g. asthma, cholesterol measurement, immunisations). This may then be an opportune time for community pharmacy to create their own control over drug use and offer an alternative to the general medical practitioner. The roles of the medical and pharmaceutical professions may be about to converge again, and the public will have an expectation and choice of either approaching the pharmacist or the general practitioner for advice and treatment.

Health care is delivered by a range of professions who share a commitment to the welfare of their patients and clients and a prohibition on exploiting their dependency. However relations between these professions are often strained because of the dominance of medicine over the other professions. This dominance is attributed to the fact that medicine was the first profession to develop within the nineteenth century's rapidly expanding health care sector. Thus, although many of the allied professions such as nursing, have many of the core features of a profession, they have not achieved all the benefits such as autonomy, remunerative rewards or equity of status. This pattern is replicated in varying degrees in other professions such as physiotherapy, chiropody and pharmacy (see also Chapter 12).

The profession of community pharmacy was said by Hamilton and Dunn (1985) to be held in low esteem because:

- The commercial side of the work leads to a store keeper-like image
- Pharmacists can, if they wish, do no more than dispense, which is essentially a technical activity
- Community pharmacy is seen as the career option for pharmacists for whom hospital or industry is not to their liking

However, whilst the functions of the community pharmacist and the general medical practitioner may often overlap, the community pharmacist should be seen as providing a complementary rather than a competitive service to the general public. General medical practitioners should welcome the contribution that community pharmacy could make to a reduction in workload, and the improved overall service that is made available to patients. Notwithstanding this, the response of the medical profession to an extended role for the community pharmacist has not always been totally supportive, and their ability to deliver it has been questioned. One survey of general medical practitioners indicated that whilst formalisation of traditional roles, such as counselling and advice on medicine storage may be supported by doctors, more innovative areas such as pharmacist managed total parenteral nutrition were not (Begley et al. 1994).

Separation of hospital and community pharmacy

It has been said that pharmacy differs from many, although not all professions in that it is divided into two major areas of practice on the basis of location rather than activity. Thus the community and hospital branches of pharmacy have become almost mutually exclusive, and their practice paths have increasingly diverged. Within the hospital category, several further sub-groups have emerged each with a different professional status. Of these, the clinical pharmacist who has a greater involvement with both patients and medical prescribers, as opposed to the more technically oriented compounding and distribution tasks, may be perceived to have the higher rank.

Until recently, there has not been a sufficient range of tasks offered in community pharmacy for any similar differentiation to emerge. However the *'extended'* role provides an opportunity both for specialised sub-groups of community pharmacy to develop, and for a new category of pharmacy itself to develop, namely *primary care pharmacists*, based on those pharmacists working directly within the general practice setting. Different models of delivering pharmaceutical care should be encouraged to facilitate the maximum contribution of pharmacy to health care.

The primary health care team and pharmacy

The *primary health care team* was first described in 1979 by the Royal Commission on the NHS. In 1988, Professor Michael Drury Department of General Practice Birmingham wrote: *'one thing that can be said about team work in general practice is that there is not a lot of it about'* (Drury 1988). There is evidence that this has changed in recent years probably motivated by radical changes in the delivery of health care. However, unlike other paramedical groups and professions, the community pharmacist is still not seen to be part of the primary health care team, certainly not part of the core team, and often not part of the wider team as described in a review of the primary health care team (Martin 1992). This does not reflect the wishes of the pharmaceutical profession. A survey of a sample of pharmacists in England showed that 95% were overwhelmingly in favour of being part of a multidisciplinary primary health care team (Sutters and Nathan 1993).

CHANNELS AND BARRIERS TO EFFECTIVE COMMUNICATION

Principles of team working

Good professional communication in health care is an essential component of team working. Many professionals, each with their own specific expertise, may be involved in the care of a single patient. This approach has the potential to deliver optimum care yet, to fully realise the health care benefits, the potential pitfalls must be recognised and addressed. The key components of effective teamworking are summarised in Box 15.1.

Box 15.1 Key components of effective team working

Effective communication is central to achieving all of these components, whether it is at a superficial operational level as in the sharing of patient data, or at a deeper level focussed on an appreciation of another professional's *modus operandi* and professional standing. Openness and honesty are paramount as well as effective team management, rather than leadership. Differing levels of remuneration of different team members may cause tensions within the team. These tensions are historical and will not be changed easily. Although resolution of such tensions and differential remuneration is the ultimate goal, in the interim it is important to make all team members feel equally valued in other ways.

Inter-professional communication

Of the health professionals interacting with community pharmacy, general medical practitioners are probably most involved with the pharmacist. The extended role features fairly regularly in journals read by the large majority of general medical practitioners. In general, such articles support a wider community pharmacy role, although there are those that express reservations. Surveys have also indicated that general medical practitioners are generally supportive of an extended role for the community pharmacist, although they tend to favour its more traditional, as opposed to its more innovative aspects. In one survey a mismatch was found as to why community pharmacists and general medical practitioners did not collaborate (Sutters and Nathan 1993). Seventy seven per cent of community pharmacists thought general medical practitioners did not want their input, but only 17% of the general medical practitioners admitted this. Thus, lack of confidence in the potential '*professional welcome*' offered by the general medical practitioners could be a rate-limiting step to improved collaborative working practices.

The current position

A survey of London community pharmacists carried out in the late 1980s (Smith 1990), showed that 43% had some contact with primary health care personnel other than general medical practitioners. The most frequently cited professionals were the district nurse and staff of residential homes, although seventeen different professional groups were named, and the contacts were mostly initiated by the other profession, rather than the pharmacist. The frequency of contact was at least weekly, though contact with general medical practitioners was more frequent. The vast majority of these contacts were associated with prescriptions, with three quarters of these contacts initiated by the pharmacist. The study gave an important insight into interaction with the primary health care team. Sixty per cent of the responding pharmacists felt that in spite of the level of contact, their contribution to the team was not acknowledged.

Some community pharmacists have a dispensing base within a health centre and it has been shown that these pharmacists have good communication with the local general medical practitioners. When the community pharmacists are based in health centres, there is more collaboration and communication between the two professions than when the pharmacist is more traditionally based in the '*high street*'. One of the medical participants in such a health centre commented that such pharmacists were '*in a privileged position in that none of their advice need be commercially orientated*' (Harding and Taylor 1990).

Examples of good practice

Published work demonstrates an increasing number of examples of the community pharmacist being integrated into the health care team. For example, drug misuse is increasingly prevalent and the care of drug misusers has increasing resource implications. This problematic group of patients are not always welcomed by the professionals or their other clients, and their planned management is particularly important (see also Chapter 21). In this regard, in Scotland in the 1990s two shared care schemes (between general practitioners and pharmacists) emerged independently (Gruer *et al.* 1997; Bond and Bunn 1998). In such schemes, general practitioners prescribe substitute methadone to drug misusers, following agreed principles of good prescribing but also including agreed communication with the pharmacist regarding the dispensing of the daily dose, encouraging professional feedback and making the drug misuser aware that this is all part of their formal programme of care. These schemes invoke a common purpose, acknowledge specific roles, and involve sharing of information and responsibility for outcomes. Similarly, on a more one to one basis, a clinical pharmacist working as part of a single practice team can run *H pylori* eradication clinics and make recommendations for patient treatment (MacIntyre *et al.* 1997). These schemes demonstrate an understanding by the general practitioner of the pharmacist's clinical knowledge, a trust that it will be used well, and a shared goal of reducing expenditure on drugs which could, in practice, be offset against the pharmacist's salary.

Finally, in this evidence-based age, community pharmacists, general practice colleagues and consultants have been brought together to develop clinical community pharmacy guidelines for use by pharmacists and their assistants when recommending OTC remedies. At the first of one of these group meetings which was formally observed using standard case study methodology, there was no mutual understanding across these three professional groups about their professional perspective, and for the doctors, of the knowledge base and skills of their pharmacy colleagues. After three or four meetings of open discussion and sharing of knowledge the situation was totally changed. At the end of the final meeting the consultant was reported as saying: *'The community pharmacist is in a very useful position. I initially came to these meetings with a very negative attitude but now understand the role of the community pharmacist. These guidelines will be very important'* (Bond and Grimshaw 1995).

PRESCRIBING AND MEDICINES MANAGEMENT

An increased role for the pharmacist is inextricably linked to *'medicines management'*, a fundamental role which reflects the unique training and specialised knowledge of pharmacists. The term medicines management covers a wide range of activities including advice and recommendations for treatment to professionals and the public, and supply of medicines. Pharmacists' input into prescribing is one facet of this.

Prescribing may be defined as a recommendation for the use of a drug or remedy. However, the word prescribing is usually interpreted as the recommendation for a medicine by a doctor or dentist (or more recently selected nurses) and the vehicle through which this is mediated is the piece of paper known as the *'prescription'*. Nonetheless, in its strictest definition, a pharmacist's role in providing OTC advice to a patient in a community pharmacy, which includes the recommendation of a medication, is also prescribing. There have been moves to blur these two roles for some time, and the recently published Crown Report may provide options to facilitate this in the UK (Crown 1999).

Pharmacists' influence on general practitioners' prescribing

When the NHS was first established, and free medical advice and treatment were made available to all UK citizens, the OTC advisory role of the pharmacist appeared to be obviated. Pharmacists were utilised more as suppliers of medicines and their role became very technical. However, with the advent of potent drugs, formulated, produced and packaged by mass production methods, traditional dispensing skills became increasingly redundant:

'The pestle and mortar days of preparing medicines have been overtaken by pharmaceutical industrial technology which accurately and aseptically produces complex medicines, pills and ointments. Only occasionally, following consultant directions, are complicated medicines made up in the pharmacy. The mixing role of the chemist has thus been eliminated' (Roberts 1988).

Today the dispensing task is not just restricted to the technical formulation and compounding of a prescription. It is more concerned with verifying the prescription, taking into account patient factors, and previous drug history (as far as is available from the PMRs), and then when the dispensed medication is handed to the patient providing appropriate counselling on medication use. The actual transfer of the drugs from one bottle to another is normally only a small part of this process, although there will still be the occasion when traditional compounding skills are required. However this will become increasingly infrequent, particularly with the *'Patient Pack'* initiative, proposals for original pack dispensing, and requirements for patient information leaflets.

This change in what has come to be understood by dispensing has allowed pharmacists to develop a more proactive role in the prescribing process, at the interface with the patient, and is increasingly recognised by other health care professionals. Thus, community pharmacists are expected to identify dosage errors, incorrect prescribing, and drug interactions. They are also at the forefront of the transfer of patients to CFC-free inhalers, and their potential to support patient concordance with prescribed medication is frequently cited.

A further future proactive involvement for pharmacists in the prescribing process is in the management of repeat prescribing. Repeat prescribing accounts for approximately 75% of all general practice prescribing in the UK, and many patients are on poly-pharmacy regimes. Current practices for generating repeat prescriptions, either computer or receptionist written, are generally acknowledged to provide inadequate control, resulting in over-prescribing, stockpiling of drugs and infrequent review of therapy which may lead to failure to identify issues such as drug interactions, adverse drug reactions, poor compliance, and inappropriate treatment.

Proposals have been made for increased involvement of the community pharmacist in primary health care, interfacing both with the general practitioner and directly with the general public (Department of Health and Royal Pharmaceutical Society of Great Britain 1992) and the control of repeat prescribing is an example of one such proposal. Several pilot studies have been carried out which have demonstrated that pharmacists can appropriately manage repeat prescribing with a resultant increase in the detection of problems, for instance, adherence problems, identification of adverse drug reactions and drug interactions. There is also a reduction in drug wastage and cost avoidance by patients, as well as improved clinical benefit (Bond *et al.* 2000).

In separate but parallel moves, pharmacists have also had an impact on prescribing at the professional interface. Across the developed world, drug costs have risen relentlessly and there has been a range of policy decisions and strategies introduced to address this. One such change in the UK was the introduction in 1989 of Medical and Pharmaceutical Prescribing Advisers to monitor and support the Indicative Prescribing Budgets imposed at that time on general practitioners. These Health Authority posts were generally, but not exclusively, held by doctors and pharmacists respectively. The two posts work closely together, with the remit to review general practice prescribing through interpretation of the computerised feedback provided by the prescription pricing authority. On the basis of this, subsequent advice would be given and areas of *'poor'* prescribing targeted for support and review. There is a growing body of research evidence which demonstrates that such input can influence prescribing patterns. This was one of the first examples of the formal involvement of pharmacists in advising doctors on their prescribing in primary care. This contrasts with secondary care, where clinical pharmacy became established in the early 1980s, with pharmacists' therapeutic knowledge utilised in a formal way.

This move has arguably paved the way for pharmacists to become associated with general practice on an individual basis. One of the first such reported collaborations was a feasibility study in the early 1990s (Burton *et al.* 1995) in which a pharmacist was placed in a general practice setting and, using her own initiative, asked to suggest roles for the pharmacist in this context. Examples identified at that time included review of computerised prescribing records to introduce both cost effective and clinically effective changes (e.g. generic substitution, drug therapy changes), face to face interviews with patients to discuss medication use and the introduction of a practice formulary and prescribing policies. Other less prescribing-related roles were also identified and/or piloted. Further arguments for such a *'consultant community pharmacist'* have also been published, and their feasibility and cost-effectiveness demonstrated.

Devolving of primary care budgets to fundholding general medical practitioners in the UK allowed these types of initiative to be explored and enabled community pharmacists to take their place in *'the practice-based team'* as opposed to the wider team, primarily to provide prescribing advice. In some cases, the local community pharmacist can fulfil this. In other cases, the pharmacist may have moved from a hospital post, or may be looking to return to a flexible part-time and challenging post after taking a career break. There are some ethical problems if the community pharmacist advising a doctor on prescribing is also the pharmacist who dispenses the prescription. Historically, the prohibition of links between community pharmacists and general medical practitioners, in order to separate the two parts of the prescribing/dispensing process, has favoured the development of

the pharmaceutical profession. It has now become a professiona'
liability and is inhibiting links being made which are not centred or
the distributive dispensing process.

Primary care pharmacists

Pharmacists working in general practice are increasingly referred to as
primary care pharmacists and a separate arm of the pharmacy professior
is emerging. This has probably been beneficial with respect to education
training and support. Pharmacists in both community and genera'
practice settings are isolated from their fellow professional peers and
this should be countered by peer support wherever possible. Pioneers of
this new branch of the pharmacy profession were largely employed by
fundholding practices, but more recently health authorities have
identified funds to support the role. Evaluation of this has been largely
on the basis of case study reports but more recently rigorous evaluations
have also been carried out which clearly demonstrate the benefits of the
primary care pharmacist approach.

Most recently there has been a further boost to pharmacists'
contribution to prescribing in the UK general practice setting. The
reconfigured NHS introduced on April 1st 1999 is focussed on primary
care. Within the primary care trusts, health care is delivered on a
locality basis though Primary Care Groups (PCGs), or Local Health
Care Co-operatives (LHCCs) in England and Scotland respectively. In
Scotland particularly, there is a clear budget for each LHCC, which is
cash limited, for prescribing. Pharmacists are being appointed to each
LHCC to provide strategic advice at LHCC level, as well supporting
individual primary care practice pharmacists and community
pharmacists within the LHCC.

The recently published UK Crown Review (Crown 1999) of the
prescribing, supply and administration of medicines, has facilitated the
further involvement of pharmacists as both dependent and independen'
prescribers. The review recommends that individual groups of
professionals should be able to apply for the authority to prescribe
certain medicines. This could facilitate drug selection by a pharmacist for
individual patients after initial diagnosis by the general medical practitioner, or greater autonomy in managing repeat prescribing after the
initial prescribing decision has been made. Such activities would need to
complement and not threaten the emerging role of the nurse practitioner
who is also seen as contributing to more efficient use of primary health
care services. A triumvirate of doctor, nurse and pharmacist could be a
very powerful and efficient combination for providing a previously
unparalleled level of service to patients.

Influences on changes in OTC prescribing

It may be that the prescribing pharmacist will become the focus of the
'*extended*' profession; this is consistent with the recommendation of the

Nuffield Inquiry into Pharmacy (1986) that the core function of the pharmacist is the sale and supply of medicines and with Sogol and Manasse (1989) who have said that: *'Pharmacy is a professional service that promotes and assures rational drug therapy in order to maximise patient benefit and minimise patient risk.'*

As well being involved in the prescribing of drugs by medical practitioners as described above, and in a possible extension of this role as dependent prescribers, pharmacists also have a role as independent prescribers. This is through their sale of OTC drugs as recommended treatments for patients who seek advice for the management of symptoms in community pharmacies. This role has been made more effective in recent years through the change in status of a range of previously Prescription Only Medicines (POM). This change in status from 'POM' to 'P' (Pharmacy Medicine) or even GSL (General Sales List) is variously called *'reregulation'*, *'switching'* or *'depomming'*! Although of benefit to the pharmaceutical profession, the main driving force has been the meeting of several agendas, which includes the pharmaceutical profession, but also the pharmaceutical industry and the government. The move has been supported both by the pharmaceutical profession and the industry, but has had a mixed reception from the medical profession (see Chapter 9).

First, the pharmaceutical industry has been suffering as a result of the moves to curb NHS spending on drugs and is looking to the OTC market to extend the brand life of existing products. Second, governments worldwide are looking at ways to reduce drug costs. In the UK, the cost of general practitioner prescriptions has risen by 52% in real terms over the past decade, although they have remained a constant three-quarters of all drug costs and 10% of the total health budget. The average *'real'* cost per prescription has increased by 16.7%, and the number of prescriptions written by 30%. Reasons proposed for this are the ageing population, an increased rate of diagnosis and the increased use of drugs in preference to other treatments. It is thought that increased self-medication, supported by community pharmacists, will help reduce the drugs bill.

However, the full potential for self medication has been limited because of legal restrictions on the range of drugs which are available for sale. There have been worldwide moves to change this by the reclassification of a range of drugs. Hence European directive 92/26/CEE states that medicines should only be POM if they are dangerous when used other than under medical supervision, frequently used incorrectly, new and need further investigation or are normally injected. The consensus criteria for deregulation are currently said to be that the drug should be of proven safety, of low toxicity in overdose, and for the treatment of minor *'self-limiting'* conditions.

In 1989, Denmark was amongst the first of the Northern European countries to deregulate a large number of medicines including cimetidine. The process started slowly in the UK with the deregulation of ibuprofen and loperamide (1983), terfenadine (1984) and hydro cortisone 1% cream (1985) but it has continued steadily with the support of the government, the Royal Pharmaceutical Society of Great Britain, and, to a limited extent, the Royal College of General Practitioners. Other target preparations for future deregulation include oral contraceptives and the 'morning after' pill, which has the support of both the Royal College of General Practitioners and the General Medical Services Committee of the British Medical Association.

If costs are defined to include both monetary and non-monetary elements, it has been shown that the OTC availability of topical 1% hydrocortisone saved patients in the UK £2 million pounds in 1987 alone (Ryan and Yule 1990) and the NHS is said to save money too. Savings from the deregulation of loperamide were estimated to be £0.13 million in 1985, £0.15 million in 1986, and £0.32 million in 1987 (Ryan and Yule 1990). Standard models of supply and demand can also be employed to demonstrate the theoretical economic advantages of deregulation (Ryan and Bond 1994).

The extension of the OTC prescribing role of the community pharmacist under the current system, through increased availability of a wider range of medicines has caused some concerns because of the potential for the masking of serious disease, the increase in likelihood of adverse drug reactions (ADRs) and drug interactions. Pharmacists and their staff therefore need to be trained for this increased responsibility and one way of addressing this increased responsibility has been through the development of guidelines by multidisciplinary groups, which should include community pharmacy representation as well as general practitioners, relevant consultants and pharmacologists. Examples of such guidelines have been published and the educational benefit reported.

With such potent medicines now more widely used, it would be advantageous if they could be added to a central patient drug record which could be accessed by both general practitioner and community pharmacist. For general practitioners, this would provide information on the treatments already tried/being taken by the patient, underpin future prescribing decisions, and increase their awareness of the potential for drug interactions or therapeutic duplication. For pharmacists, access to a central medical record would inform their OTC prescribing decisions.

Government funding for the provision of a restricted formulary of products would support the development of pharmacists' advisory role. It would also reduce the number of general medical practitioner consultations, wherein patients seek a prescription for a medicine for which they are exempt from payment, but which can also be bought from a pharmacy, though the cost may be prohibitive. Whilst this move would possibly be against the main rationale of the deregulation trend, since it would transfer costs back to the NHS, it would have considerable savings in general medical practitioner time. Mechanisms, based on means testing, could also be introduced to restrict those eligible for such pharmacy-generated prescriptions. The full economic effect of various options such as these would need to be evaluated.

Information technology

The use of information technology in the health service is currently relatively small compared to other industries such as banking and tourism. However, recent initiatives in the UK have linked all general practitioners to the NHS-net. In Scotland there are clear signs that community pharmacists will also soon be linked in. This should open up the possibility for *'read and write'* access for all health professionals to an electronic patient record, which would facilitate many of the innovative developments described above. Obviously full requirements specification will need to be carried out with wide consultation, including professionals and patients' groups to ensure appropriate levels of read and write access are agreed and to define the data fields. Such a mechanism to improve communication and information flow, in a controlled but relevant way, will support the greater involvement of pharmacists in multidisciplinary patient care. It should also make possible delivery of some aspects of the role described previously from the community pharmacy base, rather than by a primary care pharmacist based in surgeries. This could avoid the total partitioning of the profession into three main groupings and would actually promote a range of different models of involvement.

CONCLUSION

Pharmacists have an opportunity to extend their role in multidisciplinary health care, because of external factors resulting from the agendas of Government and the pharmaceutical industry. Reclassification of drugs has contributed significantly to that opportunity, but has also created conflicts between successful self-care, the profit motives of individual community pharmacists, and the commercial opportunism of the pharmaceutical industry.

One scenario for an extended pharmacy role would be for a *'community'* pharmacist to be based full-time in a general medical practice, developing a range of services which could include activities such as advice on formulary development, patient medication review and asthma clinics, as well as pain and warfarin clinics. Development of a role for pharmacists within the general medical practice base would not obviate the need for *'high street'* pharmacies. Rather, it would be an additional model for delivering pharmaceutical care which would allow utilization of a wider range of pharmacists' skills.

The development of a wider role for the community pharmacist within the general medical practitioner's own territory may seem unlikely given the historical problems of hierarchy and competition. Other issues may have contributed more to these problems than has previously been acknowledged. Removal of community pharmacists from the commercial setting would allow them to provide advice untainted (imagined or otherwise) by possible commercial pressures. General medical practitioners have shown that they can work with the nursing professions, although it has been said that this is because the nursing profession is still within the control of medical doctors (Eaton and Webb 1979). However, they also work with many other professions, including health visitors, midwives, opticians, chiropodists, clinical psychologists and dentists, who are independent practitioners within the NHS. It therefore seems unlikely that collaboration with pharmacists is as much of a problem as has been speculated. Historically, this sort of major boundary change has occurred for a variety of reasons, but the driving force has most often been external circumstances such as war or an economic crisis (Kronus 1976). In the current scenario, governments are contributing to the boundary change by a general review of health care delivery, and specifically drug expenditure; this latter has major implications for the pharmaceutical industry. The future for the community pharmacist is therefore probably more dependent on political and commercial expediency than professional competence. However, the opportunities are there and the barriers can be overcome.

FURTHER READING

Adams, T. (1999) Dentistry and medical dominance. *Social Science and Medicine*, **48**, 407–420.

Ashley, J. (1992) Pharmacists and the 'D' word. *Pharmaceutical Journal*, **248**, 375.

Blane, D. (1991) Health professions. In: G. Scrambler (Ed.) *Sociology Applied to Medicine*, Balliere Tindall, London.

Bond, C.M. and Grimshaw, J.M. (1994) Clinical guidelines for the treatment of dyspepsia in community pharmacies. *Pharmaceutical Journal*, **252**, 228–229.

Bond, C.M., Grimshaw, J.M., Taylor, R.J. and Winfield, A.J. (1998) An evaluation of clinical guidelines for community pharmacy. *Journal of Social and Administrative Pharmacy*, **15**, 33–39.

Bond, C.M., Sinclair, H.K., Taylor, R.J., Williams, A., Reid, J.P. and Duffus, P. (1995) Pharmacists: an untapped resource for general practice *International Journal of Pharmacy Practice*, **3**, 85–90.

Bond, C.M. (1999) The pharmacist in the Primary Health Care Team In: J. Sims (Ed.) *Primary Health Care Sciences: a Reader*, Whurr London.

Comptroller and Auditor General (1993) *Repeat Prescribing by General Medical Practitioners in England*, HMSO, London.

Comptroller and Auditor General (1994) *A Prescription for Improvement*, HMSO, London.

Cotter, S.M., Barber, N.D. and McKee, M. (1994) Professionalisation of hospital pharmacy: the role of clinical pharmacy. *Journal of Social and Administrative Pharmacy*, **11**, 57–66.

Crown, J. (1999) *A Review of the Prescribing, Supply and Administration of Medicines*, Department of Health, London.

Cunningham-Burley, S. (1988) Rediscovering the role of the pharmacist. *Journal of the Royal College of General Practitioners*, **38**, 99–100.

Department of Health (1987) *Promoting Better Health*, CM249, HMSO, London.

Department of Health (1989) *Working for Patients*, CM555, HMSO, London.

Department of Health (1997) *The New NHS – Modern, Dependable*, CM3807, HMSO, London.

Dowell, J., Cruickshank, J., Bain, J. and Staines, H. (1999) Repeat dispensing by community pharmacists: advantages for patients and practitioners. *British Journal of General Practice*, **48**, 1858–1859.

Drury, M. (1991) Doctors and pharmacists-working together. *British Journal of General Practice*, **41**, 116–118.

Earles, M.P. (1991) *A History of the Society in 150 Years of a Science Based Profession. Supplement to the Pharmaceutical Journal*, April 1991.

Edwards, C. (1992) Liberalising medicines supply. *International Journal of Pharmacy Practice*, **1**, 186.

Ford, S. and Jones, K. (1995) Integrating pharmacy fully into the primary care team. *British Medical Journal*, **310**, 1620.

Freidson, E. (1972) *Profession of Medicine*, Mead and Co, New York.

Harris, C.M. and Dajda, R. (1996) The scale of repeat prescribing. *British Journal of General Practice*, **46**, 643–647.

Jepson, M. and Strickland-Hodge, B. (1993) Patients' choice of pharmacy, the importance of patient medication records and patient registration. *Pharmaceutical Journal*, **251**, R35.

Macarthur, D. (1992) Professions at war: a look at the uneasy relationship between dispensing doctors and pharmacists in the UK. *The Australian Journal of Pharmacy*, **73**, 870–871.

Marsh, G.N. and Dawes, M.L. (1995) Establishing a minor illness nurse in a busy general practice. *British Medical Journal*, **310**, 778–780.

Matheson, C. and Bond, C.M. (1995) Lower gastrointestinal symptoms. *Pharmaceutical Journal*, **253**, 656–658.

Matthews, L.G. (1980) *Milestones in Pharmacy*, Merrell Division, Egham.

Porteous, T., Bond, C., Duthie, I. and Matheson, C. (1997) Guidelines for the treatment of hayfever and other allergic conditions of the upper respiratory tract. *Pharmaceutical Journal*, **259**, 62–65.

Porteous, T., Bond, C.M., Duthie, I., Matheson, C. (1998) Guidelines for the treatment of self-limiting upper respiratory tract ailments. *Pharmaceutical Journal*, **260**, 134–139.

Reilly, P. and Marinker, M. (1994) Rational prescribing: how can it be judged. In: M. Marinker (Ed.) *Controversies in Health Care Policies: Challenges to Practice*, BMA Publishing, London.

Rogers, P.J., Fletcher, G. and Rees, J.E. (1992) Recording of clinical conditions by community pharmacists in patient medication records. *Pharmaceutical Journal*, **249**, 723–727.

Scottish Office Department of Health (1997) *Designed to Care – Renewing the National Health Service in Scotland*, CM3811, HMSO, London.

Spencer, J. and Edwards, C. (1992) Pharmacy beyond the dispensary: general practitioners' views. *British Medical Journal*, **304**, 1670–1672.

Taylor, R.J. (1986) Pharmacists and primary care. *Journal of the Royal College of General Practitioners*, **36**, 348.

Wain, C. (1992) The primary care team. *British Journal of General Practice*, **42**, 498–499.

Welsh Office (1997) *Putting Patients First*, CM3841, HMSO, London.

Whitehouse, C.R. and Hodgkin, P. (1985) The management of minor illness by general practitioners. *Journal of the Royal College of General Practitioners*, **35**, 581–583.

REFERENCES

Begley, S., Livingstone, C., Williamson,V. and Hodges, N. (1994) Attitudes of pharmacists, medical practitioners and nurses towards the development of domiciliary and other community pharmacy services. *International Journal of Pharmacy Practice*, **2**, 223–228.

Bond, C.M. and Bunn, D. (1998) Shared care for drug misusers *Innovations in Primary Care Conference*, Edinburgh.

Bond, C.M. and Grimshaw, J.M. (1995) Multidisciplinary guideline development: a case study from community pharmacy. *Health Bulletin*, **53**, 26–33.

Bond, C.M., Matheson, C., Williams, S., Williams, P. and Donnan, P. (2000) Repeat prescribing: a role for community pharmacists in controlling and monitoring repeat prescriptions. *British Journal of General Practice*, **50**, 271–275.

Brodie, D.C. (1981) Pharmacy's societal purpose. *American Journal of Hospital Pharmacy*, **38**, 1893–1896.

Burton, S.S., Duffus, P.R.S. and Williams, A. (1995) An exploration of the role of the clinical pharmacist in general medical practice. *Pharmaceutical Journal*, **254**, 91–93.

Crown, J. (1999) *A Review of the Prescribing, Supply and Administration of Medicines*, Department of Health, London.

Department of Health and Royal Pharmaceutical Society of Great Britain (1992) *Pharmaceutical Care: the Future for Community Pharmacy*, Royal Pharmaceutical Society of Great Britain, London.

Drury, M., (1988) Teamwork: the way forward. *Practice Team*, **1**, 3.

Eaton, G. and Webb, B. (1979) Boundary encroachment: pharmacists in the clinical setting. *Sociology of Health and Illness*, **1**, 69–89.

Gruer, L., Wilson, P., Scott, R., Elliott, L., Macleod, J., Harden, K., Hinshelwood, S., McNulty, H. and Silk, P. (1997) General practitioner centred scheme for treatment of opiate dependent drug injectors in Glasgow. *British Medical Journal*, **314**, 1730–1735.

Hamilton, D.D. and Dunn, W.R. (1985) *Report Submitted to the Post Graduate Education Committee of the Royal Pharmaceutical Society of Great Britain. Paper 1*, Royal Pharmaceutical Society of Great Britain, London.

Harding, G. and Taylor, K. (1990) Professional relationships between general practitioners and pharmacists in health centres. *Journal of the Royal College of General Practitioners*, **40**, 464–466.

Kronus, C.L. (1976) The evolution of occupational power. *Sociology of Work and Occupations*, **3**, 3–37.

MacIntyre, A.M., Macgregor, S., Malek, M., Dunbar, J., Hamley, J. and Cromarty, J. (1997) New patients presenting to their GP with dyspepsia: does Helicobacter pylori eradication minimise the cost of managing these patients. *International Journal of Clinical Practice*, **51**, 276–281.

Martin, C. (1992) Partners in practice: attached, detached, or new recruits. *British Medical Journal*, **305**, 348–350.

Merrison, A.W. (1979) *Royal Commission on the National Health Service*, CM7615, HMSO, London.

Nuffield Committee of Inquiry into Pharmacy (1986) *Pharmacy: a Report to the Nuffield Foundation*, Nuffield Foundation, London.

Roberts, D. (1988) Dispensing by the community pharmacist: an unstoppable decline? *Journal of the Royal College of General Practitioners*, **38**, 563–564.

Ryan, M. and Bond, C. (1994) Dispensing doctors and prescribing pharmacists. *Pharmacoeconomics*, **5**, 8–17.

Ryan, M. and Yule, B. (1990) Switching drugs from prescription-only to over-the-counter availability: economic benefits in the United Kingdom. *Health Policy*, **16**, 233–239.

Smith, F.J. (1990) The extended role of the community pharmacist: implications for the primary health care team. *Journal of Social and Administrative Pharmacy*, **7**, 101–110.

Sogol, E.M. and Manasse, Jr. H.R. (1989) The Pharmacist. In A.I. Wertheimer and M.C. Smith (Eds.) *Pharmacy Practice: Social and Behavioural Aspects*, Williams and Wilkins, Baltimore, p 59.

Sutters, C. and Nathan, A. (1993) The community pharmacist's extended role: GPs and pharmacists' attitudes towards collaboration. *Journal of Social and Administrative Pharmacy*, **10**, 70–84.

Self-assessment questions

Question 1:   What are the key factors affecting the relationship between the professions of medicine and pharmacy today?

Question 2:   What are the key principles of team working? Give a pharmacy related example to illustrate each of these.

Question 3:   In which two discrete ways do pharmacists have an input into prescribing decisions?

Key points for answers

Question 1:

- Common ancestry
- Medical monopoly over prescribing
- Pharmacy monopoly over dispensing
- Competing medical specialisation (e.g. pharmacology)
- Commercialisation of pharmacy
- Recent government moves
- Physical isolation from the rest of the primary care team

Question 2:

- Sharing a common purpose (e.g. shared care of drug misusers)
- Having a clear understanding of one's own role and recognising common interests (e.g. review of general practice prescribing)
- Understanding the roles and responsibilities of others (e.g. *H. pylori* eradication clinics)
- Pooling knowledge and resources (e.g. guideline development)
- Sharing a responsibility for outcomes (e.g. prescribing and dispensing a prescription)

Question 3:

a) For prescription only medicines:

- Advice to general practitioners within the general practice setting
- Review of patients' notes
- Face to face patient review
- Formulary development
- Management of repeat prescribing
- Support to primary care groups
- Future IT links with practices

b) For OTC medicines:

- Increased role regarding minor ailments due to pressures on drug budgets
- Increased role regarding minor ailments because of number of drugs re-regulated to pharmacy sale
- Liaison across primary groupings for managed care networks for minor ailments
- Clinical pharmacy OTC guidelines
- Future IT links with practices

PART FIVE

Meeting the Pharmaceutical Care Needs of Specific Populations

16 Ethnic Minorities

Mohamed Aslam, Farheen Jessa and John Wilson

INTRODUCTION	274
ETHNIC DIFFERENCES IN DISEASE MORBIDITY AND MORTALITY	274
PROVIDING CULTURALLY SENSITIVE HEALTH ADVICE	275
The public's perception of the pharmacist	275
Language and communication	275
Use of family and friends	276
TRADITIONAL SYSTEMS OF HEALTH CARE	276
Traditional medicine from the Indian subcontinent	277
The philosophical background of Asian medicine	277
Ayurvedic System	277
Unani System	278
Conflicts with allopathic medicine (hot/cold theory conflict)	278
Hazards of traditional practice	279
Dual treatment	279
Toxicity	279
Drug interactions	279
Compliance	280
Adulteration	280
RAMADAN	280
Effect of Ramadan on specific disease states	281
Gastrointestinal disorders	281
Asthma	281
Diabetes	282
Pregnancy and breast feeding	282
Drug compliance and Ramadan	283
Cessation of therapy	283
Change in dosage intervals	283
Antacids	283
Fruit juices and carbonated drinks	283
Pharmacists' role in patient compliance during Ramadan	284
Information resources	284
CONCLUSION	284
FURTHER READING	285
REFERENCES	285
SELF-ASSESSMENT QUESTIONS	286
KEY POINTS FOR ANSWERS	287

INTRODUCTION

Ethnicity refers to variations in the human species created by the interplay of geography and heredity. Each ethnic group can be defined as a
social group with a distinctive language, values, religion, customs and
attitudes (Hillier 1991). In the United Kingdom there are a wide range
of these groups including Turks, Greeks, Irish, Jews and West Indians.
But those groups with a significant number of people include Chinese
(mainly from Hong Kong), Afro-Caribbean and large numbers originating from the various countries of the Indian subcontinent including
Hindus, Sikhs and Muslims. For the purpose of this chapter the term
'Asian' will be used to cover people originating from India, Pakistan,
Bangladesh and East Africa.

The problems of complying with/adhering to a medication regime
are common, and not specific to ethnic minorities. However, within
this group, culture and religious faith, as well as literacy problems, are
additional factors which may affect compliance. Culture refers to a
group's religious values, attitudes, rituals, family structure, language
and social structure (Rothschild 1981). In order to deliver optimal
pharmaceutical care, pharmacists need to be aware of patients' culture
and religion as well as their medical condition. Cultural differences
can affect perception of illness, treatment-seeking behaviour, and
response to health care. This chapter will discuss the pharmaceutical
implications of some religious and cultural beliefs, an understanding
of which will help the pharmacist respect the unique needs of clients
from ethnic minorities, and provide a more appropriate service.
Failure to respect or be aware of these differences may well result in a
failure of medications.

ETHNIC DIFFERENCES IN DISEASE MORBIDITY AND MORTALITY

Epidemiological studies have shown that there are distinct variations
in mortality and morbidity between ethnic minority groups and the
indigenous population due to their different genetic and cultural backgrounds, suggesting different health service needs. For instance,
Asians and Afro-Caribbeans have relatively high mortality rates for
strokes and hypertension. Diabetes is very high in immigrants from
the Indian sub-continent, whilst Asian women are at higher risk of
osteoporosis. These are a few examples of which there are many more
Marmot (1989) suggests that:

'*These variations may occur due to a variety of reasons; the conclusion may be
that we should pay great attention to the social and economic position of
immigrants but these are unlikely to be the only factors that determine their
pattern of disease.*'

By focussing on cultural/lifestyle features there is the prospect for
enhancing the understanding of disease aetiology and for disease pre-

vention. Social, cultural and dietary customs for example, may directly contribute to some of the diseases suffered by Asians, such as rickets and osteomalacia. There are also instances where morbidity and mortality amongst an ethnic minority are lower than the national average. Inflammatory bowel disease, for example, is rare amongst Indian migrants, whilst multiple sclerosis is rare amongst migrants from Asia and Africa to Britain.

In the United Kingdom, the government's concerns about disadvantages which may affect all racial minority groups was acknowledged in a report, in which they set out to aim for an improvement in the rights and standards available to all patients: '... *all health services should make provision so that ... your privacy, dignity, religious and cultural beliefs are respected*' (Department of Health 1991). Additionally, the Commission for Racial Equality's Code of Practice in Primary Healthcare Services (1992) urged community pharmacists to ensure that services are delivered in a way that is both appropriate and accessible to ethnic minorities. Pharmacists therefore require an awareness of the ethnic population(s) they serve together with an epidemiological grounding in the culturally diverse patterns of disease.

Providing culturally sensitive health advice

The public's perception of the pharmacist

Ethnic minorities' expectations of health care may influence their use of pharmaceutical services. Those originating from countries with little access to Western style medicine may, for instance, not regard the pharmacist as an appropriate source of health care advice. In order to try and overcome this, promotional campaigns are required to inform ethnic minorities of the pharmacist's advisory function.

Language and communication

Pharmacists should identify sub-groups with particular health needs or communication difficulties. Literacy rates and dialects vary between ethnic groups, and hence will affect the types of problems experienced in providing a pharmaceutical service to those groups. The problem of communication could be addressed by employing staff from the local community.

Some people from ethnic minority groups may not be able to read English. Those who have difficulty in English usually also have difficulties in reading their '*mother*' language. However, it is equally important to realise that a leaflet in English is likely to be understood by at least one member of the family, even if the patient is unable to read it. Therefore it is better to provide a leaflet written in English rather than none at all.

Providing translated material from the pharmacy requires careful consideration because of the large number of languages which may be spoken by ethnic groups. Leaflets written in English generally relate to the indigenous lifestyle and do not translate readily to meet the specific needs of ethnic minorities. To overcome the language and cultural barriers that are present in existing health promotion requires the production and dissemination of culturally sensitive and linguistically appropriate materials. Such materials should be made readily available to health and community workers and also distributed to community and religious centres. They might also include audio or videotapes in addition to written information.

An alternative approach to disseminating health advice, is the use of suitable media coverage such as Asian satellite television and radio or magazines and newspapers read by ethnic minorities, which routinely feature items on health issues.

Use of family and friends

Pharmacists may be able to marshal family and friends in promoting pharmaceutical care among ethnic groups. A pregnant woman, for instance, will receive a lot of support from other members of her family, especially her mother, mother-in-law or an equivalent elder, who will feel that it is their responsibility to advise the younger women about pregnancy.

Folic acid consumption by women pre-conception, and in the first trimester of pregnancy, is recommended to reduce neural tube defects in infants, a condition particularly prevalent among infants of mothers born in Pakistan and India. A recent campaign targeted women contemplating pregnancy (Health Education Authority 1996). Instead of targeting only child-bearing women, the pharmacist would be wise to include family members when giving health education and promotional advice. By informing the mother-in-law or husband for example, about the importance of folic acid, the patient can be actively encouraged to follow the advice provided.

TRADITIONAL SYSTEMS OF HEALTH CARE

All cultures have a system of health beliefs that explains how illness occurs, how it can be treated or cured, and who should be involved in the healing process. Sensitivity to patients' health beliefs and cultural differences is important in delivering health care. Traditional medicine, its preparations and practices, plays a major role in the health care of the ethnic community. Strong ties to the traditional diets and religions brought from the mother country remain. Not surprisingly comparable ties exist for health care and medicine. Ethnic minorities demonstrate pluralistic patterns of health care consumption. That is, the traditional health beliefs are integrated with those of the indigenous health care system. For example, consumers from ethnic minorities may adopt OTC (over the counter) medication. However the same consumers simultaneously maintain many of the cultural health beliefs of the culture of origin, such as the use of traditional remedies for ailments.

In many parts of the world, the only health care available to people is provided by traditional healers. Many groups of people now living in the UK retain their belief in traditional medicine to varying degrees, regarding it as an integral part of their culture, affecting diet and social behaviour.

Traditional medicine from the Indian subcontinent

The indigenous system of medicine in India is called the Ayurvedic system, whilst in Pakistan it is known as Unani-Tibb or Unani for short. Both systems of medicine employ crude herbal drugs and these are normally administered in the form of pills, syrups, confectionery or alcoholic extracts. Ayurvedic medicine is solely of Hindu origin, whilst Unani derives from Ancient Greece, and that practised today has been influenced by Persian, Egyptian and African medicine.

The central figure in both systems of medicines is the traditional healer known as the Hakim. There are also associated pharmacopoeias akin to the British and European Pharmacopoeias. The Hamdard pharmacopoeia, for example, lists over 3,000 different preparations supplied by a flourishing pharmaceutical industry based on traditional medicine.

The philosophical background of Asian medicine

It is important that pharmacists are aware of the theory of Ayurvedic and Unani medicine. This section illustrates the importance of knowing about patients' belief systems in facilitating communication and support between patient and health professional, which in turn enhances patients' confidence in their treatment.

Ayurvedic system

The basis of all treatments in the Ayurvedic system is the balancing of the life energies within a person. It uses meditation as a primary and fundamental tool and also employs diets, mineral substances, aromas and herbs. The components that are used in Ayurveda do not originate from scientific concepts or experiments but from '*direct observation*' of nature. There are five elements of Ayurveda; ether, air, water, fire and earth. These are meant to communicate the essential universal principle that is inherent in a particular element.

Unani system

The basis of the Unani system is humoral pathology, in which the four main humours of the body: blood, mucus, yellow and black bile are combined with the four primary qualities: warmth (or heat), cold, moisture (or dampness) and dryness. Thus the humours are categorised as blood (damp and hot), mucus (damp and cold), yellow bile (dry and hot), black bile (damp and cold). If the humours are in equilibrium, the person is healthy. If however one becomes dominant then the equilibrium is disturbed, resulting in illness. Thus, by conserving the symmetry in a patient's life and maintaining the humoral balance health will be protected. The role of the Hakim is to teach the patient how to conserve or restore symmetry.

The Chinese believe in a similar 'yin-yang' theory in that yin stores vital strength inside the body whilst yang protects the outside and corresponds to the surface of the body. Diseases occur when there is an imbalance between 'yin' and 'yang' and the fundamental principle once again, is to restore balance and harmony.

Conflicts with allopathic medicine (hot/cold theory conflict)

The hot/cold imbalance appears prominently across various different cultures, e.g. Chinese and Asian. It emphasises the importance of temperament and the humours, and places great emphasis on the concept of hot and cold applied to medicines, herbs and food. This does not refer to the temperature of the material. Broadly, hot foods are those rich in protein, cold foods are rich in vitamin C. In these traditional systems all food and medicines are classified according to their particular qualities as hot or cold, damp or dry, to varying degrees.

Treatment of disease with the Unani and Chinese medical systems is dependent on the principle that a hot disease is cured by a cold remedy, damp diseases require dry preparations and so on. This concept brings conflict with allopathic medicine, as in Unani and Ayurvedic practice it is believed that most Western medicines are 'hot' and therefore inappropriate for hot illnesses. Pregnancy, for example, is a 'hot' condition and therefore in pregnancy one should not eat too many 'hot' foods. It would therefore be considered inappropriate to take 'hot' medicines during pregnancy. This could contribute to poor compliance with, for example, folic acid tablets or iron preparations taken before and during pregnancy.

A similar philosophy is applied to disease states. In the absence of disease, the body humours are considered to be in balance; any disturbance in this balance results in morbidity. Some diseases are of '*hot*' temperament e.g. kidney ailments and warts. The body's balance is restored and the illness cured by ingestion of medicine or food of the opposite temperament.

Both the Unani and Ayurvedic systems of treatment are now available in Britain. In Britain the majority of Hakims, although offering a service to the Asian community, have no formal qualifications to practice. The holistic approach and the sympathetic ear are of undoubted psychological benefit and some remedies do appear to work. Patients of alternative healers tend to rate highly the interpersonal skills of these healers and report a better healer-patient relationship (Ahmad 1992). Unfortunately the benefits can often be outweighed by the potential hazards, therefore it seems that before the positive benefits of traditional healers can be appreciated the detrimental consequences of their practices must first be eliminated by imposing strict controls.

Hazards of traditional practice

Pharmacists providing a service for ethnic minorities should be aware of traditional health concepts and the possible problems and associated dangers.

Dual treatment

Patients may be receiving dual treatment from both their Western medical doctor and their traditional healer. If they are given the same drug by both this can lead to problems such as overdose.

Toxicity

There have been cases of poisoning associated with the use of Chinese herbal remedies due to the ingestion of aconitine, anticholinergic agents and podophyllin. There is also a potential risk of exposure to heavy metals. Minerals such as gold, silver, tin, mercury, lead and arsenic are commonly used in Asian medicine in uncontrolled quantities, e.g metal-containing or coated pills known as kushtay are taken by adult Asian males for sexual dysfunction and are supposed remedies for psychosexual problems. Although there is no direct evidence for adverse reactions to the use of these materials, it is clear that the ingestion of materials containing several per cent by weight of arsenic, mercury, lead and other heavy metals cannot be beneficial.

Drug interactions

Interactions may occur between Western drugs and biologically active substances present in traditional medicines. An example of this is the use of the fruit Karela (*Momordica charantia*) which is used in curries, but is also used by the Hakim to lower blood sugar. It can interact with chlorpropamide and may produce hypoglycaemia in an otherwise stabilised diabetic patient.

Compliance

Patients may be poorly compliant if a prescribed Western drug is not compatible with the traditional concept of disease, e.g. pregnant women and 'hot' medicines.

Adulteration

Western medicines may be present in uncontrolled quantities in 'traditional' remedies. Adulteration of Chinese herbal remedies with synthetic substances has also been reported.

RAMADAN

During the month of Ramadan, the ninth month of the Islamic year, all adult Muslims are expected to fast between the hours of sunrise and sunset. The actual date for commencement of this fast varies from year to year depending on the phase of the moon. During this period all food and drink and, except in special cases, all medicines are excluded. When fasting, no food or water is consumed and smoking is prohibited. No medicines of the following forms are used: oral medications, injections, ear and nose drops, pessaries or suppositories and inhalations. Following sunset, the family meet together and the fast is broken with a light snack and a lot of fluid, often fizzy drinks (Aslam and Wilson 1997).

After about twenty minutes prayers are said and a large main meal 'Iftar' is served. A further light meal, 'Suhur' is eaten early in the morning before dawn prayers, after which the fast continues until the evening. Fasting involves major changes in the pattern of physical activity and sleep patterns as well as an alteration in the normal pattern of intake of food and fluid.

The Qur'an (the Muslims' Holy Book), says that health is promoted by fasting. Complete fasting is seen as a way of combining spiritual, physical and individual needs, whilst at the same time establishing a greater awareness of God, self-discipline and an empathy with the poor and needy.

Those who have acute or chronic disease are exempt from the fast as well as menstruating, pregnant or lactating women. Individuals travelling long distances, would be expected to make up the fast at a later date. Children and the elderly may or may not be expected to fast depending on their age and health. Normally children do not fast until they reach the age of puberty. Some devout Muslims still fast despite their pregnancies and ill-health. Abstaining from fasting is difficult when the rest of the family observes the fast, due to feelings of isolation or social pressure to keep the fast.

In people who are fit and well, the fast seems to create no particular difficulties and the body's normal homeostatic mechanisms will usually cope. Urinary volume, electrolytes, pH and nitrogen excretion tend to remain within normal limits. Some studies however, have indicated that some biological functions do change. Arousal, vigilance and memory may decrease during Ramadan, especially during the first few days. Studies of hormonal changes have given inconsistent results. Hakkou *et al.* (1994) concluded that even though Ramadan has been practised for fourteen centuries and is followed by perhaps one billion people worldwide, there have been few well conducted studies on its impact on health and disease.

Effect of Ramadan on specific disease states

Fasting during Ramadan has particular implications for health care workers, since in some cases fasting can result not only in general lethargy, but also in problems with drug compliance (Box 16.1). This highlights the need for pharmacists' awareness of the particular needs of these patients during this month.

Box 16.1 Problems of drug compliance and lethargy during Ramadan

A study of accident and emergency attendances showed a significant increase in the number of Muslims attending during Ramadan compared to non-Muslims (Langford *et al.* 1994). It was suggested that this increase was due to non-compliance and general fatigue resulting from fasting, leading to a lowered threshold for help-seeking advice.

Gastrointestinal disorders

Fasting would logically be expected to cause problems for patients with peptic acid disease, particularly ulceration (Box 16.2).

Asthma

Studies have shown that there are no chronobiological effects on the pharmacokinetics of sustained release preparations of theophylline (Box 16.3).

Box 16.2 The effect of fasting on peptic acid disease

Endoscopic examination conducted in the Kashmir Valley, an area with a prevalence of 4.7% for peptic ulcer, showed that it was not uncommon for patients to have both duodenal and gastric ulcers (Malik *et al.* 1995). During Ramadan 1995, patients with peptic ulceration were instructed to take ranitidine twice daily, at 'Suhur' and at 'Iftar'. While patients with acute duodenal ulcer showed signs of healing during Ramadan those with chronic peptic ulcer did not. Indeed, several patients with chronic peptic ulcer suffered bleeds during the study period. Ramadan fasting was concluded to be hazardous to patients with acid peptic disease in general and those with chronic peptic ulcer in particular.

Cherrah et al. (1990) showed that the area under the plasma concentration time curve (AUC) and maximum plasma concentration (C_{max}) for sustained release theophylline (Armophylline-R) did not vary significantly with the time of administration, indicating that the drug could be taken outside daylight hours and still provide asthmatic control. In a study of a small group of men with stable asthma who wished to fast, sustained release theophylline (Euphylline CR) was given before dawn (0300 hours) (Daghous et al. 1994). Blood samples taken over five days following dosing indicated considerable inter-patient variability. However, for individual patients there was no significant difference between plasma concentration during and following Ramadan fasting. The study concluded that asthmatic patients could be allowed to fast if they were stabilised on a sustained release theophylline preparation.

Diabetes

There have been a number of studies of the effects of fasting amongst diabetic patients (Box 16.4).

Salman et al. (1992) observed 21 insulin dependent diabetic children aged between 9 to 14 years during Ramadan fasting. Doses of insulin were carefully adjusted and the insulin given both before the evening meal and the pre-dawn meal. There were no significant complications and none of the patients developed symptomatic hypoglycaemia, indicating that Ramadan fasting is feasible in older and long standing diabetic children, and does not alter short-term metabolic control. Nevertheless fasting should only be encouraged in children with good glycaemic control whose blood glucose levels are regularly monitored at home.

One study has concluded that most adult patients with type II diabetes can fast (Beshyah et al. 1990), but it is necessary to increase the dosage of hypoglycaemic medication in the evening to combat hyperglycaemia and reduce it in the morning to prevent hypoglycaemia. However, other studies have reported considerable problems with diabetic control during the fast (Tang and Rolfe 1989), whilst Barber and Wright (1979) found no convincing evidence to suggest that it is safe for all Muslims with diabetes to fast.

Pregnancy and breast feeding

Pregnant women who fast have a lower glucose and insulin concentration and higher triglyceride levels at the end of Ramadan. Women who fast during breastfeeding lose on average 7.6% total body fluid during the day and the milk concentration of lactose, sodium and potassium is changed (Rashed 1992).

Pregnant, breast-feeding and menstruating women are exempt from fasting during Ramadan. However they are often unaware of these exemptions. If informed of these exemptions, evidence suggests they choose not to fast (Reeves 1992).

Drug compliance and Ramadan

Cessation of therapy

Complying with prescribed medication may present problems during Ramadan, and evidence suggests that the majority of patients will modify their treatment (Aslam and Assad 1986), whilst some will stop medication completely or take all their doses in a single intake (Aslam and Healy 1986). Stopping medication completely is potentially dangerous, for example epileptic attacks have been reported in patients who ceased their medication whilst fasting (Aslam and Wilson 1992). Likewise, patients with chronic respiratory disease, normally managed with steroids and bronchodilators, have been admitted into intensive care as a result of not taking their medication during daylight hours (Wheatly and Shelly 1993).

Change in dosage intervals

If doses are omitted during daylight hours there is an increased likelihood that patients on multiple therapy will take medications together in a single dose increasing the risk of drug interactions. As the plasma half-life is unaffected by dose size, the time period for which the blood concentration is above the minimum effective level will increase if multiple doses are taken together, whilst toxic adverse effects may be produced. To overcome this, sustained release preparations are preferable as they produce the required therapeutic effect without excessive high blood concentrations which may lead to adverse effects. Similarly, drugs with a long half-life in the body will have a longer action and can therefore be taken less frequently. For instance, the non-steroidal anti-inflammatory drugs (NSAIDs) vary in half-life from 2–3 hours for ibuprofen up to 36–38 hours for piroxicam.

Antacids

Gastrointestinal disorders ranging from constipation to peptic ulcers are frequently treated by antacids. However, if, during Ramadan, they are taken immediately after breaking the fast with large quantities of milk, or directly after the main meal, their efficacy will be substantially impaired.

Fruit juices and carbonated drinks

The large quantities of orange juice and carbonated drinks consumed at the conclusion of the fast may affect the bioavailability and pharmacokinetics of a number of drugs. Such drinks have a markedly acidic pH, in the order of 2 to 4. Consumption of large quantities, of up to a litre at one time, will affect the pH of the gastro-intestinal tract, which may in turn interfere with dissolution of enteric coated preparations, such as prednisolone, and affect the action of antibiotics such as erythromycin base and ampicillin. The activity of such antibiotics may also be reduced as they are frequently taken with meals during Ramadan.

Pharmacists' role in patient compliance during Ramadan

The implications of Ramadan for pharmacy and patient health are valid throughout the Muslim world. Pharmacists require an awareness of the potential difficulties Ramadan poses with respect to prescribed medication regimens. Pharmacists have a key role, not only in counselling patients on their medication, to ensure patient concordance with dosage regimens, but also in recommending to prescribers, products such as slow release preparations and drugs with longer half-life, which enable continued treatment during fasting.

Faced with a fasting patient, for whom one has just dispensed a medicine with a frequent dosing schedule, what does one do? Many patients will wish to fast even though they are technically exempt, and attempts to persuade them to break their fast by taking the medication may well prove futile. In such a situation, the pharmacist could, in addition to informing the patient's general practitioner, have recourse to religious advice from the local mosque.

Information resources

Pharmacists should be aware of Muslim patients' informational needs during Ramadan. This requires an awareness of when Ramadan starts and finishes each year. This information can be obtained from the local mosque along with the exact timings that the fast starts and finishes for each day for the whole month. Larger mosques, like Christian cathedrals, are fully staffed during office hours, and a mullah would be pleased to offer advice to pharmacists and patients.

Given the implications of Ramadan to patient health, we believe that this information should also be published in appropriate medical and pharmaceutical journals.

CONCLUSION

The concept of pharmaceutical care requires pharmacists to assume responsibility for ensuring optimal therapeutic outcomes for patients. To achieve this requires a flexibility to respond to patients' individual needs, which in turn requires pharmacists' awareness of the multicultural population they serve, promoting appropriate use of medicines.

A cultural and religious sensitivity is central to adoption by pharmacists of a holistic model of primary care encompassing health promotion, health maintenance and disease prevention. Misunderstandings stemming from differences in language or cultural perspective can result in sub-optimal care and poor therapeutic outcomes.

FURTHER READING

Apter, A.J., Reisine, S.T., Affleck, G., Barrows, E. and Zuwallack, R.L. (1998) Adherence with twice daily dosing of inhaled steroids. Socioeconomic and health-belief differences. *American Journal of Respiratory Critical Care Medicine*, **157**, 1810–1817.

Bhugra, D. and Bhui, K. (1998) Psychotherapy for ethnic minorities: issues, context and practice. *British Journal of Psychotherapy*, **14**, 310–326.

Hawthorne, K., Mello, M. and Tomlinson, S. (1993) Cultural and religious influences in diabetic care in Great Britain. *Diabetic Medicine*, **10**, 8–12.

Jesson, J., Sadler, S., Pocock, R. and Jepson, M. (1995) Ethnic minority consumers of community pharmaceutical services. *International Journal of Pharmacy Practice*, **3**, 129–132.

REFERENCES

Ahmad, W.I.U. (1992) The maligned healer. The 'Hakim' and Western medicine. *New Community*, **18**, 521–536.

Aslam, M. and Assad, A. (1986) Drug regimens and fasting during Ramadan: a survey in Kuwait. *Public Health*, **100**, 49–53.

Aslam, M. and Healy, M.A. (1986) Compliance and drug therapy in fasting muslim patients. *Journal of Clinical and Hospital Pharmacy*, **11**, 321–325.

Aslam, M. and Wilson, J.V. (1992) Medicines, health and the fast of Ramadan. *Journal of the Royal Society of Health*, **112**, 135–136.

Aslam, M. and Wilson, J.V. (1997) Pharmacists, medicine and the fast of Ramadan. *Pharmaceutical Journal*, **259**, 973–975.

Barber, S.G. and Wright, A.D. (1979) Muslims, Ramadan and diabetes mellitus. *British Medical Journal*, **2**, 675.

Beshyah, S.A., Jowett, N.I. and Burden, A.C. (1990) Metabolic control during Ramadan fasting. *Practical Diabetes*, **9**, 54–55.

Cherrah, Y., Aadil, N., Bennis, A, Bechekroun, Y., Gay, J.P., Soulaymani, R., Hassar, M., Brazier, J.L. and Ollagnier, M. (1990) Influence of the time of administration on the pharmacokinetics of an SR preparation of theophylline during Ramadan. *European Journal Pharmacology*, **183**, 2122.

Commission for Racial Equality (1992) *Race Relations Code of Practice in Primary Health Care Services*, Commission for Racial Equality, London.

Daghfous, J., Beji, M., Louzir, B, Loueslati, H., Lakhal, M. and Belkahia C. (1994) Fasting in Ramadan, the asthmatics and sustained release theophylline. *Annals of Saudi Medicine*, **14**, 523.

Department of Health (1991) *The Patients' Charter: Raising the Standard* HMSO, London.

Hakkou, F., Tazi, A. and Iraki, L. (1994) Conference report Ramadan health and chronobiology. *Chronobiology International*, **11** 340–342.

Health Education Authority (1996) *Folic Acid and the Prevention of Neural Tube Defects – Guidelines for Health Service Purchasers and Providers*, Health Education Authority, London.

Hillier, S. (1991) The health and health care of ethnic minority groups In G. Scrambler (Ed.) *Sociology as Applied to Medicine*, Bailiere Tindall, London.

Langford, E.J., Ishaque, M.A., Fothergill, J. and Touquet, R. (1994 The effect of the fast of Ramadan on accident and emergency attendances. *Journal of the Royal Society of Medicine*, **87**, 752–761.

Malik, G.M., Mubarik, M. and Hussain, T. (1995) Acid peptic disease in relation to Ramadan fasting: a preliminary endoscopic evaluation *American Journal of Gastroenterology*, **90**, 2076–2077

Marmot, M.G. (1989) General approaches to migrant studies: the relation between disease, social class and ethnic origin. In J.K. Cruickshank and D.G Beevers (Eds.) *Ethnic Factors in Health and Disease*, Wright, London, p 15.

Rashed, A.H. (1992) The fast of Ramadan. *British Medical Journal*, **304** 521–522.

Reeves, J. (1992) Pregnancy and fasting during Ramadan. *British Medical Journal*, **304**, 843–844.

Rothschild, H. (Ed.) (1981) *Biocultural Aspects of Disease*, Academic Press, New York.

Salman, H., Abdallah, M.A., Abanamy, M. and Al Howasi, M. (1992 Ramadan fasting in diabetic children in Riyadh. *Diabetic Medicine* **9**, 583–584.

Tang, C. and Rolfe, M. (1989) Clinical problems during fast of Ramadan. *Lancet*, **i**, 1396.

Wheatly, R.S. and Shelly, M.P. (1993) Drug treatment during Ramadan. Stopping bronchodilator treatment is dangerous. *British Medical Journal*, **307**, 801.

SELF-ASSESSMENT QUESTIONS

Question 1: Explain how cultural differences affect the patient' response to pharmaceutical care

Question 2: What are the cultural consequences for fasting patients, and what advice should be given to them?

Question 3: How might traditional medicines have an impact on pharmaceutical care today?

Question 4: Discuss the importance of being aware of the patient's culture when providing pharmaceutical care.

KEY POINTS FOR ANSWERS

Question 1:

- Major problems in communication with a patient who does not speak the same language as the pharmacist
- Degree of autonomy shown by the patient
- Barriers that may exist between inter-ethnic communication
- Attitudes towards the health professional
- Patients' perception of illness

Question 2:

- Fasting affects bioavailability and pharmacokinetics of some drugs
- Fasting affects drug compliance as adjustments are often made by the patient
- Important to point out that Islam allows the sick to abstain from fasting
- Islam allows exemption for pregnant, breast-feeding and menstruating women
- To reduce side effects in patients who fast, the use of 'sustained release' preparations is advocated

Question 3:

- Potential for interaction between Asian medicines and more orthodox drugs
- Adulteration of Asian medicines with synthetic substances
- Dangers concerning safety, quality and efficacy of Asian medicines
- Control and regulation of Asian medicines is required

Question 4:

- Culture affects a patient's perception of health and illness
- Differences in morbidity and mortality are evident among different ethnic groups
- Language and communication
- Awareness of the possible use of traditional systems of health care

Parents and Children

Sally Wyke, Sarah Cunningham-Burley and Jo Vallis

INTRODUCTION	290
RECOGNISING WHEN A CHILD MIGHT BE ILL	290
Normality	291
RESPONDING TO SYMPTOMS	292
Doing nothing	292
Non-medication – home nursing and remedies	293
Consultation with a doctor	293
Self-medication	294
USE OF PHARMACISTS	295
Purchasing medicines or seeking advice	295
The pharmacist – an alternative to the general practitioner?	295
CONCLUSION	296
FURTHER READING	297
REFERENCES	297
SELF-ASSESSMENT QUESTIONS	298
KEY POINTS FOR ANSWERS	298

INTRODUCTION

Parents face difficult and complex decisions in caring for their children. They work hard to keep their children healthy and happy, and to care for them when they are ill. Most people have an idea of what it is to be *a good mother* (for it is women who remain the main carers of their children despite changes in the social structure) and most mothers strive to achieve this ideal.

Current health policy in the UK calls for a patient-centred health service, in which the needs of patients are central. A reorientation of health services is demanded, with services delivered, and developed, taking into account patients' perspectives, enabling partnerships between patients and professionals to develop and grow.

Pharmacists, and pharmaceutical care, are a much valued and well-used resource for parents in caring for their children. Community pharmacists are promoted as the *first port of call* for people in their management of minor illness. However, in order to make an effective contribution to meeting the health care needs of parents of young children, pharmacists need to understand the place they, and the medicines or advice to which they provide access, hold in parents' repertoire of responses to illness in their children. They need to understand parents' actions and the wide range of views they hold in order to develop a truly patient-oriented service.

This chapter concerns parents' perspectives in the recognition and management of children's illnesses. It considers the range of ways in which parents recognise and respond to their children's illnesses, the important place held by over the counter (OTC) medicines in the repertoire of responses, and the actual and potential role of pharmacists in supporting parents in the care they provide. As an example, it draws particularly on a qualitative, sociological study undertaken by one of the authors of this chapter (SC-B) who investigated mothers' perceptions of, and responses to, minor illnesses in their children. This is referred to as *'The Cultural Context of Children's Illness'* (CCCI) study (see Box 17.1 for details of the study). The quotations in this chapter derive from the CCCI study unless otherwise stated.

RECOGNISING WHEN A CHILD MIGHT BE ILL

Recognising, identifying and interpreting symptoms and signs of illness, and deciding whether that illness is threatening to a child's overall well-being, is a complex process for parents, which is based on an intimate knowledge of their child in the context of their everyday life. It involves a welter of mundane observations and minor decisions but is a skill which mothers recognise they have. For example, one mother said: *'It's a funny thing with mothers – you can tell when they're [the children] not well.'*

Box 17.1 Methods used in The Cultural Context of Children's Illness (CCCI) study

This rather intuitive knowledge is grounded in two important aspects of their experience – perceptions of normality and certain changes in behaviour. Importantly, the meaning of these '*soft*' non-specific symptoms may be different for mothers and health care professionals.

Normality

Mothers recognise illness and symptoms in their children by using their knowledge of what is normal for their child as well as for children in general, particularly in relation to behavioural symptoms. However, what is considered normal is not a static concept. It differs according to the age of the child, and what is considered normal at different stages of development. For example, a baby not eating is a worrying deviation from normal, and a cause for concern: '*When she was a baby ... she couldn't tell you that she wasn't hungry and you used to worry because you would think there was something wrong with her.*'

By contrast, a toddler not eating may be seen as being normal toddler behaviour, and not anything to worry about: '*He is a wee bit of a picky eater ... depends what kind of mood he's in as to what he eats.*'

In addition to being related to common sense knowledge about development, mothers' concept of normality is also based on their unique knowledge of their own child or children: they know if something is wrong because the child differs from his or her normal self. Mothers also make different judgements based on their knowledge of their different children: '*She gets kind of cross if she is getting anything. C used to get off his food for a whole week and ... he was bad with eating but he went right off it if he was going to be ill. L gets fretty and under the weather, you can tell.'*

Mothers in the CCCI study used understandings of normality in a variety of ways (Box 17.2).

Box 17.2 Mothers' use of understandings of normality

- As a measure of whether or not a child was *'ill'* with a particular condition they had (e.g. the child has a cold, but is not *'ill'* with it, because s/he is still eating and sleeping properly)
- To assess whether the child was sickening with something (e.g. the child is grumpier than usual, which may be a sign that they will become ill)
- To interpret whether an illness was something to worry about or not (e.g. was it a normal childhood illness?)
- To consider whether illnesses, which frequently affected the child, were being experienced normally (e.g. was the child with frequent croup, coughing *'normally'* as he or she usually did with croup?)

RESPONDING TO SYMPTOMS

It has long been recognised that most illness does not come to the attention of health care professionals. Some form of self-care is the most common response to illness for adults caring for themselves and their children alike. Responding to symptoms and signs are a part of their everyday life, and people use past experience of similar symptoms, talk to friends and family, and draw on advice from health professionals and other sources of information (see also Chapter 7). Their decisions and actions are thus based on a range of knowledge, experience and advice. Dean (1986) has suggested four alternative forms of response once symptoms have been recognised, summarised in Box 17.3.

Box 17.3 Four alternative forms of illness behaviour once illness has been recognised (Dean 1986)

- Decisions to do nothing about symptoms
- Self-medication
- Non-medication forms of self-treatment
- Decisions to consult professional providers

Doing nothing

No action is often the first response to signs or symptoms of illness in a child. Mothers often *'wait and see'* what is going on, and whether the changes they notice amount to illness which requires a response.

Rogers *et al.* (1999) have pointed out that *'no treatment'* action can often be an effective way of managing an illness. It may be a way of coping with a set of symptoms in a child, in response to competing pressures. For example, a mother may decide to deal with a child's illness by ignoring it. Often a child feeling a little unwell, will be sent to school or nursery so that alternative arrangements do not have to be made for their care.

No action may also be taken when there is a ready explanation for the signs and symptoms, or when an illness is normalised. For example, a child with a headache and sleepy after a long day outside will be dealt with very differently from a child having a headache and being sleepy for which there is no ready explanation.

Non-medication – home nursing and remedies

Traditional home remedies are no longer commonly used as responses to illness, or they may be used only by older generations. Nevertheless, home care in terms of nursing or curtailing usual activities, for example by dealing with cuts and grazes, providing drinks, encouraging a child to eat or rest, and making a child with symptoms comfortable, and providing attention and care is a common response to illness.

Consultation with a doctor

Consultation with a doctor is the least common response to illness in children. In the CCCI study, professional consultation in response to symptoms and signs noted in the health diaries was recorded only 33 times, which represented only 7.2% of days when something was noticed, and 11.2% of days when action was taken. The advice of a doctor was sought only when symptoms did not clear up, if they worsened, or if the mother felt the child needed immediate attention. For example, one mother said: 'If it didn't clear up, I would go to the doctor, but I like to try and fix them up myself first.'

People learn from experience, and from the experience of others, whether consultation with a doctor is worthwhile (Rogers et al. 1999). Leaving with a prescription having consulted a doctor is often interpreted to mean that the condition was serious enough to consult and that similar experiences should be dealt with in the same way. A randomised controlled trial (Little et al. 1997) found that prescribing antibiotics for sore throats did little to alleviate symptoms, but enhanced patients' belief that they were an effective treatment and their intention to consult again with similar symptoms. Similarly, learning that a doctor may respond to some symptoms and not others when mothers were evaluating whether or not to consult with a set of symptoms was evident in a study carried out in the north-west of England (Rogers et al. 1999). A mother of young children in that study explained: 'I don't take the children to the doctor if they have "bright eyes", because the GPs don't bother as long as they are bright-eyed.'

Thus self-care is a much more common response to children's illness than consulting general practitioners or health visitors. The most frequent response to illness is to self-medicate (or in the case of children, for parents to provide medicines).

Self-medication

Taking, or providing, OTC medicines is the most common response to illness. For example, in a recent, all age, study of lay management of illness and use of services, 549 people in 215 households completed a health diary for up to 28 days (Hassell *et al.* 1998). During that time 53% took an OTC medicine for at least one day. Similarly, in the CCCI study, providing OTC medicine was the commonest response to children's symptoms.

Some mothers did not see themselves as '*medicine takers*' but nevertheless used OTC medicines from time to time, even when they felt cynical about their efficacy. For example:

'Well, I'm not a person for medicines or anything like that. I just let them keep it until it's better. I don't bother ... I never run with medicines or anything like that ... I don't believe in them. I think if you give them too much medicine they cannot fight things ... [but] I've seen me get a bottle of Calpol. I've got a bottle of that a couple of times.'

Only four of the mothers in the CCCI study did not mention medicines or community pharmacists at all. Most mothers felt that had to do *something* for their sick child, even if they did not feel it would do much good. They would hope to relieve their symptoms yet, importantly, would also feel they were being '*good*' mothers by responding *actively* to the situation and *doing something* other than going to see a doctor.

It has been argued that the tangible and consumable nature of medicines gives them symbolic significance. Van der Geest and Whyte (1989) suggest that medicines enable people to help themselves and reduce reliance on professionals. They refer to the '*charm*' of medicines; their charm lying in their very '*concrete*' nature. Through the consumption of medicines, healing itself is objectified. Thus responding to children's illness through providing medicines can be seen as objectifying both the children's healing process and mothers' effort to help the child.

However, it is clear that medicines are not all viewed in the same way. People use a range of OTC preparations in response to a range of symptoms. Vallis (1998) showed that as well as keeping many medicines in their homes and being familiar with wide ranges of brand names, respondents in her study were familiar with the application of different medicines for different symptoms. Medicines kept in the house fell into three, overlapping, categories: basic and special standby medicines; once-off medicines; and regular supplies. Box 17.4 details how these distinctions were used.

It is important to remember that self-medication practice does not mean that people *consult* community pharmacists. We have seen that self-medication is often the first response to the active management of illness, but most people already have a range of medicines in their homes. These include those left over from

Box 17.4 Different medicines viewed in different ways

prescriptions, as well as OTC preparations bought either at a pharmacy or other retail outlet.

USE OF PHARMACISTS

There has been a great deal of interest in the public's use of pharmacists as a *'first port of call'* in their response to minor ailments. Reasons for this include a desire to reduce the NHS drugs bill and to look for cheaper providers of health care. The pharmacy profession itself has also been drawing attention towards the potential and strategic importance of pharmacists as part of the primary health care system. It is therefore important to consider the place that community pharmacists currently hold in the repertoire of responses used by parents in their response to children's illnesses.

Purchasing medicines or seeking advice

From the extent of self-medication in response to illness, it is clear that the *potential* for community pharmacists to interact with parents of young children is great. A study on the nature and process of advice-giving in community pharmacy (Hassell *et al.* 1996) showed that pharmacies are mainly used as a supply source for medicines and other goods. Researchers observed interaction between pharmacy staff and customers: most of the interactions concerned the dispensing of prescription medicines. Only 5% of interactions concerned symptoms being presented to pharmacy staff for consideration.

THE PHARMACIST – AN ALTERNATIVE TO THE GENERAL PRACTITIONER?

In both the CCCI study and the *'Pathways to Care'* study reported by Hassell *et al.* (1998) and Rogers *et al.* (1999), visiting the pharmacist either for advice or to buy medicines was sometimes seen as an alternative to a general practice consultation. A common reason for this in both studies, for adults and children, was to avoid 'bothering the doctor'.

Cunningham-Burley and Maclean (1987) have shown that mothers with young children use community pharmacists in a range of ways:

- For differential diagnosis; as an alternative to the doctor
- As a stepping stone to the doctor
- For the purchase of OTC medicines for self-care

Such varied use suggests dilemmas as well as opportunities for community pharmacists. It also demands that the pharmacist is aware of the expectations of the parent of a young child consulting them, has knowledge of their understandings of illness, and is conscious of what the parent may have already done for their child.

CONCLUSION

This chapter has shown that parents, particularly mothers, actively observe their children and manage their symptoms and signs of illness. They use their intimate knowledge of their children to assess the risk of illness in terms of perceptions of normality and behaviour change. If a child is ill, a wide range of strategies to manage and contain the symptoms are used, including doing nothing (watching and waiting); home nursing and the use of OTC medication. A consultation with a general practitioner may be a rare response.

Community pharmacies, on the other hand, are a valued resource, as a source of OTC medication, and occasionally of advice. Community pharmacists can be seen as an alternative to the doctor, mainly because parents are concerned not to 'bother the doctor', but they may also act as a route into more formal primary care services.

However, whilst pharmacists are seen as experts in drugs, they are not necessarily seen as an alternative to a GP for *diagnostic advice* (nor do pharmacists want that role). Vallis *et al.* (1997) suggest that community pharmacists are held in high regard, but that people have low expectations of them. Pharmacists are not expected to be a '*primary care resource*', rather they are expected to be available for the purchase medicines and other goods, and to be available for advice or medicines as and when required.

In many ways, pharmacists are viewed as an alternative source of *medicines* rather than an alternative source of *advice*. Thus, pharmacists are not necessarily viewed as part of formal primary care services

(Hassell *et al.* 1998), but are a valued element of lay responses to illness. They operate at the *interface* between lay people and other health care professionals, supporting lay responses to illness.

FURTHER READING

Rogers, A., Hassell, K. and Nicolaas, G. (1999) *Demanding Patients? Analysing the Use of Primary Care,* The Open University Press, Buckingham.

Wyke, S. and Hewison, J. (1991) *Child Health Matters,* Open University Press, Buckingham.

REFERENCES

Cunningham-Burley, S. and Maclean, U. (1987) The role of the chemist in primary health care for children with minor complaints. *Social Science and Medicine,* **24,** 371–377.

Dean K. (1986) Lay care in illness. *Social Science and Medicine,* **22,** 275–84.

Hassell, K., Harris, J., Rogers, A., Noyce, P. and Wilkinson, J. (1996) *The Role and Contribution of Pharmacy in Primary Care.* Summary Report, National Primary Care Research and Development Centre, Manchester.

Hassell, K., Rogers, A., Noyce, P. and Nicolaas, G. (1998) *The Public's Use of Community Pharmacies as a Primary Health Care Resource,* The Royal Pharmaceutical Society of Great Britain, London.

Little, P., Gould, C., Williamson, I., Warner, G., Gantley, M. and Kinmonth, A.L. (1997). Reattendance and complications in a randomised trial of prescribing strategies for sore throat: the medicalising effect of prescribing antibiotics. *British Medical Journal,* **315,** 350–352.

Rogers, A., Hassell, K. and Nicolaas G. (1999) *Demanding Patients? Analysing the Use of Primary Care,* The Open University Press, Buckingham.

Vallis, J. (1998) *Consumers' Views of Community Pharmacists in a Scottish Commuter Town.* Ph.D. Thesis, Queen Margaret College, Edinburgh.

Vallis J., Wyke S. and Cunningham-Burley, S. (1997) 'She's good that one down there'. Views and expectations of community pharmacy in a Scottish commuter town. *Pharmaceutical Journal,* **258,** 457–60.

Van der Geest, S. and Whyte, S. (1989) The charm of medicines metaphors and metonyms. *Medical Anthropology Quarterly*, 3 345–367.

SELF-ASSESSMENT QUESTIONS

Question 1:   What has research told us about some of the ways in which parents recognise and respond to illness in their children?

Question 2:   What place have community pharmacists had in parents' responses to children's illness?

Question 3:   How could community pharmacists develop patient centred services for parents of young children?

KEY POINTS FOR ANSWERS

Question 1:

- Parents base their response on an intimate knowledge of their child, through a welter of mundane observations and minor decisions
- Parents' knowledge is grounded in perceptions of what is normal for their child, and in observation of changes in behaviour which may be indicative of underlying illness
- Parents may respond in a variety of ways to illness: they may do nothing (they wait and see), they may also use home nursing, they may consult a doctor or they may try OTC medicines
- Consultation with a doctor is rare

Question 2:

- Pharmacies are mainly used as a source for medicines and other goods. Only rarely are they a source of solicited advice about symptoms
- Visiting the pharmacist is an alternative to 'bothering the doctor' to access medicines or rarely advice
- Pharmacists are held in high regard as experts in drugs, but people have low expectations of them in relation to advice on symptoms

Question 3:

- Pharmacists could recognise that they are not viewed as part of the formal primary health care team in the same way as doctors or health visitors
- Instead, they are a valued element of lay response to illness
- In giving advice about taking or purchasing medicines, pharmacists should recognise that parents are experts in their children's illnesses, and ground the advice in the everyday life of the family. For example, if a parent seeks a cough medicine for symptomatic relief, the pharmacist could ask when the cough is most troublesome, and advise taking the medicine accordingly

18 Pregnancy and Breastfeeding Mothers

Lolkje de Jong-van den Berg and Corinne de Vries

INTRODUCTION	302
DRUG TERATOGENICITY	302
History	302
Drugs and the unborn child	303
Drug use before pregnancy	304
Drug use during the first trimester	304
Later stages of pregnancy	304
HOW IS SAFETY DETERMINED?	305
DRUG USE IN PRACTICE	305
Prescribed drugs commonly encountered in pregnancy	305
DRUGS AND LACTATION	306
CLASSIFICATION SYSTEMS	306
THE PHARMACIST'S ROLE	308
Prevention of birth defects	308
Folic acid	308
Lactating mothers	309
CONCLUSION	310
FURTHER READING	310
REFERENCES	310
SELF-ASSESSMENT QUESTIONS	311
KEY POINTS FOR ANSWERS	312

INTRODUCTION

In the community or in hospitals, pharmacists are frequently asked questions concerning the safety of specific drugs during pregnancy. For instance, prescribers may ask them which is the least teratogenic drug when medication is essential for pregnant women who have diabetes or epilepsy, or they may consult on the use of oral contraceptives during lactation. In many cases it is difficult to obtain adequate information on drug safety during pregnancy or breastfeeding from commonly used pharmacological textbooks or formularies. Most available information for both health care workers and consumers is that on standard product information leaflets often stating: *'use in pregnancy is not recommended unless the potential benefits justify the potential risks to the foetus'*. Nonetheless, pharmacists will be required to provide appropriate information to prescribers and users of medicines. This chapter discusses drug use and safety during pregnancy and the sources of information in this field.

DRUG TERATOGENICITY

Teratogenicity or reproductive toxicity has been defined as: *'the capability of a substance to interfere with developmental and reproductive processes'*. The manifestation of these effects can vary from infertility to spontaneous abortion, intra-uterine death, premature birth, low birth weight, birth defects, pre- or postnatal growth delay, and functional disorders (Box 18.1). The effects can be seen immediately at birth or will be detected at a much later time (Rubin 1995).

Box 18.1 Teratogenic drug effects

- Spontaneous abortion
- Major structural defects
- Minor structural defects
- Functional defects
- Prenatal growth retardation
- Postnatal growth retardation
- Developmental retardation
- Behavioural disorders

History

The history of drug registration in most developed countries has been strongly influenced by the thalidomide tragedy. Thalidomide was the first drug that was recognised as teratogenic. At the end of the 1950s thalidomide was marketed as a hypnotic and anti-emetic drug which could be used safely during pregnancy. It was available in approximately 30 countries, and known by 51 different trade names. In some countries it was available as an over the counter (OTC) drug. Shortly after its launch, a dramatic increase in the frequency of a previously rare birth defect, phocomelia (severe limb reduction) was seen. In addition to limb defects, the 'thalidomide children' had a number of other malformations such as ear, eye, heart, and renal defects. Because the limb reduction was immediately visible at birth and had been seen so very rarely in the past, the link with thalidomide was made relatively easily and early in its history (McBride 1961). Nevertheless, more than 5,000 thalidomide children were born before the association was detected and the drug was withdrawn from the market in 1961.

Ten years later, problems with another drug illustrated how difficult it can be to study or detect drug teratogenicity. Diethylstilbestrol (DES), a drug that was prescribed to prevent miscarriages, was found to cause vaginal carcinomas in daughters of women who had used DES during pregnancy. This was not detected until some 15 to 25 years after their mothers had used DES (Herbst *et al.* 1971).

These unexpected adverse drug reactions prompted regulatory authorities to demand a series of extensive toxicological tests on animals and humans to be performed, prior to drug registration for market approval. While these procedures provided much information on drug safety in general, they failed to solve the problem that had led to their introduction: how to ensure the safe use of drugs during pregnancy. Clearly, there are ethical constraints with performing experiments of drug teratogenicity in humans.

Drugs and the unborn child

The discovery that a rubella infection during pregnancy can lead to blindness in the new-born, and subsequently the discovery of thalidomide's teratogenicity, have demonstrated the incorrectness of the formerly common assumption that the placenta is an impermeable barrier between mother and child. With the exception of very few examples, most drugs taken by pregnant women cross the placenta and enter the bloodstream of the unborn baby. Exceptions are insulin, heparin, and curare, all of which are drugs with an extremely bulky molecular structure (Rubin 1995).

The effect that a drug can have on the unborn baby depends on a number of issues (Box 18.2). The first three issues all determine the amount of a drug to which the unborn child is exposed. The fourth relates to the timing of the exposure.

Box 18.2 Issues influencing the effects of drugs on unborn babies

- The drug's pharmacological/physiological properties
- The amount taken by the mother
- The length of time over which the drug is taken
- The stage, or trimester, of pregnancy during which the drug is taken

Drug use before pregnancy

Some drugs can be teratogenic even if they are taken long before pregnancy occurs. For example, the anti-psoriasis drugs acitretin and etretinate are stored in the fatty tissue and can damage the unborn child, even if pregnancy does not occur until several months after the drug therapy has ended. Further, certain types of cytostatics that are taken before conception may affect the genetic material of men's semen or women's ova, causing spontaneous abortion or harm to the foetus even at this early stage (Shepard 1992; Schardein 1993).

In the first two weeks after conception, when the cells are not yet differentiated, exposure to teratogenic drugs follows the '*all-or-nothing*' principle. This means that exposure can either cause early embryonic death, or has no harmful effect at all and is followed by a completely normal (although sometimes delayed) development of the embryo (Rubin 1995).

Drug use during the first trimester

During the first trimester of organogenesis all organs and limbs are formed in the unborn child. In this first phase of pregnancy, the unborn child is most susceptible to drugs that may cause birth defects (structural malformations). In cases where structural malformations in a newborn are suspected to be a teratogenic drug effect, drug exposure has to have been within the time span of the first 18 to 55 days of pregnancy. For information about exposure to drugs, pharmacy records are very useful because they contain a great amount of detail, such as the date of dispensing a medication, the brand that was dispensed, and the prescribed dosage. Research has demonstrated that obtaining additional information from the women who were prescribed a drug may be useful in determining (non)adherence and OTC drug use.

Later stages of pregnancy and post-birth

When given in the second or third trimester, teratogenic drugs may still cause disorders of growth and function, especially in the brain. These effects are rarely fatal but they can delay growth and cause mental retardation, or behavioural effects such as hyperactivity, brief attention span, or temper outbursts. Finally, drugs taken by the mother in late pregnancy, or during breastfeeding, can cause other problems. Since the immature body systems of the newborn baby, particularly in premature infants, cannot metabolise or eliminate medicines like the mother's systems, small amounts of drug can accumulate in the baby. For example, repeated doses of diazepam taken by the nursing mother may cause sedation in her infant, especially when her baby is premature. As a consequence, drug-induced problems such as respiratory failure and sedation can occur (Bennett 1996).

HOW IS SAFETY DETERMINED?

For obvious ethical reasons there are few randomised, placebo-controlled clinical trials to evaluate the efficacy and safety of drugs in pregnancy. Studies of aspirin in the prevention of pre-eclampsia, studies of folic acid in the prevention of neural tube defects and some small studies of antihypertensive agents are exceptions to this rule. Currently, two methods are used to determine the safety of drugs when taken during pregnancy: experimental studies in laboratory animals, and observational epidemiological studies.

Experimental teratogenicity studies in laboratory animals are required by the registration authorities (EMEA, FDA and MCA) for all drugs that are submitted for market approval, to determine the effects on the reproductive system, such as male and female fertility, on conception and implantation of the embryo; development of the foetus; birth; and health and survival of the offspring. However, although animal studies can provide valuable information on a drug's pharmacological properties, they are of limited value in assessing safety during human pregnancy. A drug that is teratogenic in one species may have little or no effect in another. For example, aspirin and corticosteroids are teratogenic in animals, but not in humans. On the other hand, thalidomide is much more toxic in humans than in animals. Genetic differences may influence the teratogenic response and, therefore, the effects of many drugs in human pregnancy remain unknown when they are first given to human subjects.

It follows that, in almost every instance, new drugs are inevitably released on the market with little knowledge on their safety in human pregnancy. Consequently, knowledge about the safety and efficacy of the drug in human pregnancy has to be derived gradually from experience in practice. This information comes from epidemiological studies.

DRUG USE IN PRACTICE

Prescribed drugs commonly encountered in pregnancy

Although it is generally agreed that women should avoid using medicines during pregnancy unless it is absolutely necessary, many do take medication while pregnant. At the end of the 1980s, under the auspices of the World Health Organisation's European office, the Collaborative Group on Drug Use in Pregnancy set up an international multi-centre study to assess drug use in pregnancy across various cultural and health care settings. A total of 14,778 women from 22 countries were involved in the study (de Jong-van den Berg 1992). Results indicated that during pregnancy 86% of the women received an average of 2.9 different drugs. There were marked inter-country variations in prescribing habits. Most drug use comprised iron preparations (55% of the women) and vitamins (46%). Anti-infectives were taken by

17% of the women, followed by analgesics (15%), immunologicals (14.5%), cardiovascular drugs (13.5%), gastrointestinal drugs (11.6%), hormonal preparations (8.1%), drugs that act on the central nervous system (5.2%) and asthma drugs (3.3% of the women). From this and other studies, it is known that some drugs used during pregnancy are suspected, or known, to be teratogenic. In some of these cases, the women and the health professionals were unaware of the pregnancy at the time of treatment. In other cases, the risk may have been unavoidable because of a serious condition that requires pharmacotherapeutic treatment (such as epilepsy, diabetes, or hypertension). Alternatively, a woman who was unaware of the teratogenic risk associated with the drug, took the drug without the physician's or pharmacist's knowledge. It is important to avoid the use of potentially toxic drugs in pregnancy entirely if safer products are available, as is the case with, for example, tetracycline.

DRUGS AND LACTATION

The full consequences for the baby, of maternal drug use during lactation remain uncertain. It is well known that women use a variety of drugs, especially in early lactation. Generally, drugs that are prescribed to nursing mothers include analgesics, laxatives, vitamins, antibiotics, antiemetics, sedatives and tranquillisers. However, it is best to avoid or minimise dispensing such drugs to a nursing mother since most drugs will find their way into breast milk to some extent. The fact that some drugs (for example diazepam and metoclopramide), if taken by a breast feeding mother, can harm an infant is beyond any doubt. It must also be acknowledged that certain medicines pose no threat to the breastfed infant, and their use by the mother should not be a reason to stop breast feeding. For most drugs, however, neither safety for the infant nor the quantity excreted in the milk is known.

Some drugs may influence the process of lactation by decreasing or increasing milk yield. Oral contraceptives, which are sometimes used after birth to delay the next pregnancy, can impair the production of milk and decrease the duration of breastfeeding. On the other hand, neuroleptic and anti-emetic drugs enhance milk yield. This is recognised as an unintended side-effect of these drugs. Consequently, there is a trade-off when drugs are used during lactation, and a realistic risk assessment of the drug has to be made since breastfeeding provides the best nutrition possible for the baby and it also protects against many infectious diseases.

CLASSIFICATION SYSTEMS

As a consequence of the need for pharmacotherapy in some women of childbearing age, health care professionals and women need to be informed about the risks and beneficial effects of drug treatment during pregnancy. Since the beginning of the 1980s classification systems have been introduced in the USA, Sweden and Australia (LINFO 1993; Briggs 1998). Information from both animal, and epidemiological studies is used in these systems to classify drugs according to their safety in pregnancy (Box 18.3). The aim is to provide guidance for prescribers and pharmacists when they have to advise on drug choice in cases where pharmacological treatment during pregnancy is essential. These systems divide drugs into categories of teratogenicity, according to the degree of risk to the foetus and are primarily based on knowledge in humans.

Category A	Drugs which have been taken by a large number of pregnant women and women of childbearing age without any proven increase in the frequency of malformations or other direct or indirect harmful effects on the foetus.
Category B	Drugs which have been taken by only a limited number of pregnant women and women of childbearing age without an increased incidence of malformations or other direct or indirect harmful effects on the foetus. As experience of effects of drugs in this category in humans is limited, results of reproduction toxicity studies in animals are indicated by allocation to one of three subgroups:
Group B1	Studies in animals have not shown any evidence of an increased incidence of foetal damage.
Group B2	Studies in animals are inadequate and may be lacking, but available data show no evidence of an increased occurrence of foetal damage.
Group B3	Studies in animals have shown evidence of an increased occurrence of foetal damage, the significance of which is considered uncertain in humans.
Category C	Medicinal products which, by their pharmacological effects, have caused, or must be suspected to cause, harmful effects on the human foetus or neonate without being directly teratogenic. These effects may be reversible.
Category D	Medicinal products which have caused an increased incidence of foetal malformations or other permanent damage in humans. This category comprises drugs with primary teratogenic effects.
Category X	Drugs that have such a high risk of causing permanent damage to the foetus that they should not be used in pregnancy or in women who may become pregnant.

Box 18.3 The concept of a risk classification system

Box 18.4 summarises the Swedish classification system for drug safety during breastfeeding (LINFO 1993). Nursing mothers who need to use drugs can be advised to use drugs from group I or II.

Group I	The substance is not excreted into breast milk
Group II	The substance is excreted into breast milk but is not likely to influence the child when therapeutic dosages are used
Group III	The substance is excreted into breast milk in such quantities that there is a risk of influence on the child when therapeutic dosages are used
Group IVa	It is not known whether the substance is excreted into breast milk
Group IVb	Information on the excretion of the substance into breast milk exists but is insufficient for assessment of the risk to the child

Box 18.4 Categories of drug safety during lactation (Swedish system)

The pharmacist's role

Pharmacists play a distinct role in advising women of childbearing age on drug use. Since they dispense and sell medication and are in contact with the users and prescribers of medicines, they can help to prevent birth defects, advise on drug use during pregnancy and lactation, and provide information regarding the (timing of) drug exposure in epidemiological teratogenicity studies.

Prevention of birth defects

Primary prevention of birth defects can be defined as the use of methods to eliminate the origin of a birth defect, in contrast to secondary prevention, which focuses on the prevention of the birth of a child that has been diagnosed with a birth defect. The primary prevention of birth defects can be achieved when a drug is identified as a teratogenic agent and is not approved, is restricted in use, or is removed from the market. When thalidomide was recognised as the probable causal factor of the increased prevalence of phocomelia, removal of this drug from the market resulted in the disappearance of these specific birth defects. Other drugs that are known to be teratogenic, such as vitamin A derivatives and some anti-epileptics, are very beneficial to specific patient groups, and consequently, remain on the market. In these cases, health care professionals such as pharmacists have to prevent pregnant women, or even better, women of childbearing age, from using these drugs. Changing or, in some cases, stopping treatment temporarily may help to avoid risks of drug-induced birth defects. Pharmacists have the tools available to them to provide prescribers, as well as fertile and pregnant women, with sound advice on drug use in pregnancy, using their knowledge of drugs' pharmacological properties, the international classification systems, and teratology information centres.

Folic acid

We have discussed how drugs can cause birth defects and what possible preventive measures are available. However, sometimes a drug can actually reduce the risk of birth defects. A recent example is the discovery that folic acid use from one month before conception and until the third month of pregnancy can reduce the risk of neural tube defects (NTDs) in the new-born. It has been estimated that, if 0.4 mg of folic acid is taken daily during this time period, the risk of NTDs decreases approximately sevenfold. Since folic acid is in fact a vitamin (vitamin B11) that is present in our daily food intake (albeit in lower quantities than 0.4 mg daily), it has been suggested that food be fortified with folic acid. However, in many countries there are legal constraints to doing this (theoretically, taking large quantities of folic acid may mask symptoms of pernicious anaemia, which would then impose a risk on another part of the population). In these countries, women are advised to take folic acid supplements from one month before conception up to and including the first two months of pregnancy.

Since future mothers are such a healthy group and since they have to be informed so specifically and typically just before they get pregnant, it has been difficult to inform women about this health advice. Pharmacists can play a role here. Typically, health care workers including midwives and physicians are not aware of a (possible) pregnancy until the end of the first pregnancy trimester, or even later. At that time, it is too late to provide advice on folic acid use. Women should be informed of the beneficial effects prior to pregnancy. While this can be done by physicians, pharmacists can also play a role, for example, through information leaflets or label information on dispensed (oral) contraceptives (Box 18.5). Other examples of preventive effects from drug use during pregnancy are: adherence to asthma treatment, treatment of diabetes, and treatment of epilepsy. In these cases, the disease actually bears more risk than the treatment, and adequate treatment reduces the risk of birth defects in these populations.

Box 18.5 Printed text on the box of oral contraceptives	'If you decide to discontinue using the pill and to become pregnant, before your pregnancy please ask your pharmacist about folic acid use'

Lactating mothers

Most drugs cross over into breast milk to some extent, but in most cases this is no reason to discontinue breastfeeding. Pharmacists can advise the nursing mother as well as the general practitioner that mothers who are breastfeeding should avoid a few drugs, such as benzodiazepines, tetracyclines, and aspirin. In other cases, advice regarding the dose of a drug or the timing in relation to breastfeeding is sufficient to avoid any adverse effect.

CONCLUSION

In summary, for most drugs, little is known about effects on offspring of their use during pregnancy and lactation. As a consequence, health care workers have to be cautious with the use of pharmacotherapy in fertile and pregnant women, and question the need for medication use during pregnancy. This includes drug use before and during labour. Initially, one should look for non-drug solutions for discomfort or pain during pregnancy and lactation.

In this chapter, information sources that can be consulted for teratogenicity information have been indicated. In cases where medication use is a necessity, these information sources will provide guidance on the choice of drugs that have been used widely and that are proved safe during pregnancy (category-A drugs or if these are not available, category-B drugs). In addition, if a pregnancy occurs unexpectedly, these sources can provide information regarding potential teratogenic effects of drugs that have been taken before or during the first trimester. If needed, such effects can be specifically monitored for. To prevent such situations from occurring, pharmacists can play a role by regarding every woman of reproductive age as a potentially pregnant woman. When dispensing category-D (and X) drugs, they should give the following warning on the (inner) medication box: *'If you are intending to become pregnant, please consult your physician for an alternative treatment for this medication'*.

FURTHER READING

Bennett, P.N. (1996) *Drugs and Human Lactation* (2nd Edn.) Elsevier Amsterdam.

Briggs, G.G., Freeman, R.K. and Yaffe, S.J. (Eds.) (1998). *Drugs in Pregnancy and Lactation. A Reference Guide to Fetal and Neonatal Risk* (5th Edn.) Williams and Wilkins, Baltimore.

Gilstrap, L.C. III and Little, B.B. (1988) *Drugs and Pregnancy* (2nd Edition). Chapman and Hall, London.

Koren, G., Pastuszak, A. and Ito, S. (1998) Drugs in pregnancy. *New England Journal of Medicine*, **338**, 1128–1137.

Rubin, P.N. (Ed.) (1995) *Prescribing in Pregnancy* (2nd Edn.) BMJ Publishing Group, London.

Schardein, J.L. (Ed.) (1993) *Chemically Induced Birth Defects* (2nd Edn.) Marcel Decker Inc., New York.

REFERENCES

Bennett, P.N. (1996) *Drugs and Human Lactation* (2nd Edn.) Elsevier, Amsterdam.

Briggs, G.G., Freeman, R.K. and Yaffe, S.J. (Eds.) (1998) *Drugs in Pregnancy and Lactation. A Reference Guide to Fetal and Neonatal Risk* (5th Edn.) Williams and Wilkins, Baltimore.

Herbst, A.L., Ulfelder, H. and Poskanzer, D.C. (1971) Adenocarcinoma of the vagina. Association of maternal stilbestrol therapy with tumor appearance in young women. *New England Journal of Medicine*, **284**, 878–881.

Jong-van den Berg, L.T.W. de (1992) *Drug Utilisation Studies in Pregnancy: What Can They Contribute to Safety Assessment (Dissertation)*. Styx, Groningen.

LINFO (1993) *Classification of Medicinal Products for Use During Pregnancy: The Swedish Systems*. LINFO, Drug Information Ltd, Kungsbacka, Sweden.

McBride, M.G. (1961) Thalidomide and congenital abnormalities. *Lancet*, **2**, 1358.

Rubin, P.N. (Ed.) (1995) *Prescribing in Pregnancy* (2nd Edn.) BMJ Publishing Group, London.

Schardein, J.L. (Ed.) (1993) *Chemically Induced Birth Defects* (2nd Edn.) Marcel Decker Inc., New York.

Shepard, T.H. (Ed.) (1992) *Catalog of Teratogenic Agents* (7th Edn.) The Johns Hopkins University Press, Baltimore.

SELF-ASSESSMENT QUESTIONS

Question 1: A woman enters your pharmacy with a question: what are the risks of enalapril (an antihypertensive drug) use during pregnancy? What is your response?

Question 2: You dispense acitretin (a drug for psoriasis) to a 25-year old woman. Do you give her any advice regarding potential pregnancy?

Question 3: You receive a telephone call from a man who enquires about effects of minocyclin (a tetracycline antibiotic drug) on spermatogenesis. He uses this drug against acne, but wonders whether he should stop using it now he and his partner want to try to have children. What is your response?

Question 4: A young mother asks for advice about the use of oral contraceptives while breastfeeding her baby. She wants to know which oral contraceptive can be safely used. What is your response?

Key points for answers

Question 1: Find out why she asks the question:
– *retrospective advice* – has she been using it and is she already pregnant? In that case, there is no evidence for teratogenic effects within the first trimester, so do not alarm needlessly.
– *prospective advice* – does she want to get pregnant and does she consider discontinuing treatment? In that case, alternatives are available that are known to be safe. Additionally, advice about folic acid use could be given.

Question 2: Acitretin use should be discontinued at least 2 years before a pregnancy occurs. It is important that female users in the age group 15–45 are well aware of this and the advice should be provided when the drug is dispensed, combined with a warning label on both the inner and outer packaging.

Question 3: Tetracyclines are teratogenic due to their effects on bone and teeth development. Little is known about the effects on spermatogenesis. However, since the drugs are widely used and no alarming reports have been published regarding mutagenic effects of these drugs, there is no direct reason for potential fathers to stop using them. It could also be argued, however, that in this case the drug is used for cosmetic purposes only and that, to be on the safe side, it could be discontinued temporarily. EMEA's web site reports on drug effects on spermatogenesis, if available. Additionally, advice about folic acid use could be given.

Question 4: The use of combined oral contraceptives can decrease the production of milk especially in early lactation. Some textbooks recommend the use of progestagen-only pills, others assert that combined oral contraceptives do not influence breastfeeding when started more than 6 weeks after delivery. In some countries the use of combined oral contraceptives is recommended from the second month of delivery.

19

The Elderly and their Carers

Ruth Goldstein

INTRODUCTION	314
THE ELDERLY POPULATION	314
Elderly people and their medication: the potential problems	315
Living conditions of the elderly	315
Carers of the elderly	316
ACCESS TO PHARMACEUTICAL SERVICES	317
Accessing pharmaceutical services	318
PHARMACEUTICAL SERVICES	318
Medication management	318
Pharmaceutical services to the elderly	319
Extended pharmaceutical services to the elderly	321
Domiciliary visits	321
Repeat prescribing services	321
Pharmacy clinics in non-pharmacy premises	323
Pharmacy telephone help lines	324
Services to residential homes	324
CONCLUSION	324
FURTHER READING	324
REFERENCES	326
SELF-ASSESSMENT QUESTIONS	326
KEY POINTS FOR ANSWERS	327

INTRODUCTION

This chapter deals with the delivery of pharmaceutical services to the elderly. Elderly people deserve particular attention in the context of pharmaceutical care for two reasons. First, as the body ages it ceases to function as efficiently as previously and physical and cognitive disabilities may develop. Second, access to services may be problematic due to these physical and cognitive disabilities, so the standard service provision may not be adequate for the elderly. This chapter will cover, in general terms, the physical and cognitive effects of ageing which result in this sector of the population being 'in need'. It will then explore why access to services is particularly problematic for the elderly population. The final section will consider particular services that have been, and are being, developed for elderly people.

THE ELDERLY POPULATION

It is recognised that people aged 75 years and over are more likely than the general population to take prescribed or purchased medicines. Ageing results in altered pharmacokinetics and pharmacodynamics and consequently elderly people have a greater susceptibility to drug-related problems. Furthermore, poly-pharmacy and iatrogenic disease are more prevalent in the elderly. These factors, together with impairment of cognitive and physical function may result in their failure to use medication appropriately.

When medicines are prescribed, the intention is to improve the patient's quality of life. There is, however, always an element of risk associated with medicine taking, which may result in a diminished quality of life, or a less than optimal pharmaceutical outcome. Sub-optimal pharmaceutical outcomes often lead to hospital admission and these have been found to be most prevalent amongst elderly people living alone, those taking two or more medications or those receiving no assistance with their medication. Five main causes of sub-optimal outcome following the incorrect use of medicines have been identified (Box 19.1).

The provision of specific pharmaceutical services, such as medication reviews and domiciliary visits, can ensure that these potential problems do not lead to poor outcomes.

Box 19.1 Five main causes of sub-optimal outcome following the incorrect use of medicines (Hepler and Strand 1990)

- Inappropriate prescribing
- Inappropriate delivery (e.g. medicine not available when needed or a carer fails to administer the medicine)
- Inappropriate behaviour by the patient (e.g. compliance-related problems)
- A patient idiosyncrasy
- Inappropriate monitoring (e.g. failure to monitor the effects of the treatment regimen on a patient)

Elderly people and their medication: the potential problems

Many elderly people and their carers cannot cope with the complexity of medication regimes. Reduced visual and cognitive capacity, combined with memory loss, increase the likelihood of a medication error, whilst child resistant packaging may prove a problem among those lacking manual strength and dexterity. Additionally, the small size of printing on containers, closures and labels is a hindrance to those with reduced visual capacity. Moreover, purchased over the counter (OTC) medicines may interact with prescribed medication. Many of these factors contribute to the extent to which a carer is required to assist an elderly dependant, and whether prescribed medication instructions are followed.

It seems reasonable to assume that people are more likely to use medicines correctly if they are given information in a language they understand. Explanation and reinforcement of dosage instructions on container labels are essential to avoid the misinterpretation of instructions, leading to uneven and inappropriate spacing between doses. A carer's requirement for information about prescribed medication begins once the general medical practitioner writes a prescription. It may be worthwhile encouraging patients and carers to write down information during consultations, thereby helping them to form a mental image to recall the medication regimen. Certainly, the combination of written and oral advice, together with repetition and reinforcement, is generally considered to be a most effective method for improving the ability to recall important information.

Living conditions of the elderly

Elderly people live in a range of different types of accommodation, summarised in Box 19.2.

Box 19.2 Living arrangements for elderly people

* In own home, with or without a spouse
* In home of a relative or friend
* In supported accommodation, for example a warden-controlled flat, with or without a spouse
* In residential homes
* In nursing homes
* In hospital

The type of accommodation largely reflects an individual's physical and cognitive status. Most people who live in their own homes are generally able to cope for themselves, with possibly some daily or weekly support from family members, friends or formal carers such as home carers and community nurses. As a person becomes more frail or socially isolated, perhaps following the death of a partner, supported accommodation, such as the home of a family member or warden-controlled accommodation, provides the advantage of maintaining the elderly person's independence, but with the advantage that they have someone *'looking out for them'*. More physically and cognitively frail elderly people tend to move to more caring residential settings, where carers, including home carers, nurses and doctors will take an active role in looking after the elderly person. As frailty increases, so too do the demands on health and social services.

The domiciliary arrangements for the elderly can impact on how they receive pharmaceutical services. If a person lives at home, they are likely to control their own health care provision, although they may rely upon services which are accessible from their own home, such as domiciliary visits by health personnel. Elderly people in residential care settings tend to rely upon the staff in the institution to monitor their health care needs, and access to pharmacy services is often through a carer. The effects of this on the type and nature of pharmaceutical services provided for an elderly person are discussed throughout the remainder of this chapter.

Carers of the elderly

Most of us are reliant upon the support of carers as we go through life. Children rely heavily on their parents for all their needs, teenagers like to think they can cope alone, but most will take a parent along with them when visiting their doctors. Young married people will *'care'* for one another, for example a wife may go to the pharmacy on her husband's behalf when he has a cold, to get some treatment. Prompting one another to take medication is a familiar part of cohabiting. Older people place varying demands on carers, depending on their own health status and the care available to them. Informal carers, such as partners, siblings, children and friends fulfil a major role in supporting the elderly. However, the level and type of support are often more complex, in terms of time commitment and necessary skills such as nursing care, than informal carers can provide. Furthermore, as marriages fail and family structures break down, older people, whose partners are no longer alive, place a great demand for support on the formal care service. A summary of formal carers and services that most often support elderly people is provided in Table 19.1.

Perhaps one of the most obvious, but incorrect assumptions, is to expect all persons requiring pharmaceutical services to visit a community pharmacy. The elderly may in fact, encounter difficulty in accessing a community pharmacy. In such circumstances, pharmacists should consider the needs of carers and assess whether a domiciliary service should be provided.

Type of carer/service	Type of support provided
Home carers	Personal care, social support and domestic support
Nurses	General health care, including bathing, changing dressings, supporting incontinence problems
Chiropodist	Foot care
Counsellors	Bereavement support
Social workers	Housing issues, financial advice, social issues
Doctors	Medical care
Occupational therapists	Mobility care
Pharmacists	Medication management

Table 19.1 Formal carers supporting elderly people

ACCESS TO PHARMACEUTICAL SERVICES

There has never been an accurate figure placed on the numbers of people who access pharmacy services on a daily basis. However in the late 1980s, it was estimated that in excess of six million people visit a community pharmacy daily in the UK. This figure does not take account of the telephone enquiries received by pharmacists, nor any of the additional services pharmacists provide that result in pharmaceutical services being delivered outside the pharmacy premises.

So what services do patients and carers receive from pharmacists? Before listing these, it is important to realise that pharmacists, because they are accessible to the public, fulfil more than a health care advisory and supply role. They often become a key member of a community, whether working in a primary or secondary care environment. The familiarity that comes with being accessible, means that pharmacists serve as a friend, an expert on medicine related issues, a counsellor, and a sounding board for all health and social care issues. The main reasons patients use the services from pharmacies are listed in Box 19.3.

- To purchase over the counter medication
- To obtain medication which has been ordered on a prescription
- To seek advice about prescribed or purchased medication (including information about dosage, adverse effects, drug interactions, prices, methods of obtaining supplies)
- To gain health promotion advice (for instance on diet control, smoking cessation)
- To discuss treatments and medication advertised on television, radio, Internet etc.
- To discuss their concerns about health, finance, family matters and general social issues
- To confirm, or otherwise, information they have received from others, such as doctors, nurses and neighbours

Box 19.3 Patients' main reasons for using pharmacies

Accessing pharmaceutical services

Pharmacies are situated in every reasonably sized hospital, in some health centres, and on most high streets. So why is access a problem? It is not a problem in terms of the spread of services. In fact, in some places there is a choice of pharmacies within a very short distance. But for some people this is still not enough. Access requires patients to go to the pharmacy. The patient, carer or other professional health or social care worker is expected to physically attend the pharmacy to receive any of the services outlined in Box 19.3. People can, of course, telephone a pharmacist to receive pharmaceutical support, but this does not adequately replace face to face interaction.

Some patients and carers may have difficulty accessing pharmacy services because they are housebound, chair bound or bed bound or have a language problem. There is also a proportion of people who, although physically capable of getting out and about, have limited access as they rely upon other people to do so.

The problem of access may appear only to be relevant to a small proportion of the population, but it is important to get a perspective on the size of that proportion. In the UK, people aged 65 and over will soon account for approximately 20% of the population. It is generally this group for whom there can be such a problem, as they receive 75% of all prescribed medication and are particularly in need of pharmaceutical support, yet they may experience the most difficulty in accessing pharmacy services.

PHARMACEUTICAL SERVICES

Medication management

Medication management involves a cyclical sequence of events (Figure 19.1). A health related problem needs to be identified and then professional services and support sought. There are a series of stages following this identification that may be carried out by a patient or carer alone, though often in collaboration. Carers may only 'oversee' a situation. For example, it may be a husband and wife team, with one haranguing the other to visit their doctor, or maybe prompting them to complete the course of prescribed medication. Alternatively, a carer may take full responsibility for their dependant's medication management. Effective medication management requires a knowledge of the services available and the treatments they are receiving and access to services and treatments. A summary of the aspects of 'knowledge and usability' are included in Figure 19.2.

If an elderly person resides in a residential or nursing home or in hospital, medication management, and their pharmaceutical support is most often the responsibility of the staff. The pharmaceutical services to residential settings, such as residential and nursing homes

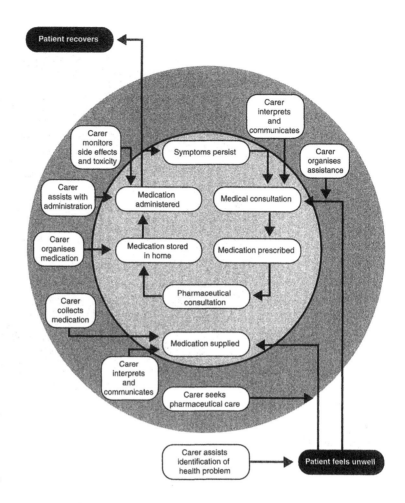

Figure 19.1 The medication management process (Goldstein *et al.* 1993)

and hospitals, are totally different to the services offered to elderly people who live more independently in the community. Pharmaceutical services to residential homes will therefore be dealt with as a separate section within this chapter.

Pharmaceutical services to the elderly

Pharmaceutical services have traditionally been supplied either from registered premises in a community environment, or from a hospital setting. The services have been limited in that everything is provided from within the building. In the community, patients and/or carers must enter the pharmacy to receive their care. In the hospital environment the nurses go to the pharmacy to collect medication and seek the advice required on behalf of their patients.

Hospital pharmacy took a lead in the early 1980s with a move towards *'ward pharmacy'*. The momentum for this change

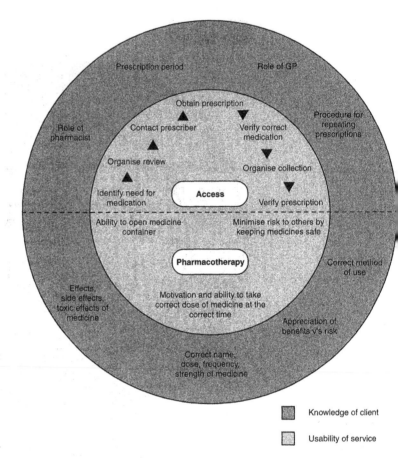

Figure 19.2 The inter-relationship between service usability and the knowledge of the client (Goldstein *et al.* 1993)

Legend in figure:
- Knowledge of client
- Usability of service

Labels in figure:
Prescription period · Role of GP
Role of pharmacist · Procedure for repeating prescriptions
Obtain prescription
Contact prescriber · Verify correct medication
Organise review · Organise collection
Identify need for medication · **Access** · Verify prescription
Ability to open medicine container · Minimise risk to others by keeping medicines safe
Effects, side effects, toxic effects of medicine · **Pharmacotherapy** · Correct method of use
Motivation and ability to take correct dose of medicine at the correct time · Appreciation of benefits v's risk
Correct name, dose, frequency, strength of medicine

was tremendous, and now all hospitals in the UK largely practice a ward-focused pharmacy service. In essence, this means that the pharmacy itself is the point at which medicines are supplied, whilst pharmaceutical advice is offered close to the patients and doctors on the wards.

Pharmaceutical services in the community have lagged behind the hospital model and although there are examples of services being offered away from the pharmacy itself, the current position is that community pharmacies remain the focus of pharmaceutical advice and support in the community. Examples of services that are helping community practices to get closer to patients are provided. However, it should be recognised that not all community pharmacists offer these services. There is no obligation for community pharmacists (other than maintaining their position as community-based experts) to accept the extended roles described below. However, for elderly patients and their carers, the provision of such services is advantageous.

Extended pharmaceutical services to the elderly

Domiciliary visits

The elderly who are unable to access pharmaceutical services may not have the opportunity to discuss their health and medication related issues, face to face, with a pharmacist. Rather, they must rely upon information and advice being provided through their carer. The potential problems of relying upon carers for pharmaceutical related support have been addressed in the residential care sector. In the UK, residential homes are required to register with a pharmacy, and the pharmacist in turn is mandated to visit the home to ensure that residents and carers are provided with appropriate levels of pharmaceutical care. For patients living in their own homes, there is no such formal system and yet there is evidence that carers in primary care often become involved with their clients' medication related needs.

There have been several attempts to implement domiciliary visits by community pharmacists. As awareness of the potential benefits of such services has increased, the impetus to provide domiciliary visits as a standard service has grown and culminated with a resource document being distributed across the country to assist in the establishment of such services.

Evidence suggests that although domiciliary visits may be beneficial to patients and carers there tends to be a poor uptake (Schneider and Barber 1996). Possible reasons for this are listed in Table 19.2.

Repeat prescribing services

The process of repeat prescribing allows patients, on regular treatment, to obtain a specified number of supplies of medication without

Table 19.2 Reasons patients and carers are hesitant to take up the offer of domiciliary pharmaceutical services

Reason	Further explanation
Identify need	Patients and carers have to know domiciliary services are available and have to accept that they may require such a service
Accepting support	As domiciliary services are *'new'*, patients and carers have to be willing to accept the service which may appear to be tailored for particularly *'dependent'* people. Who wants to be classed as dependent!
Non-traditional	This whole role is new to pharmacists, not all are willing to become involved with their patients outside the supportive structure of their shops
Emotion	Some people, who accept that they may benefit from the service, are deterred as they feel uncomfortable allowing the pharmacist access to their home

the necessity of seeing their doctor. This is popular amongst patients as they do not spend time making and attending appointments. Recent research indicates that nearly 50% of patients receive repeat prescriptions, and that the proportion increases with age, with more than 90% of patients aged 85 years and older receiving their medication via repeat prescriptions (Harris and Dajda 1996).

Although repeat prescribing is frequently used as a way of dealing with regular requests for prescribed medication, there is concern that the process for issuing prescriptions does not incorporate adequate controls to ensure that patients are regularly reviewed so that they always receive appropriate medication. For example, one study identified that 66% of repeat drugs were prescribed without the apparent authorisation of general practitioners, and that for 72% of drugs prescribed there was no evidence of a review by a doctor within the previous 15 months (Zermansky 1996).

In addition to clinical issues such as reviewing the appropriateness of medication, there is evidence that a considerable amount of prescribed medication is unused (Rees *et al.* 1993; 1995; Woolf 1996). Within Derbyshire, for example, 1.25 tonnes of unused medicine is collected quarterly from community pharmacies. There is, therefore, a potential anomaly between medication that is prescribed and supplied and patients' drug usage. Since it is accepted that a high proportion of medication is prescribed via the repeat prescribing process, it is a logical conclusion that a proportion of prescribed medication is not used by patients.

One way of reducing drug wastage as a result of repeat prescribing is to implement a repeat dispensing service, whereby repeat medication is obtained through a process operated by community pharmacists, rather than general practitioners. Anecdotal evidence suggests that some patients and general practitioners are in favour of such a scheme. However, implementation of the scheme requires a fundamental change in professional roles for pharmacists and general practitioners, which as yet, has not been widely accepted. An alternative to such a system is to develop existing roles by incorporating a more proactive approach by pharmacists.

A number of ways of involving pharmacists in the system have been tried, and include services such as:

- Pharmacists reviewing patients' requests for prescriptions when they are left at the doctors' surgeries
- Reviewing general practitioners' notes for patients, who are known to use the repeat process
- Using pharmacists' records to review medication supplies to patients using a repeat process

All the systems can potentially, identify patients who either may be suffering through a lack of monitoring or who have been receiving medication for several years without actually seeing their general practitioner.

There are a range of issues which may be revealed by involving the pharmacist in the repeat prescribing process (Box 19.4).

Box 19.4 Potential problems identified by pharmacists monitoring repeat prescribing

The problems listed in Box 19.4 show why pharmacists' involvement in repeat prescribing can be important, particularly for the elderly. However, such involvement has yet to become commonplace. If pharmacists are not involved in, for example, the reviewing of doctors' notes and repeat prescriptions, they may well be involved in providing *'collection and delivery services'*. This is a process whereby patients can place the order for their repeat medication at the pharmacy. The pharmacist forwards the request to surgery, then collects the prescriptions and dispenses the items. Furthermore, if the patient wishes, the pharmacist may arrange for the medication to be delivered to their home.

The advantages of such a system, for patients who have difficulty accessing services are clear. However, this service presents problems when medication is ordered that the patient does not require. Additionally, the service may be perceived as offering an inducement to patients to use a particular pharmacy for their supplies. Such a direction of business is contrary to pharmacists' professional Code of Ethics.

Pharmacy clinics in non-pharmacy premises

The supply of medicines classed as either Prescription Only Medicines (POMs) or Pharmacy Medicines (P) is restricted to pharmacy premises. However, the provision of *'pharmaceutical advice'* can occur from any site. For instance, pharmacists have occasionally offered *'clinic-like'* services to elderly persons' day centres and the offices of charities for the elderly, such as Help the Aged. The advantage of such a service is that elderly people who have limited mobility can receive pharmaceutical information and advice from a location that they regularly visit. Although there is no remuneration available to pharmacists for provision of such a service, the benefit is in the building up of goodwill and customer contact for the future.

Pharmacy telephone help lines

The advantages of a telephone service to an elderly person who is unable to attend a pharmacy, or a busy carer is obvious. Access to a health care professional without physically being present at the pharmacy can be beneficial. However, such a service is not financially viable for all community pharmacies and therefore a dedicated telephone service is offered only in a few locations. Additionally, elderly patients seeking support through this mechanism may speak to a pharmacist they do not know and who does not have access to their medication records.

Services to residential homes

Since the mid 1980s there has been a requirement in the UK for residential homes to be provided with the services of a named community pharmacist. For this, pharmacists receive an annual fee for the support they provide above and beyond the standard supply of prescribed medication. Pharmacists who serve residential homes must undergo specific accredited training prior to claiming a fee for these services. Each pharmacist determines the exact nature of services delivered. Some of the most common services are outlined in Table 19.3.

The home staff and the pharmacist negotiate the precise nature of services to be provided. As it is a competitive market, pharmacies often lobby residential home staff for their business, and it is up to the individual homes to choose the pharmacy that they feel will best suit their needs. This area of a pharmacist's service has become very competitive. Some pharmacies have specialised into providing these services and others have chosen not to offer such services.

CONCLUSION

This chapter has drawn attention to the specific needs of elderly people in terms of medicine usage and highlighted the potential for services in supporting these needs. This area of pharmacy service delivery is constantly being developed in response to research evidence. Furthermore, structural changes in health care delivery, for example the current emphasis on primary rather than secondary care specialised services, has created opportunities to develop new and innovative services.

FURTHER READING

Audit Commission (1994) *A Prescription for Improvement: Towards More Rational Prescribing in General Practice*, HMSO, London.

Type of service	Details of service
Medication reviews	Pharmacists review the actual medication being prescribed by going through the home's records and offer advice to the staff accordingly
Drug chart reviews	Pharmacists check the drug charts looking for unusual dosage, drug interactions and drugs being administered on a long term basis when not necessary
Administration reviews	Pharmacists check through the home's administration records to advise staff of any administration issues which may be causing problems, such as eye drops being administered at inappropriate times or sedatives being given too early in the evening
Medication storage review	Pharmacists review how medication is stored to ensure that drugs are stored at correct temperature and light conditions. They also check that potential for drugs to be mixed up between patients is avoided
General practitioner clinics	Pharmacists attend GP consultations with residents in the homes and offer advice at the point of prescribing (similar to ward rounds in the hospital environment)
OTC clinics	Pharmacists offer advice sessions to residents and staff to discuss OTC medication. Purchases are not possible, but information and guidance is given
Repeat prescription services	Pharmacists organise, with home staff and GP surgery, that they will take responsibility for the ordering and supply of repeat medication for residents
Staff training	Pharmacists provide educational programmes for staff covering issues such as identifying side-effects, correct administration procedures and common OTC preparations

Table 19.3 Range and description of services pharmacists provide to residential homes

Buetow, S.A., Sibbald, B., Cantrrill, J.A. and Halliwell, S. (1996) Prevalence of potentially inappropriate long term prescribing in general practice in the United Kingdom, 1980–96: systematic literature review. British Medical Journal, **313**, 1371–1374.

Goldstein, R. and Rivers, P. (1996) Informal carers medication role. *Health and Community Studies*, **4**, 142–149.

Goldstein, R., Rivers, P. and Close, P. (1993) Assisting elderly people with medication – the role of home carers. *Health Trends*, **25**, 135–139.

McDermott, D., Carter, P., Deshmukh, A., Carter, D. and Schofield, J. (1997) General practitioners' attitude to additional services by community pharmacists. *Pharmaceutical Journal*, **259**, R39.

Raynor, D.K. (1992) Patient compliance: the pharmacist's role. *International Journal of Pharmacy Practice*, **1**, 126–135.

Secretary of State for Health (1996) *Choice and Opportunity. Primary care: The Future*, HMSO, London.

References

Goldstein, R., Rivers, P. and Close, P. (1993) Good quality pharmaceutical care – implications for carers with elderly dependants. *International Journal of Pharmacy Practice*, **2**, 65–70.

Harris, C.M. and Dajda, R. (1996) The scale of repeat prescribing *British Journal of General Practice*, **46**, 640–641.

Hepler, C.D. and Strand, L.M. (1990) Opportunities and responsibilities in pharmaceutical care. *American Journal of Hospital Pharmacy*, **47**, 533–543.

Rees, J.A., Collett, J.H. and Asher, D.M. (1993) Quantifying the costs of repeat prescribing on multiple item prescription forms *Pharmaceutical Journal*, **251**, 636–638.

Rees, J.A., Collett, J.H. and Asher, D.M. (1995) Cumulative costs of inadvertent excess prescribing on multiple item prescription forms. *International Journal of Pharmacy Practice*, **3**, 209–212.

Schneider, J. and Barber, N. (1996) Provision of a domiciliary service by community pharmacists. *International Journal of Pharmacy Practice*, **4**, 19–24.

Woolf, M. (1996) *Residual Medicines: A Report on OPCS Omnibus Survey Data*, OPCS Social Survey Division, HMSO, London.

Zermansky, A. G. (1996) Who controls repeats? *British Journal of General Practice*, **46**, 643–647.

Self-assessment questions

Question 1: Why are the elderly considered to be '*at risk*' in terms of their ability to manage their medication?

Question 2: Who are the main sources of care for elderly people, and what factors might make these carers have difficulties with their medication roles?

Question 3: What are the key issues pharmacists should think about when devising services for elderly people and their carers?

Question 4: List the advantages and disadvantages of the following services:
a) Domiciliary pharmacy visiting scheme
b) Repeat prescribing scheme
c) Pharmacy telephone hot-line

KEY POINTS FOR ANSWERS

Question 1:

- Physical disability
- Cognitive disability
- Pharmacokinetic and pharmacodynamic changes
- Lack of support
- Lack of motivation
- Poor compliance rates
- Lack of access

Question 2:

Sources of care:
- Nurses
- Home carers
- Family members and friends
- Problems due to access

Factors creating difficulties for carers:
- Inability to comprehend situation
- Having to transfer information
- Time commitments
- Training
- Accepting the role

Question 3:

- Access to service
- Usability of medication regimen
- Simplifying service
- Considering physical and cognitive needs of patients and carers
- Understanding patient's support systems and developing services to compliment these services

Question 4:

a) Domiciliary pharmacy visiting scheme:
   Advantages: patient can be seen in their own environment, pharmacist can spend time concentrating on the needs of each patient without distractions, a full picture can be developed of patients' medication needs.
   Disadvantages: time consuming, patients may not like pharmacists visiting them at home, pharmacists' safety.

b) Repeat prescribing scheme:
   Advantages: saves patients' time, synchronises medication supplies, gives a chance for medication reviews to rationalise supplies.
   Disadvantages: time consuming, open to abuse by pharmacists, may be seen as unethical as it could be considered as an inducement.

c) Pharmacy telephone hot-line:
   Advantages: access to pharmaceutical expertise
   Disadvantages: miss out on non-verbal communication, requires novel communication skills.

20

People with Mental Health Problems

Sally-Anne Francis

INTRODUCTION	330
MENTAL HEALTH SERVICES	330
Treatment	331
Policy guidance on services for people with mental health problems	331
Living with mental health problems	333
Social isolation	334
The stigma of mental health problems	334
Medication adherence	335
Insight and medication adherence	336
Meeting the needs of people with mental health problems	336
Examples of pharmacists meeting the needs of people with mental health problems	337
Developing current services	339
CONCLUSION	340
FURTHER READING	340
REFERENCES	341
SELF-ASSESSMENT QUESTIONS	343
KEY POINTS FOR ANSWERS	343

Introduction

Mental health problems are common in the general population. An international study of 14 countries, that investigated mental health problems in general health care, reported that 24% of the study population had a mental disorder (Üstün and Sartorius 1995). On average, disability levels among primary care patients with mental disorders were greater than disability levels among patients with other common chronic diseases such as hypertension, diabetes and arthritis. In addition, they found a low to moderate correlation between recognition of mental disorder by a primary care physician, and research diagnosis according to standardised criteria, claiming that patients with mental disorder were neither recognised, nor treated sufficiently.

Mental disorders are responsible for little more than 1 per cent of deaths, but account for almost 11 per cent of disease burden worldwide (Murray and Lopez, 1996). The limitations of using mortality statistics as an indicator of a population's health is discussed elsewhere (See Chapter 24). By 2020, it is expected that unipolar major depression will be the leading cause of disease burden for females and throughout the developing regions of the world (Murray and Lopez 1996).

In a national survey in Great Britain (Meltzer *et al.* 1995), one in six adults aged 16–64 years had experienced a mental health problem in the week before being interviewed, most commonly anxiety or depression. Less than 1 per cent of the population had experienced a more severe and complex psychotic mental health problem, such as schizophrenia. Between 1994 and 1996, there was a reported 15% increase in the proportion of women and 19% increase in the proportion of men aged 15 years or more who were prescribed antidepressant medication (Department of Health 1998a).

In the UK, the majority of people with mental health problems are looked after by primary care services. About one in 10 people who consult their general practitioner with a mental health problem, will be referred to specialist services for assessment, advice or for treatment.

Mental health services

Mental health services available in the UK, range from primary care services (including the general practitioner, community nurse and community pharmacist) to the highly specialised hospital services. The primary care services provide the majority of mental health care. People with mental health problems consult general practitioners more frequently than other patients, and about 40% of general practitioner consultations involve mental health problems (Davies 1997).

The most common mental health problems are depression, eating disorders and anxiety disorders. Many will be treated effectively in primary care, and others will require referral to specialist services. Medication and psychological approaches to treatment are used, either alone, or in combination. Annually, depression will affect one woman in every 15 and one man in every 30, and every GP will see between 60 and 100 people with depression, while the majority of the 4,000 suicides committed in England each year, are attributed to depression (Meltzer *et al.* 1995; Department of Health 1999a).

Most people with severe mental health problems such as schizophrenia will be in contact with specialist services. However, about one quarter of patients with psychosis are managed entirely within general practice (King 1992). One study has shown that people who have schizophrenia have a mortality rate 1.6 times greater than the general population and are at nine times the risk of suicide (Harris and Barraclough 1998).

Treatment

In Britain, most psychotropic drugs are prescribed by general practitioners, and most moderate anxiety and depressive disorders are entirely and successfully managed in primary care using medication.

A range of psychological treatments (e.g. cognitive behavioural therapy, anxiety management techniques) have also been shown to be effective in the treatment of mental health problems. Evidence indicates that this therapeutic approach is effective in relieving symptoms and improving functioning. However, a survey of local authorities in the UK who had completed a comprehensive assessment of need, reported that there were unacceptable variations in access to a range of psychological interventions and that there were significant variations in the availability of newer antipsychotic medication (Department of Health 1998b).

Policy guidance on services for people with mental health problems

In the UK, the shift of care for people with mental health problems from large institutions to the community has been ongoing for about 50 years. Lelliott *et al.* (1997) suggested that there have been five influential factors (Box 20.1).

Box 20.1 Factors influencing the shift of people with mental health problems from institutions to the community (Lelliott *et al.* 1997)

- The less restrictive social climate of the 1960s and 1970s
- The exposure of poor conditions and standards of care in some of the large institutions
- Social psychiatry and the impact of psychosocial interventions
- The advent of drug therapy
- The (mistaken) political assumption that community care would be cheaper

A number of policy and guidance documents have been published in recent years, aimed at improving the community care received by people with mental health problems in the UK (Box 20.2).

Box 20.2 Policy documents aimed at improving the community care of those with mental health problems

When the *Care Programme Approach* (Department of Health 1990) was first introduced, critics debated whether the scheme provided increased support to an individual or whether it was just a paper exercise. Others criticised the supervision registers for the vague inclusion criteria and the ill-thought through legal consequences for those included on, or excluded from, the register. The basis of the criticisms was that an increased demand was being placed on services without an adequate increase in resources. However, anecdotally, clinicians have claimed that because of these policies, services have been focused on the more needy patients and have improved the quality of care and supervision of patients in the community.

More recently, the UK government has published the White Paper *Saving Lives: Our Healthier Nation* (Department of Health 1999b), where mental health remains a key focus and the *National Service Framework for Mental Health* (Department of Health 1999a) which proposes a coordinated programme for improving mental health services.

- *Saving Lives: Our Healthier Nation* identified mental health problems as one of its key areas. The main target is to reduce the suicide rate by at least 20% by the year 2010. The document also promotes the ideal of individuals taking responsibility and making decisions about their own and their families' health.
- *The National Service Framework for Mental Health* has set seven standards for the delivery and monitoring of mental health services. *Standard one* is concerned with mental health promotion, reducing discrimination experienced by people with mental health problems and promoting social inclusion. *Standards two and three* address the identification, assessment and meeting the needs of individuals with mental health problems in primary care. *Standards four and five* focus on the care and needs of people with severe mental health problems. *Standard six* addresses the needs of individuals who provide care for people with severe mental health problems (carers). *Standard seven* summarises the action required to meet the target reduction in suicide rates as set out in *Saving Lives: Our Healthier Nation*.

Living with mental health problems

Many adverse factors seem to contribute to, and result from, mental health problems. These may be additive and may interact with genetic vulnerability. Such factors may include family problems, childhood sexual abuse, domestic violence, stress, loss, social isolation and a variety of social and economic pressures. Illicit drug taking and excessive intake of alcohol can exacerbate mental health problems.

Consistently, people with severe mental health problems, and their relatives, have reported preferring community to hospital care. However, one disadvantage of living in the community is the absence of social contacts that had been previously available in the larger long-stay hospitals. Other issues such as coping with the potential stigma of mental health problems and acknowledging their illness, are also pertinent to individuals living in the community. For many severe mental health problems, drug therapy is the most common form of treatment and patients have to cope with managing their medication and the potentially quite disabling adverse effects. Consequently, current providers of care are challenged to develop suitable services in the community to address these concerns.

Social isolation

Many studies have illustrated the social isolation experienced by people with mental health problems living in the community and the subsequent association with a poor outcome. For example, isolation in the home, as well as poor housing, polluted neighbourhoods, crime and inadequate benefits have been factors associated with depression and anxiety in women (Payne 1991).

Many people with serious mental health problems experience disintegration of family relationships, but greatest effects are evident with other social contacts. The size of social networks have been shown to diminish with continued readmissions to hospital.

The stigma of mental health problems

In the UK, there has been wide media coverage of events where people with serious mental health problems have committed public acts of violence, crime or 'deviant' behaviour. Such incidents have questioned the success of community care and resulted in the instigation of crucial reviews and recommendations concerning the care of people with mental health problems in the community (e.g. Ritchie et al. 1994). However, sensationalist publicity can reinforce negative attitudes towards people with chronic mental health problems and enhance the stigma experienced by sufferers. Failure to understand the causes of mental health problems and the associated stigma can result in discrimination and social exclusion.

Stigma is an aspect of a patient's self-conception represented by feelings that other people think less of them, avoid them or feel uneasy with them because of their illness (Hyman 1971). The social order defines stigma by imposing its values of what is deemed acceptable or deviant and such criteria of stigma may vary over time and between cultures (Scambler 1984). Today, psychiatric illness continues to have a negative image, impacting considerably on the lives of people with mental health problems.

'Stigma is thus a social phenomenon that implies a person, an audience, and a set of powerful negative images that connect the two. There is no measurement procedure ... that allows one to establish stigma and differentiate it from social undesirability' (Fabrega 1990).

Although discharge from hospital may remove an initial 'label', it still promotes the individual as having a psychiatric history and therefore not 'normal'. Equally, sufferers in the community who are socially isolated and do not have the opportunity for social interaction with others, have limited means by which to rationalise feelings of suspicion, hostility and anxiety that may develop. It has been claimed however, that the stigmatized person can use the label to their benefit by adopting it as an explanation for their misfortunes in life, hence protecting themselves from social responsibilities (Goffman 1963).

Box 20.3 The stigma of mental health problems

Stigma is a major issue for those suffering mental health problems and their families (Box 20.3). A study of adults in the United Kingdom, revealed that 60% would be embarrassed to consult their general practitioner for depression (MORI 1992). Educational programmes such as the *Defeat Depression* Campaign and *Changing Minds: Every Family in the Land* have been launched with the aim of changing practices and to:

'*Increase public and professional understanding of mental disorders and related mental health problems; thereby to reduce the stigmatisation and discrimination against people suffering from them; and to close the gap between the differing beliefs of health care professionals and the public about useful mental health interventions*' (Crisp et al. 1998).

Medication adherence

One of the most common reasons cited for nonadherence with antipsychotic medication is a high incidence of extra-pyramidal side-effects (EPSE). Sexual disturbance and weight gain have also been reported as important predictors of patients discontinuing their medication. However, not all literature supports a relationship between the presence of adverse effects and nonadherence. Other studies have found that mild side-effects were not associated with nonadherent behaviour. Therefore, simply substituting therapy with an atypical antipsychotic drug, with an improved side-effect profile, may not be sufficient to guarantee complete adherence with drug therapy.

It has been estimated that up to 50% of patients are nonadherent with their oral antipsychotic medication within a few months of discharge from hospital (Weiden and Olfson 1995). A double-blind controlled study also showed that patients with schizophrenia who defaulted on oral medication were also very likely to default on depot (intramuscular injections) medication and that both forms of maintenance medication had similar rates of relapse (Falloon et al. 1978). Box 20.4 illustrates the factors associated with drug nonadherence (see also Chapter 11).

Box 20.4 Factors associated with nonadherence

Poor adherence with antipsychotic medication is related to personal variables such as culture and ethnic group, the patient's experiences, severity of illness, attitudes to treatment, insight into illness, poor relationship between patient and professionals, compulsory admission to hospital and a lack of social support.

Nonadherence does not only represent a patient that resists or lacks the motivation to accept the medication or treatment plan that a clinician offers. Nonadherence may also represent the failure of the practitioner to offer an appropriate clinical intervention that allows a better therapeutic outcome for that individual (See Chapter 11). Nonadherence can be an expression of independence and a judgement about the utility of an intervention.

'The quality of one's life is a personally defined concept and so too are the reasons why a patient refuses to do what is recommended. Appropriate health behavior should be thought of as a behavior that meets the person's goals and achieves some mutually definable outcome' (Liang 1989).

Insight and medication adherence

Lewis (1934) rejected the assumption that those people with mental health problems who had greater insight were more likely to accept treatment. He suggested that a lack of insight may be indicative of a negative view of ill health or disease that may be an advantage in treatment. In a long-term follow-up study of people with schizophrenia, McEvoy et al. (1989) found that patients who were supported by people with an interest in the patients' treatment were more likely to be medication adherent, whether or not they had insight, i.e. whether they perceived themselves as ill or not.

Meeting the needs of people with mental health problems

Due to the heterogeneity within specific mental disorders, patients may present with widely different symptoms and may experience different outcomes despite the treatment prescribed. Therefore, it is recommended that treatment programmes should be individualised for patients so that they receive the most appropriate care. When measuring the outcome of drug therapy, Marder and May (1986) warned that using 'not relapsed' as an indicator of functioning in the community is unacceptable. Many patients experience severe impairment in the community due to personality and environmental influences which reflect the need for other therapeutic approaches alongside drug therapy (e.g. psychotherapy, vocational rehabilitation, family therapy, social skills training). They recommend that drugs should only be used where they are demonstrably effective for an individual and at the minimum effective dose. Psychosocial and pharmacological approaches used together have been shown to have cumulative effects.

It has been suggested that patients, and their carers, should be more involved in their drug therapy and that the role of medication, and the goals of treatment, should be understood. Similarly, the limitations of drug therapy should be clearly explained, i.e. they do not always cure the illness and they do not necessarily alleviate psychosocial and interpersonal difficulties.

Donoghue (1993) investigated the problems, concerns and needs that 81 patients with mental health problems experienced with their medicines while living in community settings. Most patients reported that they received inadequate information concerning their medicines, and that greater access to information would improve their confidence in their medicines. The most frequently cited sources of information were friends or other unqualified people. Patients had reservations concerning their medicines, and more than half reported having stopped their treatment in the past, most frequently because of adverse or unexpected effects that had affected their quality of life. It was recommended that pharmacists could address these needs through providing information and advice, promoting adherence to treatment, encouraging patients to become involved in prescribing decisions, liaising with members of the community mental health team to contribute to prescribing decisions and medication review, improving the continuity of supply, providing compliance aids where appropriate, and providing information and support to patients and carers on obtaining, storing and the administration of medicines.

The United Kingdom Psychiatric Pharmacy Group (UKPPG) has published guidance for pharmacists providing pharmaceutical care for people with enduring mental health needs. The key points of the guidance focused on the differing pharmaceutical care needs of patients depending on the place of care: hospital, at the interface of hospital and community care, and in the community. Box 20.5 shows the pharmacist's roles in providing pharmaceutical care to those with mental health problems.

Examples of pharmacists meeting the needs of people with mental health problems

Kettle *et al.* (1996) reported on the positive contributions of a pharmacist to the pharmaceutical care of patients, as a member of a hospital-based community mental health team. During the 4-month project, clinicians actioned 120 of the 185 recommendations made by the pharmacist. The pharmacist also liaised between the carers of a supported

Box 20.5 Key roles for pharmacists providing pharmaceutical care to people with enduring mental health problems (UKPPG 1995)

residence and their community pharmacist, resulting in the introduction of compliance aids for residents' medication. The results of this project led to a change in the provision of clinical pharmacy services at the hospital with pharmacists consequently participating as members of nine community mental health teams. This has involved these pharmacists taking on the following roles:

- Provision of drug information to all prescribers
- Contributing to drug treatment plans and regular medication review
- Liaison where necessary with community pharmacists
- Provision of information and training on drug-related issues to other health care professionals
- Provision of information and counselling on medicines to individuals and their carers where appropriate

Watson (1997) reported on two local initiatives that had been designed and evaluated to address the pharmaceutical care needs for people discharged from psychiatric hospitals. During this study community pharmacists completed a training programme prior to providing extended services. One of the most valued outcomes of this project were the advisory sessions held by pharmacists in mental health day centres. Taking the advisory role away from the pharmacy was perceived to have additional benefits. The pharmacist did not have to contend with distractions, more reticent members of the group could be encouraged to participate and people were less inhibited in their discussions. Also, the pharmacist was viewed as *'independent'* from the psychiatric team, which was deemed an additional advantage.

The above examples are local projects where enthusiastic pharmacists with a particular interest in meeting the needs of people with mental health problems have demonstrated the positive contribution that they can make to this client group. However, evidence is limited on service models that may be implemented on a wider scale

Maslen *et al.* (1996) investigated the routine involvement of a sample of community pharmacists with people with schizophrenia and their perceived competence in advising this client group. Few pharmacists reported being routinely asked for medication-related advice. The pharmacists also reported being significantly less confident about advising patients with schizophrenia about their medication compared with other chronic illness groups such as asthma, diabetes, hypertension, depression or drug addiction.

Developing current services

A first step for all health care professionals in addressing the needs of people with mental health problems would be to correct stigmatizing attitudes by separating the person from the illness, i.e. by talking about a *'person with schizophrenia'* rather than a *'schizophrenic'* (White 1998).

Health care professionals have a major role in helping individuals with mental health problems, and their families, to understand their illness and its treatment, and to enable individuals to seek local self-help groups, e.g. SANE, MIND, Depression Alliance. As the earlier examples illustrated, it is possible for pharmacists to have a greater role in informing individuals, their carers and other health care professionals about medicine use and its management, for people with mental health problems.

Specialist mental health pharmacy services have initiated innovative services for the provision of medication information for patients and carers. In 1997, the UKPPG instigated a confidential telephone-based service for patients and carers to access information concerning their medication. Also, a specific information web site has been set-up so that information is available 24 hours daily (www.users. zenet.co.uk/nmhe).

The National Pharmaceutical Association (1998) described a number of obstacles that needed to be addressed before an extended community pharmacist role could occur: professionals involved need to accept a sharing of responsibilities, the opportunity must be made available to exchange information, further training must be undertaken in interpersonal skills and identifying medication-related problems.

Maslen *et al.* (1996) acknowledged that while community pharmacists are likely to be in frequent contact with people having mental health problems, they are also likely to have received little formal education or training since registration that focuses on the treatment of people with mental health problems. As part of the UK Government's drive to ensure that all people receive effective treatment, they state that professionals need to be aware of the evidence about what works for whom, that the outcomes of treatment must be assessed properly and reviews of long term drug treatment and psychological interventions must be carried out. Professionals need ready access to the most up to date evidence about cost-effective treatment strategies and the training, education and support to deliver these in an environment where quality matters and it is checked regularly. In the UK, recent plans have been announced by the UKPPG to establish a College of Mental Health Pharmacists. This aims to address the specialist education and training needs of pharmacists to contribute to the care of people with mental health problems at the highest standard.

CONCLUSION

Mental health problems contribute to a large proportion of disease burden worldwide. The majority of people with mental health problems live in the community and are in contact with primary care services. The community pharmacist is one of the primary health care professionals who is in a position to contribute to the care of this client group. About one in 10 people who consult their general practitioner with a mental health problem will be referred to specialist services, where specialist pharmacists may also be in a position to contribute to the care of this client group.

People living with mental health problems may have to contend with problems such as social isolation and stigma. Health care professionals can contribute to reducing the impact of these factors through forging positive relationships with this client group. Medication is a common form of treatment for many people with mental health problems. Studies have demonstrated strategies that pharmacists may adopt to help this client group with their medication, such as monitoring of drug therapy, the provision of information and the opportunity for discussion to help people and their carers understand their medication and cope with adverse effects.

FURTHER READING

Davies, T. (1997) ABC of mental health: mental health assessment. *British Medical Journal*, **314**, 1536–1539.

Pathare, S.R. and Paton, C. (1997) ABC of mental health: psychotropic drug treatment. *British Medical Journal*, **315**, 661–664.

Turner, T. (1997) ABC of mental health: schizophrenia. *British Medical Journal*, **314**, 108–111.

White, K., Roy, D. and Hamilton, I. (1997) ABC of mental health: community mental health services. *British Medical Journal*, **314**, 181–187.

REFERENCES

Crisp, A.H., Kendell, R.E., Bailey, S. and Shooter, M. (1998) *'Stigma' Campaign: Every Family in the Land*, Royal College of Psychiatrists, London.

Davies, T. (1997) ABC of mental health: mental health assessment. *British Medical Journal*, **314**, 1536–1539.

Department of Health (1989) *Caring for People. Community Care in the next Decade and Beyond*, HMSO, London.

Department of Health (1990) *The Care Programme Approach for People with a Mental Illness Referred to Specialist Psychiatric Services*, Joint Health/Social Services Circular HC(90)23/LASSL(90)11, HMSO, London.

Department of Health (1992) *The Health of the Nation. A Strategy for Health in England*, HMSO, London.

Department of Health (1998a) *On the State of the Public Health. The Annual Health Report of the Chief Medical Officer of the Department of Health for the Year 1997*, HMSO, London.

Department of Health (1998b) *Modernising Mental Health Services: Safe, Sound and Supportive*, Department of Health, London.

Department of Health (1999a) *A National Service Framework for Mental Health*, Department of Health, London.

Department of Health (1999b) *Saving Lives: Our Healthier Nation*, The Stationary Office, London.

Donoghue, J. (1993) Problems with psychotropic medicines in the community. *Pharmaceutical Journal*, **251**, 350–352.

Fabrega, H. (1990) Psychiatric stigma in the classical and medieval period: a review of the literature. *Comprehensive Psychiatry*, **31**, 289–306.

Falloon, I., Watt, D.C. and Shepherd, M. (1978) A comparative controlled trial of pimozide and fluphenazine decanoate in the continuation therapy of schizophrenia. *Psychological Medicine*, **8**, 59–70.

Goffman, E. (1963) *Stigma. Notes on the Management of Spoiled Identity*, Englewood Cliffs, Prentice-Hall Inc, New Jersey.

Harris, E.C. and Barraclough, B. (1998) Excess mortality of mental disorder. *British Journal of Psychiatry*, **173**, 11–53.

House of Commons (1990) *National Health Service and Community Care Act*, HMSO, London.

Hyman, M.D. (1971) The stigma of stroke. *Geriatrics*, **May**, 132–141.

Kettle, J., Downie, G., Paln, A. and Chesson, R. (1996) Pharmaceutical care activities within a mental health team. *Pharmaceutical Journal*, **257**, 814–816.

King, M.B. (1992) Management of schizophrenia-the general practitioner's role. *British Journal of General Practice*, **42**, 310–311.

Lelliott, P., Audini, B., Johnson, S. and Guite, H. (1997) London in the context of mental health policy. In: S. Johnson, R. Ramsay, G Thornicroft, L. Brooks, P. Lelliott, E. Peck, H. Smith, D. Chisholm, B. Audini, M. Knapp and D. Goldberg. (Eds.) *London's Mental Health. The Report for the King's Fund London Commission*, King's Fund, London, pp. 33–44.

Lewis, A.J. (1934) The psychopathology of insight. *British Journal of Medical Psychology*, **14**, 332–348.

Liang, M.H. (1989) Compliance and quality of life: confessions of a difficult patient. *Arthritis Care and Research*, **2**, S71–S74 (Abstract).

Marder, S.R. and May, P.R.A. (1986) Benefits and limitations to neuroleptics-and other forms of treatment-in schizophrenia *American Journal of Psychotherapy* **XL(3)**, 357–369.

Maslen, C.L., Rees, L. and Redfern, P.H. (1996) Role of the community pharmacist in the care of patients with chronic schizophrenia in the community. *International Journal of Pharmacy Practice*, **4** 187–195.

McEvoy, J.P., Freter, S., Everett, G., Geller, J., Appelbaum, P. Apperson, J. and Roth, L. (1989) Insight and the clinical outcome of schizophrenic patients. *Journal of Nervous and Mental Disease*, **177** 48–51.

Meltzer, H., Gill, B., Petticrew, M. and Hinds, K. (1995) *OPCS Survey of Psychiatric Morbidity in Great Britain. Report 1*, HMSO, London.

MORI (1992) *Attitudes Towards Depression*, Royal College of Psychiatrists, London.

Murray, C.J.L. and Lopez, A.D. (Eds.) (1996) *The Global Burden of Disease: A Comprehensive Assessment of Mortality and Disability From Diseases, Injuries and Risk Factors in 1990 and Projected to 2020 Summary*, World Health Organisation, Geneva.

National Pharmaceutical Association (1998) *Medication Management Everybody's Problem*, NPA, St. Albans.

Payne, S. (1991) *Women, Health and Poverty*, Harvester Wheatsheaf London.

Ritchie, J.H., Dick, D. and Lingham, R. (1994) *The Report of the Inquiry into the Care and Treatment of Christopher Clunis*, HMSO London.

Scambler, G. (1984) Perceiving and coping with stigmatizing illness In: R. Fitzpatrick, J. Hinton, S. Newman, G. Scambler, and J Thompson (Eds.) *The Experience of Illness*, Tavistock Publications London, pp. 203–226.

United Kingdom Psychiatric Pharmacy Group. (1995) Community care: pharmaceutical care for people with enduring mental health needs. *Pharmaceutical Journal*, **255**, 501–503.

Üstün, T.B. and Sartorius, N. (Eds.) (1995) *Mental Illness in General Health Care*, Wiley, Geneva.

Wahl, O.F. and Harman, C.R. (1989) Family views of stigma. *Schizophrenia Bulletin*, **15**, 131–139.

Watson, P.J. (1997) Community pharmacists and mental health: an evaluation of two pharmaceutical care programmes. *Pharmaceutical Journal*, **257**, 419–422.

Weiden, P.J. and Olfson, M. (1995) Cost of relapse in schizophrenia. *Schizophrenia Bulletin*, **21**, 419–429.

White, P.D. (1998) 'Changing minds': banishing the stigma of mental illness. *Journal of the Royal Society of Medicine*, **91**, 509–510.

Self-assessment questions

Question 1: What are the five main factors which have been suggested to have contributed to people with mental health problems being cared for in the community?

Question 2: What contributions can the pharmacist make to the care of people with mental health problems?

Question 3: What factors have been associated with nonadherence to drug therapy in patients with mental health problems?

Key points for answers

Question 1: Lelliott *et al.* (1997) suggested the following factors:

1. The less restrictive social climate of the 1960s and 1970s
2. The exposure of poor conditions and standards of care in some of the large institutions
3. Social psychiatry and the impact of psychosocial interventions
4. The advent of drug therapy
5. The political assumption that community care would be cheaper

Question 2: Through the provision of information and advice, helping people to understand their illness and its treatment, provision of compliance aids and help in the daily management of drug therapy, monitoring of medication and help in minimising adverse effects, and providing contact details of local self-help groups.

Question 3:

- Features of the medication – form, type, regimen, adverse effects
- Features of the patient – culture, ethnic group, experiences, expression of independence, judgement of the utility of the drug therapy
- Illness severity
- Function of health care professionals – attitudes, relationship with patient
- Features of the patient's environment – living independently, living with family, support available
- Function of therapeutic setting – compulsory treatment, self-treatment programme

21

Injecting Drug Users

Janie Sheridan and Trish Shorrock

INTRODUCTION	346
WORKING IN PARTNERSHIPS WITH OTHER PROFESSIONALS	346
HARM REDUCTION AND HARM MINIMISATION	347
HEALTH NEEDS RELATED TO THE ROUTE OF DRUG ADMINISTRATION	349
Injecting	349
Skin/vein problems	349
Viral infections	349
HIV/AIDS	349
Treatment	351
Hepatitis B	351
How to avoid contracting or transmitting Hepatitis B	351
Harm reduction measures for chronic Hepatitis B sufferers	352
Hepatitis C	352
How to avoid contracting/transmitting Hepatitis C	352
Treatment of Hepatitis C	353
Harm reduction measures for those with Hepatitis C	353
Non-Injection routes of administration	353
HEALTH NEEDS RELATED TO THE DRUG BEING USED	354
DRUG INTERACTIONS	355
POLY-DRUG USE	355
PREMATURE DEATH	355
Overdose	356
PSYCHOLOGICAL AND PSYCHIATRIC MORBIDITY	356
LIFESTYLE-RELATED HEALTH NEEDS	357
Poor nutritional status	357
Poor dental health	357
Respiratory problems	357
Diabetes	358
Epilepsy	358
Hepatic and renal failure	358
SPECIAL GROUPS	358
Pregnant heroin users	358
The homeless	359
THE COMMUNITY PHARMACIST'S ROLE	359
CONCLUSION	360
FURTHER READING	361
CONTACTS	361
REFERENCES	361
SELF-ASSESSMENT QUESTIONS	362
KEY POINTS FOR ANSWERS	362

Introduction

Between September 1999 and March 2000, 31,815 drug users in England presented for treatment, and 40% of them reported having injected drugs in the previous four weeks (Department of Health 2000). This obviously only repesents a proportion of the total number of people who are misusing one or more of a number of illicit drugs, either on a regular basis or in a more *'recreational'* manner, for example occasionally at weekends. Whilst considering illicit drug use then, it is important to remember that not all drug users inject drugs and not all injectors suffer from the health-related consequences of injecting which are described in this chapter.

Drugs may be taken in a number of ways – by mouth, by inhalation (smoking), intranasally (*'snorting'*) or by injecting. Injecting drugs intravenously is the route of administration associated with the greatest risk: the effect is immediate, there is more risk of physical harm and there is increased risk of an overdose. A number of health-related issues arise from injecting substances which are not intended for this purpose, as they are frequently non-sterile and may be contaminated with adulterants (often insoluble), although adulterants are rarely implicated in overdoses. Additionally, the purity of illicit substances varies increasing the risk of overdose. It should be noted that some illegally used drugs are in fact prescribed drugs which have been diverted onto the illicit market. These are often tablets which end up being crushed for injection. Sharing used injecting equipment also carries with it a risk of contracting bloodborne viruses (BBVs) such as Human Immuno deficiency Virus (HIV) and hepatitis B and C.

While injecting drug users (IDUs) will have the same health care needs as the general population, they may also incur health-related problems either due to the drug itself, through injecting, or through lifestyles associated with illicit drug use (Table 21.1).

Most of the drug misusers in contact with community pharmacists are likely to be opiate (e.g. heroin, methadone) or stimulant users (e.g. cocaine, amphetamine). Because the community pharmacy is a conve nient source of sterile injecting equipment, it is likely that many inject ing drug misusers will visit pharmacies to obtain such equipment, so this chapter will focus largely on their needs.

This chapter is by no means exhaustive, but rather focuses on those issues particularly pertinent to UK pharmacists, though the issues covered here will also be applicable to other countries and other health care systems.

Working in partnerships with other professionals

The management of drug misuse in the context of health care involves a multi-professional, multidisciplinary approach. An obvious partner

Health care issues of IDUs	Examples
Those which arise out of the route of drug administration (injecting)	• Those relating to BBVs (HIV, hepatitis), abscesses, phlebitis, cellulitis • Venous and arterial damage
Those which are related to the drug being used	• Respiratory problems in opiate users • Constipation • Poor dentition • Drug interactions • Drug overdose • Psychological or psychiatric problems
Those which relate to the lifestyle of many drug users including poly-drug use	• Poor general health status • Poor nutritional status • Poor dentition • Liver function • Overdose
Special groups	• Pregnancy and contraception • Homelessness

Table 21.1 Health care issues of IDUs

ship is between the pharmacist and the IDU's general practitioner. In the UK, the government has recommended that all IDUs should be encouraged to register with a general practitioner. However, there have been reports of general practitioners not wanting to have drug users on their list (Glanz 1986), in much the same way as some pharmacists prefer not to provide services for this group of patients (Sheridan *et al.* 1996). Nonetheless, all general practitioners are required to provide general health care for all their patients, as should pharmacists.

Drug misusers are often stigmatised in society and sometimes by health care professionals, so an important aspect of health care provision is a non-judgmental, professional service. Pharmacists should develop good working relationships with general practitioners, especially where they are prescribing treatments for the management of drug misuse. Interprofessional feedback is to be encouraged. In addition, a knowledge of local agencies and professional groups is a basic essential, and where appropriate, closer working links should be encouraged. Some of these agencies are listed and described in Table 21.2

HARM REDUCTION AND HARM MINIMISATION

Many individuals who use drugs may be unwilling or unable to stop using them. *Harm reduction* and *harm minimisation* are philosophies which underpin much of the treatment and advice given to drug misusers, i.e. to minimise the harm that drug misusers may incur while continuing to use drugs. Harm reduction has been defined as:

Agency/professional	Description/example
Drug treatment centres	Often known as drug dependency units (DDUs), community drug teams (CDTs). Provide assessment of drug problem and support. May also provide a prescribing service
General practitioners	Provide primary health care, and in some cases management of drug dependence often in 'Shared care' arrangements with DDU's and CDT's
Street agencies	Provide a *'drop-in'* service for people with drug problems. They may be targeted at specific groups such as young drug users, women, steroid users, stimulant users, etc.
Outreach workers	Go out into communities to make contact and provide help for those who would not normally contact traditional services, such as ethnic minorities, prostitutes, steroid users
Social services	e.g. housing support, child care issues
Probation services	e.g. counselling through probation services
Needle exchange	May be offered by pharmacies, but also by other agencies
Self-help groups	e.g. Narcotics Anonymous, family support groups

Table 21.2 Agencies and health professionals involved in the care of IDUs

'*The process of gradually reducing the psychological, social, medical and legal problems to a safer overall level in the context of continued drug misuse. It is an important intermediate and practical goal for drug misusers not able to achieve abstinence. It includes safer injecting and sexual practice to reduce the risk of HIV infection transmission by injecting drug misuse. Harm reduction can lead to harm minimisation and ideally ultimately to abstinence*' (Department of Health 1996).

Providing clean needles and syringes, and a facility for the safe disposal of used equipment through needle exchange programmes, is a harm reduction approach which attempts to reduce the need to share used injecting equipment and therefore reduce the risk of contracting BBVs. Prescribed methadone contributes to harm reduction, in that heroin injectors are given an oral dose of methadone (a substitute opiate) to prevent withdrawal symptoms. This reduces the need to inject, and moves the drug user away from the cycle of criminality, and reduces the risks associated with injecting drug use.

HEALTH NEEDS RELATED TO THE ROUTE OF DRUG ADMINISTRATION

Injecting

There are many hazards associated with injecting drug use. Those covered here are, for the most part, related to intravenous injecting. However, it should be noted that not all injecting drug use is intravenous, possibly due to poor venous access. Some users inject intramuscularly (e.g. for steroid use), while others inject small amounts just beneath the skin surface ('*skin popping*'). Whilst this method does not carry the same risks as intravenous use (such as damage to veins), there remains the risk of acquiring viral or bacterial infections. Pharmacists should be familiar with, and recognise the possible hazards/conditions associated with injecting drug use, as they may be the only primary health care worker who has regular contact with the IDU. They should also be aware of the dangers of injecting in certain areas of the body such as the groin (near the femoral nerve and artery) and the different sizes of needles which are used.

Skin/vein problems

A number of skin and vein problems result from injecting and these are summarised in Table 21.3.

Viral infections

BBVs such as HIV and hepatitis B and C may be contracted by sharing contaminated needles and syringes, as infected blood may remain in the syringe when it is passed between users. IDUs should be discouraged from sharing not only needles and syringes, but also other 'injecting paraphernalia' such as spoons, filters or water used in the preparation of the drug for injecting, as these are possible sources of infection of BBVs, especially of hepatitis C.

HIV/AIDS

Acquired Immune Deficiency Syndrome (AIDS), first recognised in 1981, is caused by HIV. For the UK as a whole, it is estimated that approximately 9% of those known to be infected with HIV (i.e. HIV positive) are injecting drug users (PHLS 2000). Estimates of the proportion of IDUs who are HIV positive, range from less than 1% outside London to 2–8% in London in 1998 (Unlinked Anonymous HIV Surveys Steering Group 1999). Drug misusers as a group are already stigmatised and, in addition to this, a diagnosis of being HIV positive can further increase a feeling of isolation.

Drugs, prescribed or illicit, may have a detrimental effect on the immune system, an important consideration for HIV positive drug users. However, not all IDUs who are diagnosed HIV positive will

Condition	Cause	Signs/symptoms	Treatment
Phlebitis (can lead to 'track marks')	Painless inflammatory response to injecting	Inflammation	Use of different injecting sites gives veins change to recover
Thrombophlebitis	Inflammatory response to injecting	Swollen vein. Possible fever and malaise	Seek treatment
Cellulitis	Bacterial infection of skin and subcutaneous tissues	Reddening of limb, swelling, heat, pain	Seek medical attention
Collapsed veins	Repeated use of same vein, inappropriate injecting technique	Injectors seek other veins. Dangerous if use femoral vein as is near artery and nerve	If artery hit by accident, remove needle, apply pressure, seek medical attention
Gangrene	Impaired blood supply. Can lead to amputation	Pain, loss of feeling in the area, swelling and discoloured skin, coldness, especially fingers and toes	Urgent medical attention needed
Abscesses	Injection of irritant substances and non-sterile injection	Raised lumps in skin – may be sterile or infected	Seek medical attention
Ulcers	Defective blood supply (repeated venous trauma). Impaired vascular supply	Craters of unhealed skin	Seek medical attention
Deep vein thrombosis	Caused by injecting into femoral vein. Periods of immobility e.g. during periods of unconsciousness	Blood clots formed – may end up in lungs and can lead to heart attack. In leg – hot, red and swollen. Soreness	Urgent medical attention needed
Emboli	Due to unfiltered particles being injected	Can end up in the eye, and in the lung leading to breathing difficulties	Urgent medical attention needed
Septicaemia	Injection of bacteria into blood stream	Malaise with unexplained fever	Urgent medical treatment

Table 21.3 Skin and vein problems associated with intravenous injecting

either want, or be able, to cease using either their illicit (or in some cases – prescribed) drugs. What is important is that advice and practical help is available to enable these individuals to practise safer drug use and safer sex. The use of sterile injecting equipment and condoms should always be recommended to prevent the spread of the virus.

Other concerns for HIV positive drug users include the possibility of interactions between drugs taken for treatment of HIV infection and other medication. Both protease inhibitors and non nucleoside reverse transcriptase inhibitors (NNRTIs) are metabolised in the liver and can cause either induction or inhibition of the cytochrome P450 enzyme system, with possible drug interactions occurring with other drugs affected by this route of metabolism, e.g. methadone.

Treatment

Antiretrovirals attack HIV itself and delay or prevent the damage HIV causes to the immune system. They include: nucleoside analogues, NNRTIs and protease inhibitors. Clinical trials have demonstrated that using more than one drug (combination therapy) is more effective. Triple or even quadruple therapy regimens appear to be the treatment schedules of the future. Pharmacists have a role to play in helping patients to comply with complicated medication regimes.

Treating, or trying to prevent, opportunistic infections which occur due to the immune system damage, and restoring or boosting the immune system are other methods used to manage HIV infection. More information, leaflets and advice can be obtained from the Terrence Higgins Trust and Mainliners (see below for details).

Hepatitis B

The term hepatitis means '*inflammation of the liver*', and hepatitis B is an inflammation and infection of the liver caused by the hepatitis B virus. Infection may occur following vaginal or anal intercourse, or as the result of blood to blood contact. The latter can occur by sharing blood-contaminated injecting equipment or by vertical transmission from mother to child.

Generally with an acute attack of hepatitis B, the person feels unwell, tired and loses their appetite, although some people have no symptoms, and infection can only be detected using serological testing. Jaundice occurs in some, but by no means all cases, and many cases may not be diagnosed at all.

In the majority of people, the virus is inactivated by the body's immune system. However, in about 5–10% of individuals the virus persists and these individuals became chronic carriers of the virus. About 15–25% of such carriers may develop progressive liver disease, leading in some patients to cirrhosis.

How to avoid contracting or transmitting hepatitis B

- Avoid unprotected sex
- Use new sterile equipment (as attempts to clean used equipment may not kill the virus)
- Avoid sharing any paraphernalia associated with injecting (e.g. water, cups, spoons, filters, swabs etc.)
- Infected individuals should cover up cuts and clean up any blood spillage safely using bleach
- Do not share implements such as toothbrushes or razors as these might provide direct contact with blood, e.g. through bleeding gums
- There is now a vaccine that protects against hepatitis B which involves a course of three injections. In the UK, government policy allows anyone in a *'high risk'* group to get vaccinated free, although this is often not widely implemented, and drug misusers often find it difficult to comply with the treatment regimen

Harm reduction measures for chronic hepatitis B sufferers

- Keep generally healthy and maintain a balanced diet
- Refrain from drinking alcohol at all, or keep intake to an absolute minimum
- Take precautions to avoid contracting other BBVs, as prognosis is poorer with co-infection
- When taking any drugs, whether prescribed, over the counter or illicit, advice should be sought about the possible effects these might have on the liver

Hepatitis C

Intravenous drug users have emerged as a particularly high risk group for contracting hepatitis C through the sharing of blood-contaminated injecting equipment. It has been estimated that between 50 and 80% of IDU's are hepatitis C positive (British Liver Trust). Sexual transmission of the virus is believed to occur, but risk is considered very low.

The acute phase (1–26 weeks after infection) is a time when few, if any, symptoms are experienced. A minority of sufferers (about 5%) will have jaundice, and some may experience loss of appetite and feel sick and lethargic. However, some may exhibit no symptoms. Approximately 20% of those with acute hepatitis C become virus free and make a full recovery. Eighty per cent go on to the chronic phase, when the virus grows in the liver. A very small minority of those with chronic hepatitis C appear to overcome the infection.

Estimates indicate that 10–20% of those with chronic hepatitis C go on to develop cirrhosis and, in certain cases, cancer of the liver, both of which can prove fatal. No vaccination is currently available against hepatitis C.

How to avoid contracting/transmitting hepatitis C

All the measures covered for hepatitis B apply to hepatitis C and even though the risk of transmission of hepatitis C sexually is believed to be extremely low, the practice of safer sex is still advisable. The main issue involves preventing risky injecting practices, in particular preventing the sharing of injecting paraphernalia. Drug users should also be encouraged to inject in a clean environment, free from blood spillages. Equally important is trying to prevent initiation into injecting. Some studies suggest that the majority of injectors become infected in the first three months of their injecting career.

Treatment of hepatitis C

Acute hepatitis C: A course of Interferon alpha is given for 4–12 weeks. This reduces the risk of progression to chronic infection. However, many people are not aware of being infected during the acute phase and will not receive treatment at this point.

Chronic Hepatitis C: Interferon alpha is given subcutaneously three times a week for an initial six month course. It is believed to slow or stop viral replication. Efficiency varies from nil to sustained remission (the best case scenario). Relapsers usually respond to re-treatment. A combination of Interferon alpha and Ribavirin is now being used on relapsers and those who have a poor response to Interferon alone.

A further development is the possible use of pegylated interferon, which maintains a steady level of interferon in the body for a longer period of time and requires only once a week administration.

Harm reduction measures for those with hepatitis C

- Avoid alcohol consumption altogether. This may be very difficult as it may require major changes in a person's lifestyle
- Avoid paracetamol consumption altogether, if possible
- Avoid co-infection with other BBVs (including other genotypes of hepatitis C and hepatitis D)
- Encourage clients to get vaccinated against hepatitis A and B
- Check use of other drugs: prescribed, over the counter and illicit. As with hepatitis B, certain drugs should be avoided in cases of impaired liver function

More information about all forms of hepatitis, leaflets and advice for IDUs can be obtained from the British Liver Trust (see below).

Non-injection routes of administration

Drug misusers may choose to use alternative routes of administration which carry a number of associated risks as outlined in Box 21.1.

Box 21.1 Risks associated with non-injecting routes of drug administration

Intranasal:	Nose bleeds, ulceration, rhinitis, septal perforation, risk of transmission of hepatitis C if equipment is shared
Inhalation:	Asphyxiation, aspiration, peri-oral dermatitis
Smoking:	Respiratory infection, cough, cancer, accidental burns, chronic lung disease
Oral:	Gastric irritation

HEALTH NEEDS RELATED TO THE DRUG BEING USED

While it is accepted that IDUs are generally less healthy than the general population, not all IDUs suffer serious health-related consequences. Health-related issues may arise from the drugs being used. Complications/problems associated with the specific drug taken may be idiosyncratic or dose-dependent. Idiosyncratic reactions are unpredictable, whereas dose-dependent reactions may be controlled. The purity of illicit drugs can be extremely variable, which makes accurate dosage estimates difficult.

Some specific health problems associated with two groups of drugs – opiates and stimulants – are summarised in Box 21.2 and Box 21.3 respectively.

Box 21.2 Health problems associated with opiates

Respiratory:	Opiates suppress the cough reflex, leading to increased risk of aspiration and bacterial infection. They also depress the respiratory centre in the brain and respiratory depression is the main cause of deaths due to heroin or other opiate overdose. Also, foreign body embolisation (caused by fibres from, for example, cotton wool filters – used to filter out particles before injecting, or particles mixed with the drug such as talc) is also a potential hazard.
Gastrointestinal:	Nausea, vomiting and constipation are all side-effects of opiate use. Tolerance develops to all of these and other dose-related effects, with the exception of constipation.
Cardiac:	Right sided infection – tricuspid endocarditis – has been linked to injection of opiate (and other) drugs. The symptoms include fever, weakness and general fatigue and can also include headaches, night sweats and weight loss. Medical attention should be sought immediately.
Other:	Methadone suppresses saliva production. This, coupled with lifestyle factors such as poor diet, can lead to dental problems. Clients should be encouraged to rinse mouth with water after taking methadone. They should be encouraged to register with a dentist if possible. Amenorrhoea, decreased libido

Cardiorespiratory:	Stimulants activate sympathetic autonomic activity resulting in increased blood pressure and force of myocardial contraction (and vasoconstriction with cocaine) so demand on the heart is increased, whilst the amount of blood it can receive is decreased. These drugs may also cause arrythmias, and may precipitate tachycardias and myocardial infarctions.
Neurological:	Due to raised blood pressure, headaches, strokes and cerebral bleeds may occur. Association with convulsions has been suggested. Amphetamine can also induce a psychotic state in some users.
Respiratory:	Cough, airway burns, problems with nasal septum, sinus infections, shortness of breath, possible worsening of asthma, interference with gaseous exchange.

Box 21.3 Health problems associated with stimulants (cocaine and amphetamine)

DRUG INTERACTIONS

Psychoactive drugs, such as opiates and stimulants, have a number of drug interactions. These drugs may interact in a number of ways, for example CNS depressants (e.g. alcohol, benzodiazepines and tricyclic antidepressants) may increase sedation in those on opiates and decrease respiration, increasing the risk of overdose. Interactions may also occur which alter methadone plasma levels through metabolism, e.g. rifampicin, which causes raised plasma levels. Drugs may affect the excretion of methadone by altering the urine pH. Details of drug interactions with methadone can be found in the new guidelines on clinical management of drug misuse (Department of Health 1999). Drug interactions involving illicit drugs are seldom well detailed (if reported at all), so it is often difficult to obtain accurate information.

It is essential that pharmacists are aware of potential drug interactions when dispensing prescriptions for known or suspected drug misusers. Patients who access a needle exchange scheme or who purchase injecting equipment from a pharmacy are easily identified as potential injectors. However, they may not have informed their doctor about their illicit drug taking. Discreet questioning by the pharmacist may be required in order to ascertain what other drugs they are using, and an appropriate intervention made, being mindful of maintaining confidentiality.

POLY-DRUG USE

Many injecting drug users will be using more than one drug. In a national treatment outcome study, nearly 92% of the initial cohort were poly-drug users (Department of Health 1996). There may be additional complications associated with the combined adverse effects of using the drugs. For example, heroin users may also use benzodiazepines and drink alcohol. Such combinations put the client at greater risk of accidental overdose (see below). While one drug will probably be the primary drug of misuse, the use of other drugs must be taken into account when managing drug users' problems.

PREMATURE DEATH

Injecting drug users are at greater risk of death than those who do not use drugs (ACMD 2000). Death may be due to a number of causes including intentional or unintentional overdose (see below), blood borne viruses, accidents whilst intoxicated.

Overdose

While opiate-related overdoses often prove to be fatal, many are not. In an Australian study, one quarter of a sample of heroin users had experienced a non-fatal overdose in the previous 12 months (Darke *et al.* 1996). These overdoses may be intentional (attempted suicide) or accidental. A number of factors are related to overdose, such as:

- Variable drug purity
- Mixing the drug with other sedating drugs (e.g. benzodiazepines, other opiates, tricyclic antidepressants) and alcohol (see above)
- Loss of tolerance to the drug's effects, due to a break in drug taking, for example while in prison, or after a detoxification

Because of drug users' poor physical health and often poor psychological health, they are particularly at risk of intentional overdose. The number of suicidal and undetermined deaths involving heroin or methadone increased in the UK by 900% between 1974 and 1992 (Neeleman and Farrell 1997). The signs of overdose include those shown in Box 21.4.

Box 21.4 Signs of opiate overdose

- Pinpoint pupils unreactive to light
- Shallow respiration and/or snoring
- Low pulse rate and hypotension
- Varying degree of reduced consciousness/coma

An ambulance should always be called if there is a suspected overdose, and the patient should be placed in the *'recovery'* position. Treatment for opiate overdose is with naloxone. Patients will normally be required to remain in hospital, since the half-life of naloxone is only 60–90 minutes compared to 4–6 hours for heroin and 24–36 hours for methadone. Unless hospitalised, they may slip back into overdose once the effects of naloxone have worn off.

PSYCHOLOGICAL AND PSYCHIATRIC MORBIDITY

There is a high incidence of psychological and psychiatric problems amongst drug misusers, (often known as 'dual diagnosis'), particularly those with chaotic drug-taking habits. However, the direction of causality is often difficult to determine. Many drug users will have turned to illicit drugs as a form of *self-medication* for conditions such as depression. On the other hand, certain drugs such as cannabis, cocaine and amphetamine are associated with psychotic episodes in some individuals. Psychological problems such as depression are also associated with the *'come down'* after chronic use of cocaine, and chronic amphetamine use is associated with negative effects on social functioning. Community pharmacists may be ideally placed to refer individuals with such problems to specialist agencies.

LIFESTYLE-RELATED HEALTH NEEDS

Drug users may suffer from a variety of conditions, such as asthma, diabetes, epilepsy, high blood pressure or hepatic or renal failure. Many drug users are not in contact with primary care professionals, often due to a lack of access. They are sometimes suspicious of health professionals, fearing social service intervention. They are a needy, but under-resourced group. IDUs may be homeless and susceptible to heath problems related to *'rough sleeping'*, e.g. tuberculosis, hypothermia, skin conditions and infestations.

Poor nutritional status

One of the contributing factors to the poor health status of drug users is poor nutrition and the failure to prioritise healthy eating above drug use. They often have limited financial resources, poor access to cooking facilities and a lack of knowledge about nutrition, with many obtaining most of their calorific intake from alcohol. Additionally, stimulant use reduces appetite. It is very important to take the time to discuss nutrition, persuade drug users to register with a general practitioner (if necessary) and to get a health checkup. Opiate users are also likely to be suffering from constipation, so advice on increasing the intake of fibre and fluids (not alcohol), and taking exercise is appropriate.

Poor dental health

Opiates reduce the amount of saliva produced. This has a negative effect on teeth. Coupled with this, methadone preparations may have a high sugar content (depending on the formulation), and be of a low pH, which has a detrimental effect on dental health. In all cases, encouraging IDUs to look after their teeth and register with a dentist is important.

Respiratory problems

IDUs may also take drugs by other routes. Smoked or inhaled drugs are most likely to cause respiratory problems, and hypersensitivity to any drug of misuse (including adulterants) can result in bronchospasm. Smoking cannabis and tobacco impairs gaseous exchange, deposits tar in the lungs and is carcinogenic. Suppression of the cough reflex due to opiate use can predispose individuals to respiratory tract infections. 'Crack' cocaine may produce chronic lung changes, impairing gaseous exchange. This condition is known as 'crack lung'.

Diabetes

Stimulant drugs such as amphetamine, cocaine and ecstasy can all cause a decrease in appetite, which can result in hypoglycaemia if insulin levels are not reduced. Conversely, cannabis may increase appetite and consumption of food (sometimes referred to as 'the munchies'). Diabetic drug users should ideally be referred for specialist advice.

Epilepsy

Convulsions may occur after benzodiazepine withdrawal, although this is rare and usually only takes place with shorter acting benzodiazepines. Cocaine misuse has also been linked with seizures, and convulsions are a known symptom of cocaine overdose. Sudden withdrawal of alcohol in heavy drinkers may also induce fits. Several studies indicate that cannabis may have a protective effect against convulsions.

Hepatic and renal failure

Well-documented cases of hepatotoxicity have occurred with alcohol, ecstasy and anabolic steroids. As most illicit drugs are metabolised by the liver, hepatic failure may allow them to accumulate. Exceptions which are not metabolised wholly by the liver include ecstasy, cocaine and volatile solvents (except toluene).

A metabolite of heroin and morphine is known to accumulate in patients with renal failure. Transferring heroin users to prescribed methadone is strongly advised.

SPECIAL GROUPS

Pregnant heroin users

While IDUs suffer stigma, this is accentuated for pregnant IDUs. Many may experience guilt and concern about the effect of their drug use on their baby. They may also have concerns about their child being taken into care. In the UK, a parent being an IDU is not in itself sufficient reason for a child to be taken into care, and many IDUs are good parents and successfully raise children.

Pregnant heroin users are generally not advised to stop using opiates abruptly, because withdrawal in pregnancy can be dangerous, possibly leading to miscarriage or premature birth. Methadone may be prescribed for those in contact with treatment agencies. Stopping injecting drugs and moving to orally administered drugs is advisable in order to minimise the risks of BBVs, and other injecting-related harms. Pharmacists may want to refer pregnant drug users to drug treatment centres.

One important consideration is that pregnant IDUs may not be in contact with other health care professionals. Pharmacists are in an ideal position to start a dialogue about antenatal care, the need for folic acid intake and good nutrition, and may also help a pregnant IDU to become registered with a general practitioner, where necessary.

The homeless

Research indicates that homeless people experience more health problems than the general population and that they also find the greatest difficulty in obtaining appropriate health care (Bines 1994). Homeless people who are also drug users are even more prone to health problems (Morrish 1993) and those who inject drugs run additional risks of acquiring BBVs, the problems being compounded by the lack of safe and private places to inject.

Drug misuse may have contributed towards an individual becoming homeless, or the drug problem may have occurred or been exacerbated as a result of homelessness, as many people use drugs or alcohol to escape the stress and misery of their situation.

Lack of a fixed address is not a barrier to registering with a general practitioner, although some clinics appear unaware of this, which can be problematic. However, some general practitioners are reluctant to register such patients and this, coupled with a reluctance by homeless people to approach services, means that many such individuals are not registered with a general practitioner. Community pharmacists are often their only contact with primary health care services. As such, pharmacists play a vital role in making contact with a hard-to-reach population. A helpful and non-judgmental attitude by pharmacists may facilitate the homeless drug user and those 'sleeping rough' to access other services.

THE COMMUNITY PHARMACIST'S ROLE

IDUs need a number of things in order to manage their drug use in a healthy manner, the most obvious being clean injecting equipment. Therefore, at the most basic level, meeting the health needs of drug injectors will involve providing them with sterile injecting equipment and a safe way in which to dispose of used injecting equipment, for example, through needle exchange schemes, many of which operate through community pharmacies. In addition, IDUs may need advice and information on how and why they should always use clean injecting equipment and paraphernalia.

Some injectors will be receiving treatment for their drug misuse, such as prescribed methadone for the management of opiate dependence. Methadone is prescribed as a substitute for opiates – usually heroin. Methadone has good oral bioavailability, has a long half-life and therefore can be given once a day. Almost half the community pharmacies in England and Wales provide a methadone dispensing service (Sheridan *et al.* 1996). The prescriber may require the drug to be dispensed daily and in some cases, pharmacists will also be asked to supervise consumption of methadone on the premises, to ensure compliance.

In the UK, community pharmacists have been involved in needle exchange schemes for over a decade. Pharmacies have proved to be ideally placed to provide this service because they are accessible, and most are open for a greater number of hours than drug agencies. Clients might also be worried about being seen entering drug agencies, but using a community pharmacy carries no stigma.

BBVs can be transmitted through unsafe sexual practises. For this reason many needle exchange packs contain advice on safer sex and free condoms. While it may be difficult in the pharmacy to broach this subject with drug using clients, pharmacists should ensure that they also have adequate printed information leaflets on open display. For those being treated for conditions such as HIV, hepatitis and tuberculosis, pharmacists have an important role in monitoring and encouraging compliance. They may also have to explain complex medication regimes, and will have to be vigilant for drug interactions.

Pharmacy-based services should complement those of drug agencies. In some cases it may be appropriate to refer on to such agencies, e.g. if IDUs require advice on safer injecting techniques. Pharmacists should ensure they are aware of local treatment and advice agencies and needle exchange schemes. Ideally they should make contact with such agencies and familiarise themselves with what they offer, and in turn, inform them of the services provided from the pharmacy. Pharmacists should also be aware of issues around privacy and confidentiality; more advice on this can be obtained from the Royal Pharmaceutical Society of Great Britain.

CONCLUSION

This chapters has highlighted a number of health issues relating to injecting drug misuse, which are pertinent to pharmacists. Some of these relate to drug use *per se* and others to the diverse consequences of a drug-misusing culture. These present a number of opportunities for community pharmacists, who may be responsive or pro-active in their interventions. When dealing with IDUs, pharmacists have an opportunity to provide accurate and appropriate health promotion and harm reduction advice, and to provide or display written information about HIV, hepatitis, drug misuse, where to get help, etc. On a one-to-one level, pharmacists should also be aware of the immense impact that positive feedback can have on a drug user.

FURTHER READING

Department of Health (1999) *Drug Misuse and Dependence – Guidelines on Clinical Management*, The Stationery Office, London.

Derricott, J., Preston, A. and Hunt, N. (1999) *The Safer Injecting Briefing*, Hit Publications, Liverpool.

Preston, A. (1996). *The Methadone Briefing*, Andrew Preston/ISDD, London.

Wills, S. (1997) *Drugs of Abuse*, Pharmaceutical Press, London.

CONTACTS

British Liver Trust: 01473 276326
Ransomes Europark, Ipswich, IP3 9QG, UK.
http://www.britishlivertrust.org.uk/

Mainliners: 020 7582 5434/3338.
38-40 Kennington park Road, London SE11 4RS, UK.
http://members.aol.com/linersmain/

PharMag: 0141 201 4891
c/o Kay Roberts, Area Pharmaceutical Specialist – Drug Misuse GGHB, Dalian House, 350 St Vincent Street, Glasgow G3 8YU, UK.

Terrence Higgins Trust: 020 7831 0330
52-54 Grays Inn Road London WC1X 8JU, UK.
http://www.tht.org.uk/

REFERENCES

ACMD (2000) *Reducing drug related deaths*. The Stationery Office, London.

Bines, W. (1994). *The Health of Single Homeless People*, Centre for Housing Policy, University of York, York.

Darke, S., Ross, J. and Hall, W. (1996) Overdose among heroin users in Sydney, Australia: (I) Prevalence and correlates of non-fatal overdose. *Addiction*, **91**, 405–411.

Department of Health (1996) *The Task Force to Review Services for Drug Misusers – Report of An Independent Review of Drug Treatment Services in England*, HMSO, London.

Department of Health (2000) *Statistics from the Regional Drug Misuse Databases for Six months ending March 2000.* National Statistics Bulletin 2000/30, Department of Health, London.

Glanz, A. (1986) Findings of a national survey of the role of general practitioners in the treatment of opiate misuse: views on treatment. *British Medical Journal*, **293**, 543–545.

Morrish, P. (1993) *Living in the Shadows: The Accommodation Needs and Preferences of Homeless Heavy Drinkers*, Leeds Accommodation Forum, Leeds.

Neeleman, J. and Farrell, M. (1997) Fatal methadone and heroin overdoses: time trends in England and Wales. *Journal of Epidemiology and Community Health*, **51**, 435–437.

PHLS (2000) *Communicable Disease Report, Volume 10, Number 4*, Public Health Laboratory Service (PHLS) Communicable Disease Surveillance Centre, London.

Sheridan, J., Strang, J., Barber, N. and Glanz, A. (1996) Role of community pharmacies in relation to HIV prevention and drug misuse: findings from the 1995 national survey in England and Wales. *British Medical Journal*, **313**, 272–274.

Unlinked Anonymous HIV Surveys Steering Group (1999) *Prevalence of HIV in the United Kingdom, Data to End 1998*, Department of Health, Public Health Laboratory Service, Institute of Child Health (London), Scottish Centre for Infection and Environmental Health, London.

SELF-ASSESSMENT QUESTIONS

Question 1: What are the main bloodborne viruses (BBVs) that IDU are at risk of acquiring through sharing injecting paraphernalia?

Question 2: Describe the health advice that pharmacists can give clients who are suffering from these BBVs.

Question 3: What are the physical complications associated with opiate misuse? Briefly describe how they occur.

Question 4: How is poor psychological well-being associated with injecting drug use?

KEY POINTS FOR ANSWERS

Question 1:   HIV, hepatitis B and C.

Question 2:   *HIV.* Good nutrition, advice on therapy, drug interactions, safer sex and safer injecting to prevent transmission of HIV to other individuals.

Hepatitis B and C. Keep healthy, good diet, refrain from drinking alcohol, avoid contracting other BBVs, advice on the effect of drugs on liver, drug interactions, advice on safer sex (hepatitis B), advice on not sharing any injecting paraphernalia with others. Information on hepatis B vaccination.

In addition, for hepatitis C. Avoid paracetamol, avoid co-infection with other BBVs (including other genotypes of hepatitis C) – encourage clients to get vaccinated against hepatitis A and B.

Question 3:   *Direct:* Accidental or intentional overdose, suppression of cough reflex leading to respiratory infections, nausea, vomiting and constipation, right sided infection – tricuspid endocarditis, dental problems, malnutrition.
Indirect: Problems associated with injecting drugs such as cellulitis, endocarditis, abscesses, septicaemia, BBVs.

Question 4:   Discussion should include the fact that poor psychological well-being may predispose an individual to use illicit drugs, or the use of such drugs may precipitate psychological problems. The association between homelessness, drugs and psychological problems. Suicide and intentional overdose. Poly-drug use can exacerbate these problems. Access to health care can be difficult for this client group.

PART SIX

Measuring and Regulating Medicines Use

22 Pharmacovigilance and Pharmacoepidemiology

Corinne de Vries and Lolkje de Jong-van den Berg

INTRODUCTION	368
SPONTANEOUS REPORTING SYSTEMS	370
When to report a suspected ADR	371
Establishing whether an adverse event is an ADR	371
ADVERSE DRUG REACTIONS	373
Type A	373
Type B	373
Type C	374
PHARMACOEPIDEMIOLOGY	374
What is the drug use in a specific population?	374
What are the determinants of drug use?	375
What are the outcomes of drug use (beneficial and adverse effects)?	375
Record of drug use, determinants and outcomes	375
Measuring disease frequency	378
MEASURING DRUG USE	379
STUDY DESIGN	381
Descriptive studies	381
Case-control studies	382
Cohort studies	383
Experimental studies	383
Risk estimates	384
BIAS AND CONFOUNDING	385
CONCLUSION	387
FURTHER READING	388
REFERENCES	388
SELF-ASSESSMENT QUESTIONS	389
KEY POINTS FOR ANSWERS	390

INTRODUCTION

Pharmacovigilance involves the detection of unexpected, and often undesirable, adverse effects of drugs. Pharmacoepidemiology, often considered a sub-domain in pharmacovigilance, attempts to quantify the frequency of these adverse effects, and to identify sub-populations for which there are variations in the magnitude of effects. Until recently, adverse drug effects were of limited concern as it was difficult enough to treat the disease. Reports of adverse drug effects began at the end of the nineteenth century when it was found that the use of chloroform led to an increased risk of cardiac arrest. Table 22.1 lists examples of serious and unexpected adverse effects of drugs that have subsequently been discovered (Meyboom 1998).

Year	Drug	Adverse effect
1880	chloroform	cardiac arrest
1923	cinchophen	hepatitis
1925	bismuth compounds	nicolau syndrome
1933	aminophenazone	agranulocytosis
1938	sulphanilamide (in diethylene glycol)	renal failure
1942	bismuth compounds	hepatitis and renal failure
1946	streptomycin	deafness and renal failure
1952	chloramphenicol	aplastic anaemia
1953	phenacetin	nephropathy
1958	isoniazid	hepatitis
1961	thalidomide	phocomelia
1962	procainamide	systemic lupus erythematosus
1963	gold salts	blood dyscrasias
1964	phenylbutazone and related compounds	aplastic anaemia and agranulocytosis
	aspirin and other NSAIDs	gastrointestinal ulcers and bleedings
1965	barbiturates	addiction
1966	oral contraceptives	thromboembolic disease
1970	phenacetin	urinary tract carcinoma
1971	isoniazid/rifampicin	liver injury
1972	diethyl stilboestrol	vaginal adenocarcinoma
	erythromycin	cholestatic hepatitis
1973	co-trimoxazole	Steven-Johnson syndrome
1974	practolol	sclerosing peritonitis, corneal perforation
1976	glafenine	anaphylactic shock
1979	triazolam	psychosis
1981	fenfluramine	pulmonary hypertension
1984	valproic acid	spina bifida
1996	mefloquine	central nervous system side effects
1997	indinavir	haemolytic anaemia

Table 22.1 Historical examples of ADRs

Some of the examples in Table 22.1 may be familiar. For example, most people will have heard of thalidomide. This product was advocated as safe and specifically suitable for use during pregnancy, but was found to cause limb defects in the newborn child when taken during the first trimester of pregnancy. In 1938, the revelation that diethylene glycol, used as a solvent for sulphanilamide, caused blindness, prompted authorities in many countries to develop a system for monitoring drug safety. In the USA, the Food and Drug Administration (FDA) began to collect case reports of all adverse drug reactions (ADRs) in 1960. In the 1960s, the thalidomide tragedy and, subsequently, the discovery that oral contraceptives increased the risk of thromboembolic disease, precipitated the foundation of the Committee on Safety of Medicine (CSM) in the UK and similar spontaneous reporting systems in Europe.

In the 1990s thalidomide was found to be beneficial in the treatment of leprosy and in some cases, for the treatment of Acquired Immune Deficiency Syndrome (AIDS). This demonstrates that even drugs that are known to be very toxic in certain sub-populations (foetus) can be beneficial in others (people with Human Immunodeficiency Virus (HIV) infection or leprosy).

Drug safety is central to the role of pharmacists, whether they work in a pharmacy, a pharmaceutical company, a health authority, or the government. They may have to advise on drug use or on the introduction or withdrawal of a drug from the market, or establish the likelihood that an adverse event is in fact an ADR. This chapter aims to provide insights into how ADRs are detected, how causality is established, and how studies on drug safety should be interpreted and evaluated.

Pharmacovigilance has been defined by the World Health Organisation (WHO) as '*the detection, assessment, and prevention of adverse drug effects in humans*' (World Health Organisation 1998). The major sources for pharmacovigilance are countrywide reporting systems for suspected ADRs and pharmacoepidemiology studies of specific drugs or adverse events. The major aims of pharmacovigilance are:

- The early detection of hitherto unknown adverse effects and interactions
- The detection of increases in frequency of (known) adverse effects
- The identification of risk factors and mechanisms underlying adverse effects
- To establish quantitative aspects of risks
- The analysis and dissemination of information needed for drug prescribing and regulation

The main information sources for pharmacovigilance are patients, prescribers, and pharmacists. It can be difficult to recognise an ADR.

Therefore, once suspicion has arisen that an adverse event in a patient might, in fact, be an adverse reaction to a drug, how do you decide whether or not this should be reported to a spontaneous reporting system? And how can you establish whether the adverse event is in fact an ADR?

SPONTANEOUS REPORTING SYSTEMS

Since the 1960s, many developed countries have implemented spontaneous reporting systems to perform post-marketing surveillance of drugs. These systems are mostly voluntary. Usually, report forms for ADRs are available in national drug formularies or drug bulletins. Typically, these systems will be able to detect serious and unexpected drug reactions. They can be seen as relatively inexpensive '*early warning systems*' that can signal possible problems with drugs during their entire post-marketing phase. After they are marketed, the drugs are prescribed to a population that may differ to a great extent from the population in which they were tested during the clinical trials, for instance, elderly people, people with co-morbidity patterns that differ from the trial populations, pregnant women or children.

With spontaneous reporting systems, no information is obtained about the number of people that have used a certain drug and the duration of therapy. Therefore, it is impossible to calculate the frequency of ADRs directly, and to compare risks of ADRs between drugs. For this, pharmacoepidemiological studies are needed. These are discussed later in this chapter. Unfortunately, there is a lot of under-reporting with spontaneous reporting systems: 90% of prescribers never report a suspected ADR, and reporting rates are rarely stable over time. Pharmacists report relatively more frequently, but they are less likely to become aware of an ADR because patients usually contact their prescriber and not their pharmacist about adverse events. Reasons for under-reporting have been called '*the seven deadly sins*' (Inman 1986) (see Box 22.1).

Under-reporting leads to a number of problems that are characteristic for spontaneous reporting systems. First, the frequency of ADRs may be underestimated. Second, it may lead to the delayed detection of ADRs. Third, and probably the most significant, under-reporting may not be random but is usually selective. For example, reporting rates on a new drug are usually highest during the first years after it has been introduced onto the market.

To improve reporting rates, many countries have developed ways of feedback to reporters. This feedback may comprise a preliminary evaluation of a reported adverse case, therapy advice on how to deal with the adverse event, follow-up of the report by a telephone call, a personal visit, occasional publication of a case series in scientific medical journals, or the regular publication of recently reported ADRs (Meyboom 1998).

Box 22.1 Reasons for under-reporting in spontaneous reporting systems ('the seven deadly sins')	1 *Complacency*: the mistaken belief that only safe drugs are allowed on the market 2 *Fear* of involvement in litigation 3 *Guilt* because harm to the patient has been caused by the treatment that the doctor has prescribed 4 *Ambition* to collect and publish a personal series of cases 5 *Ignorance* of the requirements for reporting 6 *Diffidence* about reporting mere suspicions which might perhaps lead to ridicule 7 *Lethargy*: a person cannot be bothered to report the ADR

When to report a suspected ADR

Specific guidelines for ADR reporting differ between countries and between spontaneous reporting systems. However, in general, all suspected ADRs should be reported if they are:

- Unexpected, whatever their severity, i.e. not consistent with product information or labelling
- Serious, whether expected or not
- Reactions to recently marketed drugs (i.e. less than five years on the market), irrespective of their nature or severity

Serious reactions are defined as a noxious and unintended response to a drug, which:

- Occurs at any dose and requires significant medical intervention such as inpatient hospitalisation or prolongation of existing hospitalisation
- Causes congenital malformation
- Results in persistent or significant disability or incapacity
- Is life-threatening or results in death

Establishing whether an adverse event is an ADR

Causality can rarely be proven when an adverse event coincides with drug use. Instead, several people have established criteria that can be applied to see how suggestive the potential association between an adverse event and drug use is of causality. Well known among these are the Bradford Hill criteria (Hill 1965) (see Box 22.2).

This is best explained using an example. Suppose an individual uses indomethacin and develops a gastric ulcer. How do we know whether that gastric ulcer occurred as a consequence of indomethacin use? The answer is that we will probably never know for sure, but the Bradford Hill criteria can be suggestive of a causal association. Taking strength (criterion 1) as an example: if the individual has a history of gastric complaints, indomethacin may have been the final '*trigger*' to developing an ulcer, but it may also be that the ulcer has developed irrespec-

Criterion	Explanation by Bradford Hill
Strength	Strong associations are more likely to be causal than weak associations because if they could be explained by some other factor, the effects of that factor would have to be even stronger than the observed association and therefore would have become evident. However, weak associations are not necessarily non-causal. Also, confounding can still be present.
Consistency	Consistency exists if the association is found repeatedly in different populations and under different circumstances. However, lack of consistency does not rule out causality.
Specificity	A true cause leads to a single effect, not multiple effects. This is not a very strong criterion: most drugs have multiple effects. This does not necessarily rule out causality.
Temporality	The cause (drug use) should precede the effect (the ADR) in time. This does not mean that the adverse effect never happens by any other cause than drug use, however (i.e. it can happen due to other causes than drug use, as well).
Biologic gradient	Is there a dose-response relationship? If there is not, there may be a *'threshold'* dose, and if there is, the association may still be confounded, but we often expect a dose-response relationship to exist in the case of causality.
Plausibility	This criterion refers to the biologic plausibility of the hypothesis, although this is often not objective or absolute, and based only on current knowledge and beliefs.
Coherence	The cause-and-effect interpretation for an association should not conflict with what is known of the natural history and biology of the disease. Here, the same concerns apply as for *'plausibility'*.
Experimental evidence	Does removal of the drug (*'de-challenge'*) lead to disappearance of the ADR, and does *'re-challenge'* lead to recurrence of the ADR? If it does, then causality is more likely.
Analogy	Is the association similar to other, well-known associations? If it is, then causality is more likely.

Box 22.2 The Bradford Hill criteria (1965) to assess causality between drugs and adverse events

tive of indomethacin use. However, the association has been found repeatedly in the literature (criterion 2), it is biologically plausible and coherent (criteria 6 and 7), and it is analogous to similar associations between other non-steroidal anti-inflammatory drugs (NSAIDs) and gastric complaints (criterion 9), for instance. The other criteria (e.g. temporality of the association) need to be established within the individual. If indomethacin use began *after* the development of the gastric ulcer, then obviously in this case it is unlikely that the gastric ulcer was an ADR.

After Hill, others developed rules for causality assessment, some of which are used at spontaneous reporting bureaux. The aim of applying such rules is to establish whether a causal association between the drug and the adverse event can be established, and to what degree (World Health Organisation 1998).

ADVERSE DRUG REACTIONS

Three different types of adverse effects are commonly distinguished on the basis of their frequency and how easily detectable they are (Strom 1994; Meyboom 1998).

Type A

These ADRs are usually detected during clinical trials, are typically dose-related, and associated with the drug's pharmacological action. Hence, they are common, predictable, and often less serious than other types of ADR. A typical example of a type A ADR is the development of extra-pyramidal symptoms ('*parkinsonism*') after phenothiazine use. These drugs have anticholinergic properties that account for the beneficial effect in the treatment of schizophrenia. However, their anticholinergic properties also affect other parts of the central nervous system, leading to extra-pyramidal symptoms. Decreasing the dosage may eliminate the adverse effects. However, in some patients this will result in a sub-therapeutic dosage and, consequently, a recurrence of schizophrenia.

Type B

These ADRs result from an allergy-type reaction to the drug. They are usually very severe, often life threatening, and they stand out because they happen very rarely. Usually, the drug must be discontinued when such an ADR happens. A typical example is the development of anaphylactic shock after penicillin use. The body develops an immune response to the drug, and therapy must be discontinued immediately. This type of event is rare and it is usually not detected at the phase of clinical trials, but only at the post-marketing phase. However, because this type of event is so rare and unexpected, the link with the drug that caused it is usually made relatively easily. Therefore, like type A ADRs, type B ADRs are relatively easy to detect. Typically, type B reactions are the type of reactions that are reported to spontaneous reporting systems and published as case reports in the medical literature.

Type C

These ADRs are the most difficult to detect. They are characterised as an increased frequency of '*spontaneous*' disease, occur at random intervals or after a long induction time, and although relatively common can be serious. The connection between the drug and the adverse event, therefore, can be difficult to prove or refute. A typical example of a type C ADR would be the possible association between breast cancer and the use of oral contraceptives. With this adverse event, the prevalence of breast cancer among the general population of women is relatively high, as is the use of oral contraceptives, there is a long time delay before the appearance of breast cancer, the effects are not experimentally reproducible, it is difficult to find a good comparator group and there are multiple causal factors.

As previously stated, spontaneous reporting systems provide early warning signals of adverse drug effects. However, despite mechanisms to assess causality, such as de-challenge (observing the effect of withdrawing a drug) and re-challenge (observing the effect of reintroducing a drug following withdrawal), for instance, suspicions of adverse effects are difficult to prove and the frequency of ADRs cannot be established directly from spontaneous reporting. Additionally, type C effects are hardly ever discovered through spontaneous reporting. To overcome these issues, pharmacoepidemiological studies are needed.

PHARMACOEPIDEMIOLOGY

Pharmacoepidemiology has been defined as: '*the study of the use and the effects of drugs in large numbers of people*'. It is based on two disciplines, clinical pharmacology and epidemiology. Pharmacoepidemiology uses the techniques of chronic disease epidemiology to study the use and effects of drugs (i.e. the content area of clinical pharmacology). Its major application is after drug marketing, to supplement any information about drug effects that is available from pre-marketing trials (Strom 1994).

Pharmacoepidemiology addresses three main issues:

- What is the drug use in a specific population?
- What are the determinants of drug use?
- What are the outcomes of drug use (beneficial and adverse effects)?

WHAT IS THE DRUG USE IN A SPECIFIC POPULATION?

Information on drug use in a population is accessed through prescribers, dispensers, and drug users. These data sources have their own benefits and limitations, such as (in)completeness of data, the (non)availability of information on adherence, of over the counter

(OTC) drug use, and the indication for which the drugs have been prescribed. Ideally, multiple information sources should be used in such a way that the data complement each other.

What are the determinants of drug use?

To achieve rational drug use, knowledge about the factors that determine drug choice or adherence to drugs is essential. For example, we could investigate why intervention methods vary in their effectiveness to influence prescribing, why women use more benzodiazepines than men, and why adolescents are less likely to adhere to their insulin therapy than other diabetic patients. With such information and with insight into underlying health beliefs, interventions in drug use can be adequately targeted.

What are the outcomes of drug use (beneficial and adverse effects)?

Finally, we are interested in the effects of drug use. Are the drugs effective in treating the disorder for which they have been prescribed, and can we establish risk estimates for the adverse effects associated with their use? Can we define sub-populations for which drugs are less appropriate? This provides the basis for decision-making at several levels of health care: prescribing, drug formularies, reimbursement policies, and market approval.

Figure 22.1 illustrates the basic approach in pharmacoepidemiology: we study the relationship between the exposure of individuals and subsequent outcome. The exposure, in pharmacoepidemiology, is usually drug use, whereas outcome is the adverse (or unexpected) effect. However, in studies of drug use determinants, drug use is the outcome whereas determinants such as age, gender, or socioeconomic status can be the exposure of interest.

Figure 22.1
The concept of pharmacoepidemiology

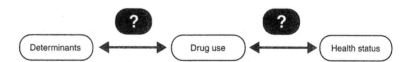

Records of drug use, determinants and outcomes

To determine drug use, several information sources can be consulted: prescribers, dispensers, and pharmacists. Each of these information sources has its strengths and limitations. This is illustrated in Figure 22.2 (Hartzema *et al.* 1998).

As seen in Figure 22.2, (in)correct information about drug use can be obtained due to missing, or incorrect information in the data source from which information about drug use is obtained. Incorrect

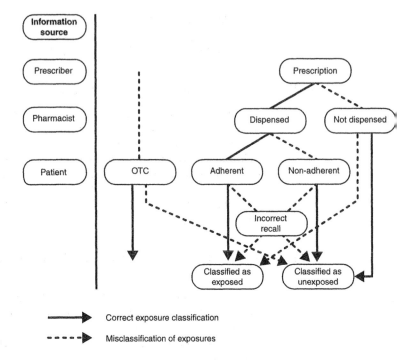

Figure 22.2
Misclassification
associated with various
information sources of
drug exposure

Correct exposure classification

Misclassification of exposures

classification of exposure status is called '*misclassification*' of exposure
The choice of information source will usually depend on the research
question. For instance, one may decide that information direct from
patients is preferable (e.g. for information about OTC drug use or
information about adherence) or that pharmacy data should be used
(e.g. if very detailed drug information is needed).

With the development of large computerised databases in the last few
decades, pharmacoepidemiology has rapidly evolved. Pharmacies,
prescribers, commercial institutions, health insurance companies, and
other health care institutions started to collect and store their health care
data electronically and this provided many opportunities for pharmacoepidemiological studies. Table 22.2 provides an overview of databases
from which pharmacoepidemiology studies have been published in the
past decades.

In most databases, the data have been collected in health care systems
for purposes other than pharmacoepidemiology research. Research with
these databases is relatively inexpensive and studies can be performed
relatively quickly after drug alerts arise, for example, from a spontaneous
reporting system. The data are already available on computer thus little
if any, extra data collection is required. However at the same time it
means that not all relevant data may be available. Also, the data may
comprise a population that is not representative for the general population, and this may introduce bias in the study. Box 22.3 summarises the
strengths and weaknesses of large computerised databases as a source
for pharmacoepidemiology research.

Database	Country	Characteristics
General Practice Research Database (GPRD)	England	population based 4,000,000 inhabitants GP and hospital data
Medicines Monitoring Unit (MEMO)	Scotland	population based 400,000 inhabitants multiple data sources
Prescription Event Monitoring (PEM)	England	first 10,000–15,000 drug users newly marketed drugs selected GP and pharmacy data
Health Maintenance Organisations (Puget Sound, Kaiser Permanente)	USA	enrolled population (large) multiple data sources; only use of formulary drugs
Health Insurance data (Medicaid, Saskatchewan)	USA, Canada	enrolled population (large) multiple data sources; only use of formulary drugs

Table 22.2 Examples of large databases used as a resource for pharmacoepidemiology research

One issue arising with these databases is patient confidentiality. Typically, for clinical research, consent is required from every subject to use their clinical details for research purposes. With these large databases, this is often not feasible because people are followed up for a long time and may be difficult to track down at the time the study is performed. However, ethical approval is often obtained for this type of study when the confidentiality of subjects is protected, because of the

Strengths

- Can quantify suspected risks relatively quickly
- Population based: no selection bias
- Can identify increased risks of rare events
- Can identify increased risks with infrequently used drugs
- Relatively inexpensive
- Cohort studies and case-control studies possible
- Little loss to follow-up
- Long follow-up period
- Delayed effects can be detected

Weaknesses

- Comparator groups difficult to define
- Residual confounding may be present
- Channelling/confounding by indication
- Misclassification of exposure/outcome
- Research is not the primary aim for data collection
- Not always representative of the general population, hence, generalisability may be a problem

These vary with database

Box 22.3 Possible strengths and weaknesses of record-linked databases in pharmacoepidemiology utility of these studies for public health. These issues regarding patient confidentiality in large health care databases have been addressed in the European Data Protection Act.

Measuring disease frequency

If we want to measure whether a drug results in an increased frequency of a disease or other adverse event, we need to compare the frequency of that adverse event in a population that has been exposed to the drug, to the frequency in the unexposed population. Two measures of frequency are commonly used in epidemiology prevalence and incidence (Hennekens and Buring 1987).

Prevalence (P) is the proportion of people in a population that have the disorder, for example the number of children with nut-allergy in a school class or the number of people with dementia in a nursing home Specifically, it is the number of *existing* cases of the disease in a defined population at a given point in time or over a defined time period, divided by the total number of people in that population. It is calculated as P which is the number of existing cases of a disease divided by the total population at a given point in time. For example, if in a nursing home with 500 residents the number of people with dementia is 175, then the prevalence of dementia in that nursing home is 175/500 = 0.35. Typically the prevalence is a proportion, and it always has a value that lies between 0 and 1. It can give us information about how common a disease is, and in that sense it can be useful in planning or budgeting for health care However, it does not give us any information about the rate at which new cases of a disease develop.

Incidence provides additional information, and may be defined as the number of *new* cases of a disease that develop over a defined time period in a defined population at risk, divided by the number of people in that population at risk in that same time period. For example, in Tayside Scotland, 799 new cases of heart failure were identified in 1995. However the denominator of the population can be defined in two ways, and this leads to two different types of incidence: the *cumulative incidence* and the *incidence density*. With the cumulative incidence (CI), the denominator is the number of people in the population at risk at the beginning of a time period. It is calculated as CI, which is the number of new cases of a disease during a given period of time divided by the total population at risk. The cumulative incidence provides an estimate of the probability, or risk, that an individual will develop a disease during a specified period of time. It assumes that the entire population at risk at the beginning of the study period has been followed for the specified time interval for the development of the outcome under investigation.

Often, however, people will enter a study population over a period of a year or several years and are then followed to a single study end-date or until they leave the study population, for example because they move to another country. With the calculation of the *incidence density*, only new cases are incorporated in the numerator, but now the actual person-time at risk is used in the denominator. Each individual's time at risk is calculated and next, the sum of each individual's person-time at risk, or the sum of the time that each person remained under observation and free from the disease. The incidence density (ID) is the number of new cases of a disease during a given time period, divided by the total person-time of observation. Example calculations for cumulative incidence and incidence density are presented in Box 22.4.

Box 22.4 Example calculations of cumulative incidence and incidence density

Consider a study of the incidence of dementia in five nursing homes from 1995–2000. At the beginning of the study period, 1,600 elderly people in these nursing homes do not have dementia. Therefore, they are 'at risk' of dementia (they have the possibility of developing it). Suppose that of these 1,600 people 400 die, of whom no-one developed dementia during the study period, and 200 develop dementia. That means that the *cumulative incidence* is $200/1,600 = 0.125$: the number of people that develop dementia divided by the number of people at risk at the beginning of the study period. Like the prevalence, the cumulative incidence is a proportion; its value always lies between 0 and 1.

The *incidence density*, however, takes into account the person-time 'at risk' that each individual contributes to the study. We assume that as soon as people in the nursing home die, other elderly people are admitted to the nursing home. Let us assume that of these 400 newly admitted people, 75 suffer from dementia at the time that they are admitted to the nursing home, and these 75 people, therefore, are *not* at risk of developing dementia. Hence, they do *not* contribute person-time at risk. The other 325 newly admitted people do not develop dementia during the study period. We also assume that on average, people who develop dementia do so at the mid-point of the 5-year study period (some of them will develop dementia before this date, others after, and we assume that this averages out). Similarly, on average the people who die do so at the mid-point of the study period. The person-time at risk, thus, becomes:

$1,600 \times 5$ person years (the complete population at risk multiplied by the study period), *minus* 200×2.5 (the number of dementia cases multiplied by the time that they contribute to the person-time at risk), *minus* 75×2.5 (the deceased elderly people who were replaced by people with dementia, who do not contribute person-time at risk) = 7312.5 person-years. The incidence density, therefore, becomes 200/7312.5 person-years. This would be expressed as an incidence density of 27 per 1000 person-years.

MEASURING DRUG USE

The frequency of drug use can be calculated in a similar manner to disease frequency. For example, if 53% of nursing home residents use laxatives for more than 10 months per year then the prevalence of laxative use is 53%, or 0.53. For longitudinal or temporal comparisons of drug utilisation between studies or between countries, a classification system was needed to systematically classify drugs within drug groups. To this end, the WHO has developed a hierarchical drug coding system (the ATC classification system) to facilitate these studies. ATC stands for Anatomical, Therapeutic, and Chemical

Groups	Level		Example	
Anatomical main group	1st level; 1 letter	M		musculo-skeletal group
Therapeutic main group	2nd level; 2 numbers	MOl		anti-inflammatory and anti-rheumatic products
- therapeutic subgroup	3rd level; 1 letter	MOlA		non-steroids
Chemical main group	4th level; 1 letter	MO1AE		propionic acid derivatives
- chemical subgroup	5th level; 2 numbers	MO1AEO1		ibuprofen

Table 22.3 The ATC classification system

and this is the hierarchy with which drugs are coded in this system (World Health Organisation 1990). An overview of the coding system plus an example is given in Table 22.3.

ATC codes are seven digit codes, enabling the user to evaluate drug use at various levels (the level of a therapeutic group such as NSAIDs, or the generic level of individual drugs). The ATC system distinguishes fourteen anatomical groups represented as the first letter of the group name. Depending on the indication for which it is used, a drug can have more than one ATC code. For example, acetyl salicylic acid is classified in main group B (Blood and blood forming organs) as an anti-thrombotic agent (B01AC06), but also in main group N (Nervous system) as an analgesic (N02BA01). To quantify drug use, the DDD measuring system was developed together with the ATC system. DDD stands for Defined Daily Dose: the recommended daily dose for adults when the drug is used for its main indication. For virtually every ATC code (with the exception of dermatological preparations and vaccines), a DDD value has been established.

An example of calculating DDDs is given in Table 22.4. This example illustrates that the use of several different drugs can be added up and compared, e.g., between people. However, in most cases the DDD is used to measure drug utilisation at the population level. Examples of the DDD as a volume measure of drug use on a population level are:

Drug	DDD value	Daily dose	mg	DDDs/ day
nitrazepam	5 mg	5 mg at night	5	1
oxazepam	50 mg	3 * 15 mg	45	0.9
flunitrazepam	1 mg	2 mg at night	2	2
paracetamol	3 g	3 * 500 mg	1500	0.5
Total	4 drugs	8 tablets	1552 mg	4.4 DDDs/day

Table 22.4 Example of quantifying drug use with DDDs

Chapter Twenty-two

- The number of DDDs/1000/day (in a country, for example)
- The number of DDDs/100 bed days (in a hospital department, for example)
- The number of DDDs/day (for example in nursing homes, or also in hospitals)
- The cost/DDD of a drug (to compare costs of this drug with other drugs that are used for the same indication)

The ATC and DDD systems have advantages in the sense that even if drug choice changes over time, or differs between countries, drug use can be compared and general trends in use can be identified. Also, they are international systems, hence it is unequivocal which drugs are, and which are not, included in a study, as soon as the ATC codes are published with such a study. However, local prescribing may of course differ from WHO guidelines on the recommended daily dose for an indication. Hence, one DDD does not necessarily indicate one treatment day for an adult. Sometimes, drugs are prescribed for indications other than the main indication for which they are registered. An example would be the use of amitriptyline (an antidepressant) for neuralgia.

Still, the systems are useful for providing overviews of drug use on a population basis. In general the ATC and DDD system are used in drug utilisation studies to monitor drug use and changes over time, to evaluate effects of market regulations, and to plan medical and health policy.

STUDY DESIGN

In pharmacoepidemiology, several epidemiologic study designs are used:

- Descriptive studies
- Case-control studies
- Cohort studies
- Experimental studies

Descriptive studies

These describe patterns of drug utilisation in relation to variables such as disease, gender, place, and time. The data that are provided by these studies are essential for health care planning as well as for epidemiologists. For health care planning, knowledge of specific subgroups of people that are most or least affected by the drugs, or most likely to use the drugs, allows the most efficient allocation of resources and the targeting of specific parts of the population for intervention programmes. For epidemiologists, next to drug alerts from spontaneous reporting systems, drug utilisation studies are often the first, hypothesis generating, step in the search for determinants or risks of drug use. Usually these studies can be performed with existing databases (see also Table 22.2) and are therefore relatively inexpensive and can be carried out relatively quickly. Typical descriptive studies in pharmacoepidemiology are case reports and cross-sectional studies of populations.

Case-control studies

These are analytical epidemiological investigations in which subjects are selected on the basis of whether they do (cases) or do not (controls) have a particular disease under study. The groups are then compared with respect to the proportion having or not having been exposed to the drug of interest. The advantages of case-control design are best illustrated using a classic example of a case-control study in pharmacoepidemiology: the discovery that diethylstilboestrol (DES) could cause vaginal cancer in women who had been exposed to DES *in utero*. In the 1960s in Boston, USA, this disease was diagnosed in eight women between 15 and 22 years old, whereas this disease occurs only very rarely in women younger than 50 years old. Prior to 1967, no-one had presented with this disease in the hospital where the physicians worked. One of the women asked her doctor whether the cancer might have been caused by her mother's use of DES during pregnancy. Because they could not find any other apparent cause, the physicians designed a structured study that would systematically compare these women – the '*cases*' – with an appropriate comparator group – the '*controls*' – to identify factors that might be associated with the disease. For each case, four female controls were found that were matched for age and the hospital ward where the cases were born, and the mothers of cases and controls were interviewed. Apart from the use of DES, cases and controls did not differ with respect to medication taken by the mothers (Herbst *et al.* 1971).

This study illustrates all the advantages of the case-control study design. It can be used to explore associations with disorders that are very rare, where there is a long lag time between exposure and outcome. This design can be used relatively quickly and inexpensively, and it can examine multiple etiological factors for a single disease. Limitations of this study design are that, unless the attributable risk is high, it is inefficient for the evaluation of rare exposures and particularly prone to bias. For example, the selection of controls can lead to bias, and also recall bias is often mentioned in association with this study design. This bias results from cases being more likely to recall prior drug use than controls. Case-control studies have a particular utility in the investigation of both rare diseases and the potential roles of multiple risk factors. Because of lower costs and relative efficiency, with careful planning and study conduct, this study design is often a useful first step in the identification of possible risk factors.

Cohort studies

In these, a group or groups of individuals are identified on the basis of the presence or absence of exposure to a drug as a suspected risk factor for the disease. At the time that exposure status is established, all subjects must be free from the disease under study. Subsequently, they are followed over a period of time to assess the occurrence of the disease. Another name for this design is *'follow-up study'*. Cohort studies are particularly suited for the evaluation of rare exposures, and they can study multiple effects of exposure. Also, because exposure status is established in disease-free individuals and these are subsequently followed up, the temporal relationship between exposure and subsequent development of the disease is easier to establish. Finally, this study design is less prone to bias in the estimation of exposure, than are case-control studies. This is particularly true if the study is prospective, when subjects are recruited and followed up prospectively rather than retrospectively. Limitations of the cohort study design are that such studies can be relatively time-consuming and, therefore, expensive, especially when they seek to evaluate rare diseases or when they involve the prospective collection of data. If they are carried out retrospectively, for example within one of the multipurpose databases detailed in Table 22.2, this requires the availability of adequate records. Finally, in cohort studies people are followed up over time. Inherent in this design is that individuals may be *'lost to follow-up'*, i.e. they withdraw from the study. This may be due to factors that are unrelated to the study, for example if they move abroad, but it may also be that this loss to follow-up is inherent to the exposure. For example, it may be that people decide to withdraw from the study because they develop serious adverse effects, and therefore refuse to cooperate further in a study of that drug. Or, it can be that the drug cures an illness so efficiently, that subjects think they are no longer needed in this study (because they are cured). If such individuals are simply excluded from the study, this type of loss to follow-up will give biased estimates of the drug's effects because only a selected population will reach the end of the study period.

Experimental studies

A special type of cohort study is the *'randomised controlled trial'* (RCT); an experimental study design that is used in the evaluation of new drugs before they can be introduced to the market. (See also Chapters 25 and 30). In RCTs, study subjects are randomly allocated to exposed or unexposed status and subsequently followed up over time. In this way, comparability of the exposed and the unexposed population is ensured which reduces the chance of obtaining biased risk estimates.

Risk estimates

In case-control studies, then, prior exposure to drug use is compared between cases and controls, whereas in cohort studies, cohorts of exposed and unexposed study subjects are followed up for an outcome. From both study types, we can calculate risk estimates of exposure and subsequent outcome (Figure 22.3).

In cohort studies, because we can estimate the true incidence of the outcome studied in the exposed and the unexposed population, a relative risk (RR) can be calculated as the incidence of the outcome in the exposed population, divided by the incidence in the unexposed population. This is calculated as follows:

$$RR = I_{exp}/I_{unexp} = CI_{exp}/CI_{unexp}$$

where: I is incidence rate, CI is cumulative incidence, exp is exposed population and unexp is unexposed population.

From this formula, it follows that if RR = 1, then the incidence is the same in both populations: there is no association between the exposure and the outcome. If RR > 1, however, then exposure is associated with an increased risk of the outcome under study. And, finally, if RR < 1, then exposure is associated with a decreased risk, or a protective effect, with respect to the outcome under study.

In case-control studies, it is usually not possible to calculate the incidence of the outcome and therefore the relative risk cannot be calculated from these studies. However, it can be estimated by calculating the ratio of the odds of exposure among cases to that among controls. Referring to Figure 22.3, this odds ratio (OR) can be calculated from:

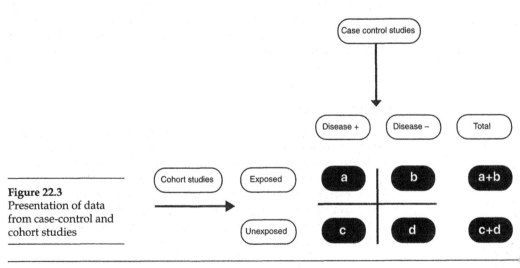

Figure 22.3
Presentation of data from case-control and cohort studies

$$OR = (a/c)/(b/d) = ad/bc$$

Under certain conditions the odds ratio approximates the relative risk (see Rothman, 1998, or Selvin, 1996).

BIAS AND CONFOUNDING

When an association between exposure and outcome has been found, we need to evaluate whether this association is valid. In other words, could this association have been found due to chance, systematic bias in the study design, or due to confounding? In this section, we shall focus on bias and confounding. Two types of bias are generally considered in epidemiology: *selection bias* and *information bias*.

Selection bias may occur in a case-control study if the selection of cases and controls is based on different criteria, and these criteria are related to the exposure of interest (Schlesselman 1982; Rothman and Greenland 1998). A classic example is a case control study in the 1960s of thromboembolism and prior exposure to oral contraceptives. Because the suspicion of this association existed, physicians were more likely to hospitalise women with symptoms of thromboembolism if these women used oral contraceptives than when they did not. As a consequence, the selection of cases from hospitals gave a case population in which oral contraceptives were over-represented compared to the underlying case population. Therefore, due to selection bias, the odds ratio was over-estimated from that study. Similarly, in retrospective cohort studies, selection bias may occur when the selection of exposed and unexposed individuals is based on different criteria that are related to the outcome of interest. In these studies, as in case-control studies, both the disease and the drug exposure have occurred at the time that individuals are selected for the study. Selection bias is unlikely to occur in *prospective* cohort studies, since in these studies, the outcome is unknown at the time of study subject recruitment (Hennekens and Buring 1987).

Information bias includes any *systematic* differences between the two study groups (cases and controls, or exposed and non-exposed individuals, respectively) in the measurement of information on exposure or outcome. This has already been alluded to in the discussion of Figure 22.2, where misclassification of exposure was discussed. If such misclassification differs between cases and controls, for example, because cases are interviewed regarding their drug use and for controls, general practitioners' records are consulted, this may lead to a biased risk estimate.

Well-known examples of information bias are '*recall bias*' and '*interviewer bias*'. An example of recall bias would be a case-control study of drug safety during pregnancy and subsequent congenital malformations. It is generally assumed that, when they are interviewed concerning drug use during pregnancy, mothers of malformed babies will be more accurate in recalling this than mothers of a healthy baby. Such recall bias will lead to over-estimated odds ratios. Sometimes researchers try to avoid this by using 'sick controls', e.g. mothers of babies with Down's syndrome. This congenital disorder is unlikely to be caused by drug use. Similarly, when interviewers know the health status of cases and controls, especially if they are aware of the exposure that is studied, it is assumed that their interview techniques may differ between cases and controls, also leading to spurious associations or overestimated odds ratios.

If the inaccuracy of data collection is the same for both groups, this will lead to a *dilution* of the effect and the risk estimate will be closer to 1 than it would have been, had the data been completely accurate. This is called non-differential misclassification (i.e. the same for both groups).

Finally, risk estimates can be over or underestimated due to *confounding*. Confounding involves the possibility that the observed association can in part, or totally, be explained by differences between the study groups *other* than the exposure under study. These differences could affect the risk of developing the outcome of interest.

The principle of confounding is represented in Figure 22.4. As can be seen from this figure, for a determinant to be a true confounding factor the following criteria must be met. A confounding factor:

- Is an independent predictor (although not necessarily a *cause*) for the occurrence of the disease
- Is associated with the exposure of interest
- Must not be an intermediate link in the causal pathway between exposure and outcome

An example of confounding is the association between the use of ulcer healing drugs and the development of lung cancer. This association is confounded by smoking. If you perform a study of lung cancer and prior exposure to ulcer-healing drugs, you may find an increased risk of lung cancer in the exposed population: there is an association between the drug and the disease (arrow 1 in Figure 22.4). However

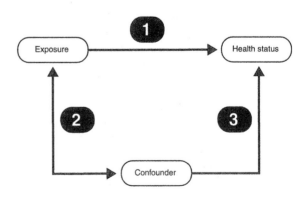

Figure 22.4 Concepts of confounding

people who smoke are more likely to have gastric complaints and, therefore, use ulcer-healing drugs (arrow 2). Also, we know that smoking is associated with an increased risk of lung cancer, which is independent of exposure to ulcer-healing drugs (arrow 3). And finally, smoking is not an intermediate link in the causal pathway: the use of ulcer-healing drugs does not cause people to take up smoking, which subsequently causes lung cancer.

Unlike bias, which is introduced by the investigators or study participants, confounding is an underlying function of relationships between exposure, disease, and other determinants. Also, unlike bias, as long as the possible confounding factors are known, they can be controlled for in the study design or in the analysis (Hennekens and Buring 1987).

However, in pharmacoepidemiology one particular kind of confounding is more difficult to control for in the analysis, and is usually dealt with at the stage of study design: confounding by the reason for prescription, or 'confounding by indication'. In some cases, it is also referred to as 'channelling'. Treated people differ from people who are not treated; e.g. new drugs are usually prescribed to the sickest patients. There is always a reason for prescribing, and especially with studies of beneficial drug effects, this reason is often associated with the outcome of interest. An example of confounding by indication is the association between the extensive use of β-agonists, or use of the newest β-agonists, and asthma mortality. This association is said to be confounded by disease severity – hence, by indication. Another example is the association between selective serotonin re-uptake inhibitors (SSRIs) and suicide rates, when the SSRIs were first marketed. Compared to classic antidepressants, suicide rates were higher among SSRI users but this was said to be entirely due to confounding by indication. It is difficult to control for this at the analysis stage in a study. People try to avoid this type of bias by measuring and controlling for disease severity or by conducting RCTs (experiments) rather than observational studies.

CONCLUSION

Pharmacovigilance is used to evaluate beneficial and adverse effects of medicines and, as such, provides an important information source for the advice that pharmacists give on drug use. This may be required for market approval, development of prescribing guidelines in general, or for the implementation of research findings locally (e.g. in their hospital, community pharmacy, peer review group, or their Drugs and Therapeutics Committee). Pharmacists, with their therapeutic knowledge and an ability to critically review outcomes of spontaneous reporting and pharmacoepidemiology studies, can contribute to the development and implementation of such guidelines. In the long run, this should result in rational drug use, so that eventually good pharmacovigilance leads to good medicine. Also, pharmaco-vigilance provides the basis for health services research and pharmacoeconomics.

FURTHER READING

Hartzema, A.G., Porta, M.S. and Tilson, H.H. (1998) *Pharmaco-epidemiology. An Introduction* (3rd Edn.) Harvey Whitney Books, Cincinnati.

Hennekens, C.H. and Buring J.E. (1987) *Epidemiology in Medicine*, Little, Brown and Company, Boston.

Hosmer, D.W. and Lemeshow, S. (1989) *Applied Logistic Regression*, John Wiley and Sons, New York.

Kleinbaum, D.G., Kupper, L.L. and Muller, K.E. (1988) *Applied Regression Analysis and Other Multivariable Methods* (2nd Edn.) Duxbury Press, Belmont.

Rothman, K.J. and Greenland, S. (Ed.) (1998) *Modern Epidemiology* (2nd Edn.) Lippincott-Raven Publishers, Philadelphia.

Schlesselman, J.J. (1982) *Case-control Studies. Design, Conduct, Analysis*, Oxford University Press, New York.

Strom, B.L. (Ed.) (1994) *Pharmacoepidemiology* (2nd Edn.) John Wiley & Sons, Chichester.

REFERENCES

Hartzema, A.G., Porta, M.S. and Tilson, H.H. (1998). *Pharmaco-epidemiology. An Introduction* (3rd Edn.) Harvey Whitney Books, Cincinnati.

Hennekens, C.H. and Buring J.E. (1987) *Epidemiology in Medicine*, Little, Brown and Company, Boston.

Herbst, A.L., Ulfelder, H. and Poskanzer, D.C. (1971) Adenocarcinoma of the vagina. Association of maternal stilbestrol therapy with tumor appearance in young women. *New England Journal of Medicine*, **284**, 878–881.

Hill, A.B. (1965) The environment and disease: association or causa-tion? *Proceedings of the Royal Society of Medicine*, **85**, 295–300.

Inman, W.H.W. (Ed.) (1986). *Monitoring for Drug Safety*, MTP Press, Lancaster.

Meyboom, R.H.B. (1998) *Detecting Adverse Drug Reactions* (disserta-tion), Benda Drukkers BV, Nijmegen.

Rothman, K.J. and Greenland, S. (Ed.) (1998) *Modern Epidemiology* (2nd Edn.) Lippincott-Raven Publishers, Philadelphia.

Schlesselman, J.J. (1982) *Case-control Studies. Design, Conduct, Analysis,* Oxford University Press, New York.

Selvin, S. (1996). *Statistical Analysis of Epidemiologic Data* (2nd Edn.) Oxford University Press, New York.

Strom, B.L. (Ed.) (1994). *Pharmacoepidemiology* (2nd Edn.) John Wiley and Sons, Chichester.

World Health Organisation (1990) *Guidelines for ATC Classification,* WHO Collaborating Centre for Drug Statistics Methodology and Nordic Council on Medicines, Oslo.

World Health Organisation (1998) *Safety Monitoring of Medical Drugs. Guidelines for Setting Up and Running of a Pharmacovigilance Centre,* World Health Organisation, Geneva.

SELF-ASSESSMENT QUESTIONS

Question 1: Describe the characteristic differences between type A, type B and type C adverse reactions. Looking at a drug's *'life'*, from initial testing in an animal model until after the drug has been 50 years on the market, in what type of studies or reports is each type of adverse reaction first recognised?

Question 2: Describe the characteristics, advantages and disadvantages of a cohort and a case-control study.

Question 3: Which study design would you prefer to detect
a) A rare ADR?
b) ADRs to an infrequently used drug?
c) ADRs to a commonly used drug?
d) The cause of a commonly found adverse event?

Question 4: Consider the following 2 × 2 table of spina bifida in the newborn and intra-uterine exposure to valproic acid:

	spina bifida +	spina bifida −	total
valproic acid +	26	49	75
valproic acid −	34	191	225
	60	240	300

a) Based on the figures in this table, which study design, do you think, has been used and why do you think so?
b) Calculate the appropriate risk estimate. What does this risk estimate tell you?

KEY POINTS FOR ANSWERS

Question 1:

Type A

- Dose-related, related to the drug's pharmacological activity
- Usually easily detectable: frequent, clear time-reaction relationship, biologically plausible, consistent, etc: all Bradford Hill criteria apply
- Detected at the stage of (pre)clinical trials

Type B

- Immunological/idiosyncratic reaction, very infrequent but usually very serious as well
- Usually easily detectable
- Detected post-marketing (because of infrequent occurrence); post-marketing surveillance/spontaneous reporting systems should be mentioned
- Background information that is relevant here: the channelling phenomenon

Type C

- Increased risk of a disease that in itself is not uncommon, and without a very clear relation between drug exposure and time of onset of the ADR
- Usually difficult to detect (case-control/cohort studies are needed and even then, detection remains difficult)
- Detected post-marketing

Question 2:

Case-control	Cohort
Usually small numbers	Usually large populations
Disease oriented	Exposure oriented
Relatively quick and inexpensive	Relatively expensive and time consuming
Multiple exposures can be studied	Multiple effects can be studied
No direct calculation of incidence	Incidence can be calculated

Prone to bias	Less prone to bias, esp. if prospective, but risk of loss to follow-up
Temporal relationship difficult to establish	Temporal relationship can be assessed
Efficient for rare diseases	Efficient for rare exposures

Question 3:

a) Case-control
b) Cohort
c) Cohort
d) Both; depending on issues listed above combined with budget and time restrictions and likelihood of bias in each design

Question 4:

a) Theoretically, any study design is possible. However, the experimental study design seems unlikely, not only because that would be regarded as unethical, but also because of the high frequency of spina bifida in the unexposed population. The high frequency of spina bifida in the study population (1 in every 5 babies) suggests that an observational cohort design and a cross-sectional study design are also unlikely although it could be possible, e.g. if the study population was taken from a clinic that specialises in problem pregnancies. However, the proportion of index and reference subjects (1:4) suggests that here, a case-control study is presented.
b) The odds ratio can be calculated as $(26 \times 191)/(34 \times 49) = 2.98$
This means that mothers who are exposed to valproic acid during their pregnancy are 2.98 times more likely to give birth to a child with a congenital anomaly than mothers who are not exposed to valproic acid during pregnancy.

23 Health Economics

Hakan Brodin

INTRODUCTION	394
BASIC HEALTH ECONOMIC CONCEPTS	394
THE SOCIAL CONTEXT OF HEALTH CARE	395
HEALTH ECONOMICS THEORY	396
Asymmetric information	396
External (interpersonal) effects	397
Risk or uncertainty	398
ECONOMIC EVALUATION OF PHARMACEUTICALS	398
The concepts of social costs and benefits	398
Opportunity cost – the alternatives	398
The discount rate	399
Productivity versus efficiency	400
METHODS FOR PHARMACOECONOMIC EVALUATION	400
Three techniques of social evaluation	401
Cost-benefit analysis	401
Cost-effectiveness analysis	402
Cost-utility analysis	403
ECONOMIC ASPECTS OF PREVENTION	403
MEDICAL ETHICS VERSUS UTILITARIAN ETHICS	404
CONCLUSION	405
FURTHER READING	406
REFERENCES	406
SELF-ASSESSMENT QUESTIONS	406
KEY POINTS FOR ANSWERS	407

INTRODUCTION

Health economics involves the application of economic theories and methods to understand and predict how the health care sector (including pharmacy) will perform from a policy perspective. It is particularly useful for optimising the use of pharmaceuticals, to promote appropriate drugs and to identify ineffective or obsolete drugs. It may also be used by health authorities and managers to organise pharmaceutical care in an efficient and resource minimising way.

Very often the terms *health economics* and *pharmacoeconomics* are used interchangeably. In this chapter *health economics* will be used for the academic discipline, theories, methodology and techniques. Health economics uses a few theories and methods, mainly from the medical and psychologic disciplines, that are not generally used in conventional economics. The term *pharmacoeconomics* may be used for health economic studies in the pharmaceutical area. There are no specific theories, methods or concepts, other than those used in general health economics, for the study of pharmaceuticals.

BASIC HEALTH ECONOMIC CONCEPTS

Economic studies focus on the use of resources. Every clinical decision taken by health care professionals has resource implications. A prescription not only impacts on a patient's health, but also on his/her purse. If the drug is subsidised, the prescription will also have consequences for how taxpayers' money is used.

In the long term, the choice of one drug over another may have positive or negative consequences for both the patient and the health care system. If a doctor asks for a second opinion from a colleague, a certain amount of time (one kind of resource) is withdrawn from the second doctor's work. If a pharmacist calls the doctor to clarify or confirm an issue on a prescription, his or her resources are spent and cannot be used for other ends. An awareness of the simple economic fact that medical work involves resources and costs is not always fully appreciated by health care organisations or the pharmaceutical profession.

Economics, including health economics, does not simply consist of concepts and definitions which are easily learned. Economics is also a way of thinking. Since the end users of health economics are often physicians and pharmacists, with little time and/or interest to invest in this way of thinking, the consequences are that economic knowledge is often used in a scattered and superficial way. An informed guess would be that a large improvement in medical outcomes, i.e. health improvement, is possible for the same amount of resources consequent upon the application of an economic perspective within health care. Pharmacists may have an important role to play in this respect.

THE SOCIAL CONTEXT OF HEALTH CARE

Modern health care is remarkably similar in different countries. The major characteristic in most countries is that it is heavily regulated by the political and administrative system. Economic markets play quite a minor part in the doctor/patient interface although there is 'normal' economic behaviour in the relationship between the health care system and, for instance, the producers of medical equipment and pharmaceuticals. Even in the most market-oriented health care systems, such as in the USA, about 40% of health care costs are financed outside of normal markets. Other countries strive to deregulate the medical system, and a common trend is to deregulate the pharmaceutical markets in favour of fewer prescription only medicines to more pharmacy (or even supermarket) sold medicines (the POM to P shift).

Across nations it is also possible to identify a single economic factor which would largely explain ($r^2 \approx 90\%$) how much resource is devoted to health care. This is the gross national product (GNP) per capita. GNP is the value of the sum total of all produced and sold goods and services in a country in one year. GNP per capita is a measure of the average output per person, but is also a measure of the average income or purchasing power of the population. Thus, it seems that differences in political systems, private or social insurance, general practitioners or hospital employed physicians etc. has less impact on the size of the health care sector than the general income level of the nation. However, public financing limits the costs to a small but significant degree when the influence from other variables is taken into account.

It also appears that health care systems in different countries will increasingly converge with time. There are two possible reasons for this. First, there is a financial need to limit the possibilities for expansion of the system, and to control costs. This is due to an increased competition in society for taxpayers' money as the health care sector expands. Second, the demands for efficiency in the health care sector have led to a global search for new technologies, especially within pharmaceuticals. This, in turn, leads to a common international health care behaviour, in that the same or similar resources will be used and the same or similar results obtained in all countries.

Different nations will encounter different epidemiological conditions. A major cause of death in one country could be of minor importance in another. Planning and monitoring health care from a public health perspective have consequently been a major issue in the health care sector, as well as at governmental levels. To this end a special branch of health economics has been established to estimate what economic consequences are attached to a certain illness: *cost-of-illness studies*. Two approaches can be identified:

- In the *prevalence approach* the (national) total annual cost of a particular illness is estimated. It answers the question '*How much money is devoted to health care of the illness this year?*'
- In the *incidence approach* the lifetime cost is estimated, i.e. '*What is the cost of the illness for patient and society?*'

Very often cost-of-illness studies provide figures of large economic burden to society, and the implied logic is that if a given disease has a large economic burden, then more resources should be devoted to it. However, it requires that (a) there is a technology/method of some kind that alters the situation and (b) that this technology is worth the invested resources.

A major part of cost-of-illness studies is usually the cost to society of lost production. Some criticisms have been directed towards the estimation of lost production. The most important is probably that it is unethical to use the contribution to GNP as a guiding rule for health care, when the sole purpose of health care should be to prolong life and maintain health-related quality of life.

HEALTH ECONOMICS THEORY

Kenneth Arrow, a well-known economist, has identified three basic 'peculiarities' or characteristics of health care that have led to massive political and administrative interference in the market structure (Arrow 1963).

Arrow's analysis of the market mechanisms led to a deeper understanding of why health care was not sold in small shops or in an unregulated marketplace alongside oven ready chickens and vegetables. He also explained why regulated health care would work better in meeting its primary goals, i.e. to create and sustain health, than a pure market approach. The basic characteristics of health care are:

- Asymmetric information between doctor and patient
- External effects
- The uncertainty of incidence of disease or injury

Asymmetric information

Much of this section is based on the work of Evans (1984). Basic economic theory tells us that in an ideal world, buyers and sellers meet and voluntarily come to agreements about exchanging goods and services according to the principles of supply and demand. However, a number of activities, especially in health care, are too complex to operate in a free market environment. They are characterised by a *principal/agent* relationship. Activity is directed by an *agent* (the pharmacist) with a special knowledge towards a *principal* (the patient/customer) who has to rely on the agent since the patient does not possess this knowledge. This is called *asymmetric information*. Clearly an agent may benefit by telling the principal of the advantages about a product and conceal the drawbacks. The agent can thus profit from the ignorance of the gullible principal.

Throughout the ages this has led to a credibility problem, such that by 400 BC Hippocrates had formulated what is widely known as the Hippocratic oath to maintain the good standards of doctors. The World Medical Association Declaration of Geneva on the Physician's Oath was adopted in 1948, amended in 1968, and is in use today. It contains most of the same elements in a modern form:

- Regulation of behaviour
- System for education
- Internal regulatory and punishment system

These provide safeguards absent from an unregulated market system. The Geneva Declaration also serves as a model for ethical pharmacy practice in many countries.

External (interpersonal) effects

The second characteristic of health care which contrasts with an unregulated market, concerns *external effects*, i.e. that someone, other than the patient, is potentially affected by the health care delivered (or withdrawn). The simplest example is the parent-child case. It is not the small child, as patient, that the doctor attempts to persuade to accept treatment, but rather the child's parents. It is also the parents that the doctor will approach for payment for treatment. This is usually termed the *altruistic external effect*. Someone is interested, by consideration and love, to pay some or all the money to ensure that another person receives health care.

An example of *selfish external effects*, is vaccination. If all the students in a class are vaccinated against polio, then the risk to the teacher of infection is considerably reduced, and he or she will, for perfectly selfish reasons, be willing to pay for the students to be vaccinated.

Another case of external effects is the tendency of governments to protect against hazardous behaviour and to promote healthy behaviour. In most countries there is extensive taxation of alcohol and tobacco, whilst health care is subsidised. This is an example of a *paternalistic external effect*. The government considers citizens, in some instances, not to be adequately responsible for their own health. It therefore attempts to persuade people, by giving them economic incentives, to consume less of some goods and more of others, relative to what they would otherwise choose in an unregulated market.

The consequences of these external effects are that health care, in general, is not only financed by the individuals themselves, but also financed by a variety of third party payments, blurring the market structure. It is difficult to separate supply from demand, and some critics of a regulated health care system claim that the health professions exert too much power and influence over governments in setting the health care budget.

Risk or uncertainty

The third characteristic that makes health care a special commodity is the presence of *risk and uncertainty* about who is going to be ill or injured. Risk and uncertainty is most often addressed by the extensive use of insurance. An insurance system leads to a departure from the simple supply and demand model because payment for service is not made at the point of delivery.

ECONOMIC EVALUATION OF PHARMACEUTICALS

The concepts of social costs and benefits

This section builds largely on the work of Drummond *et al.* (1989). Thorough evaluation of the costs and effects of health care depends on the quality of available data. Not only are quality of life issues difficult to measure, but the cost side of the analysis may also present significant problems. The concept of cost, i.e. the value of the resources used, is central to the choice and application of the study methodology. For instance, charges and other *'price-tag'* figures are not necessarily an indication of the value of resources. In the pharmaceutical area, as in many other areas of human activities, the *'welfarist'* approach should be adopted. Apart from ordinary goods and services like pharmaceutical products and pharmacy services, resources also include, e.g. energy water and the time allocated by staff in different activities. The skills of the staff and/or users involved in the activities are another kind of resource – human capital.

Consequently, monetary payment does not represent the real cost In calculating the real cost the following concepts are important.

Opportunity cost – the alternatives

When a certain amount of resources are used deliberately in one health care activity instead of another, a judgement should have been required to ensure resources are used in the best possible way Otherwise, resources will have been wasted. When resources are referred to in this way, they are called *opportunity costs*. When taxpayers' money is used in hospital care to provide a hip replacement rather than providing chemotherapy treatment, the real operating cost is what is lost in terms of chemotherapy treatment.

Applying the concept of opportunity cost to pharmaceutical technology is sometimes difficult and requires that the margina cost must be considered, instead of average cost, when estimating the resources used in a health care programme. The marginal cost quantifies how much extra resources are used when one extra unit of output is produced. This is also an expression of alternative actions and is consequently also one aspect of the opportunity cost principle.

In many cases the marginal cost can be estimated by short term operating direct costs only, excluding transferred costs for administration, rents for buildings and supply of energy and heating. This is because in most cases it is only possible to save the direct cost if a programme is not applied (opportunity cost). However, staff costs should not be excluded on the basis that staff will be fired or rendered unemployed should the service be used by fewer patients, since staff not used for one service may be used to deliver another.

The discount rate

Another important issue, especially when considering prevention activities, concerns the costs and effects at different points in time. In health care, the costs frequently occur at the commencement of a programme, whilst the benefits will often accrue some years later. In pharmaceutical care, a momentary investment in a particular activity, i.e. advice-giving to certain persons at risk, may result in reduced risk of becoming ill or being impaired for the rest of a person's life. To be able to compare costs and benefits, these must be considered as if occurring at the same point in time, normally the beginning of the activity. Both costs and benefits accruing some time in the future will be valued less than if they had occurred today. This is because it is usually advantageous to postpone costs and to advance benefits. This would be the case even in a society with no inflation or bank interest charges. In economics this is referred to as a consequence of *the personal discount rate* and varies for different people. Some people are impatient and consequently have a high rate, others, e.g. those in schools and colleges, postpone their earnings for several years, in favour of waiting for some future better living conditions. They have low discount rates.

All personal discount rates are aggregated to a *social discount rate* which is used to transform costs and benefits from different points in time into equivalent costs today. Mathematically, it resembles the interests used by banks. In health care programmes this discount rate is often around 5%, plus an extra percentage for inflation, if any. The equation for calculating the present value P from a future value F, in t years with a discount rate r is:

$$P = \frac{F \cdot 1}{(1 + r)^t}$$

An example calculation is shown in Box 23.1.

Box 23.1 Example of discount rate calculation

Productivity versus efficiency

Economic evaluation usually means evaluation of goal fulfilment. There are other types of evaluation with broader purposes, e.g. process evaluation, but economists tend to regard evaluation as specifying and valuing resources, in relation to what can be achieved in terms of the specified purpose. In health care this is typically prolonged life and increased quality of life. Figure 23.1 illustrates how the inputs/ resources are used in some process (typically unknown, or little interest for the assessment), generating outputs/outcomes of the programme.

A programme has a goal, uses resources and results in outcomes. Inputs and outputs can be compared, most often in ratios, to measure *productivity* and *efficiency*. Efficiency measures the degree of goal fulfilment (health effects) we can achieve with a certain mix and amount of resources. Productivity, on the other hand, only measures how much could be achieved in terms of customers served by the inputs used, regardless of whether health care workers do, or do not do a good job in terms of the goal, i.e. increased health among customers. Increased productivity in health care may sometimes even be detrimental to increased efficiency.

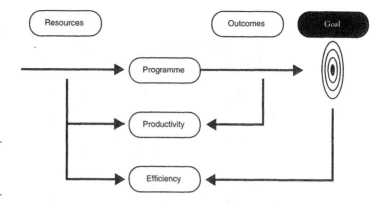

Figure 23.1
Productivity versus
efficiency

METHODS FOR PHARMACOECONOMIC EVALUATION

Private sector enterprises have little need for evaluation methods other than to measure net profits, i.e. the return on invested assets. In other words, the goal is to make money. If profit is not sufficiently high, shareholders will transfer their investment to other areas. In health care there is also a *social goal*, imposed by representatives of the population, to guarantee the provision of health care. If a hospital or pharmacy is not profitable from a business viewpoint, it may still be required to remain in business with government subsidies. In such instances a different type of evaluation is required.

Three techniques of social evaluation

Cost-benefit analysis

In cost-benefit analysis the value of the resources, measured as opportunity costs, are related to the social objective of the programme expressed in monetary terms. All possible effects, within the ethical constraints of human behaviour that affect the welfare of individuals, are estimated and valued. The most universal value of all is, of course, monetary. The increase in welfare generated by the programme should be measured by willingness-to-pay, that is, by the sum of money that an individual is prepared to pay to obtain health benefits, or as compensation for the harm inflicted on them. A programme should be undertaken if the social benefits, measured as the sum of all benefits to all individuals, exceed its social costs, measured in the same way, i.e. if the net social benefit is positive.

The expression *'within the ethical constraints of human behaviour'* is essential but implicit and sometimes overlooked. In normal activities, economists seldom have reason to discuss the ethical foundations of behaviour. Analysts do not propose illegal actions even if they would be profitable. There are always grey areas however, between the legal and illegal. When analysing programmes including personal welfare, utility and quality of life, caution should be exercised about unethical but not necessarily illegal actions. One example is the much-discussed inclusion of increased patient work-productivity as a measure of the success of a new drug.

Cost-benefit analysis is best suited for limited and well-defined projects. Projects with obscure and/or secondary effects, with consequences in many sectors of society are not well suited for cost-benefit analysis. Furthermore, in many cases market prices or charges made to individuals are inappropriate as measures of the marginal social cost or marginal social value of goods and services. For instance, the charges to users of pharmaceutical services are frequently small. The co-payments made by the consumer may however, be only a small fraction of the actual costs of those services to the insurance company or health care budget. In such cases the analyst has to consider more than the market prices: considering the *shadow prices* and scrutinising the accounts to see what the real marginal cost should be.

Cost-effectiveness analysis

As discussed previously, the effects of a social programme are typically not only marketable goods and services, but also savings in time, pain and rehabilitation of lost functioning. In such cases, cost-benefit analysis will become complex and lose its strength as a simple analytical tool. A good alternative may be cost-effectiveness analysis which measures the effects in physical units or amounts only, instead of monetary values. Cost-effectiveness analysis, on the other hand, loses one of the advantages of cost-benefit analysis, i.e. that the net result of the programme only requires to be positive in money values to tell whether a new treatment programme is to be accepted or not. Since cost-effectiveness measures physical units, it is necessary to present the result of the analysis as a cost-effectiveness ratio; e.g. dollars per saved life etc. Therefore, there is no single value that will reveal whether or not the programme is to be undertaken. The cost per unit has to be compared to other programmes estimated in the same way and the importance of the different values must then be assessed by political or administrative bodies.

In many cases the analysis can be so uncertain that it is impossible to achieve a single value representing a '*best guess*'. One way of presenting results from this kind of analysis would be to perform a *sensitivity analysis*, that is to change the values of critical variables, for instance the discount rate, and to present results in terms of maximum and minimum values.

The cost could be divided into three categories:

- *Direct costs* are resources that are used to run the programme e.g. staff costs, costs for drugs, etc. It also includes resources used by the patient or relatives/guardians to access treatment such as patient charges, travel costs and 'out of pocket' drug costs

- *Indirect costs* include the patient's lost income due to illness and treatment, and also the resulting disturbances in their workplace
- *Intangible costs* which are difficult or impossible to measure, e.g. anxiety, pain and exhaustion from treatment

Another category is often referred to as *indirect costs*. In this case it deals with secondary consequences resulting from a programme. It could be, for instance, an increase in the price of pharmaceuticals as a consequence of new laws requiring economic evaluations before product registration, which increases the development costs. This type of cost should normally not be included in a simple evaluation since the primary cost has already been included. Likewise, secondary health care effects of increased work, which are a consequence of the increased longevity or improved quality of life, should also be excluded from the evaluation to avoid double counting.

Cost-utility analysis

An appealing technique for pharmaceutical activities, which has been developed quite recently, is cost-utility analysis (CUA). The concept of utility has emerged from the utilitarian ethics, developed during the 18th century. Individuals are thought of as *'consistently attempting to achieve maximum satisfaction or well-being or utility, as the concept is variously called'* (Parkin 1997). In health care activities utility often corresponds to *'Quality of Life'*, although there are different opinions of the relationship between the two concepts. CUA is a complex and still developing technique. The different psychometric techniques to reveal the quality of life of patients/customers are particularly intriguing. The individual utility cannot be assessed by anyone other than the individual. Therefore CUA involves extensive use of psychometric questionnaires. Some user-friendly techniques of calculating so-called QALYs (Quality Adjusted Life Years) have been developed. These techniques calculate the product of the changes in length of life between alternative programmes with the quality difference of those extra years. One year of full quality is 1 QALY, as are two years with a half quality of life (see Chapter 24).

ECONOMIC ASPECTS OF PREVENTION

One of the most important contributions of health economics is to estimate the pros and cons of prohibiting illness or injuries. For many people the prevention of illness appears to be the obvious choice if possible. However, what is not considered in many instances, is the scarcity of resources, and that if resources are used for one purpose they cannot be used for another. The best use of resources has to be ascertained.

What are the actual alternatives of investing our resources? It would be strange to treat all hypertensive patients at the expense of those needing hip replacements. Instead, we need to ask what can be achieved if the cost of reducing or increasing various activities is varied by a small percentage. In prevention, the appropriate issue is to balance the costs of hypertension screening and subsequent treatment against the costs of detection and treatment of actual cardiovascular diseases when it appears in the future. When considering alternative uses of resources, a perspective across time must be adopted. It follows from the previous discussion on discount rate that it is always desirable to postpone resource use and to achieve quick treatment results. It is better to save one life today than a life in ten years (not necessarily the same life, of course). But if we can save two lives in 14 years with the same resources today used to save one life, it is slightly more favourable, if the discount rate is 5%.

If money and other resources are used for hypertension screening we must compare their value with that of the same resources used for something else, saving further resources for the future when the treatment of cardiovascular disease may be needed. For prevention activities to be favourable a few rules of thumb may be given (Box 23.2).

- Initial cost of detection of people in the risk groups should not be very high
- The fraction of people belonging to the risk group should not be very small
- The probability of prevention success should be very large
- The probability of future treatment success should be small
- The time span from identification to actual illness should not be very long

It is obvious that estimation of the costs and effects of prevention activities often requires more in terms of data and methodology than is available. We need epidemiological data about the incidence, and transition probabilities for different phases of the illness. All treatment effects such as adverse drug effects, should also be known. Additionally, the accounts of hospitals and primary care units do not generally record the resources used per individual. Therefore, the proper modelling of assumptions and consequences in terms of uncertain results are an essential element in economic evaluations.

MEDICAL ETHICS VERSUS UTILITARIAN ETHICS

Throughout this chapter ethical issues have been indicated. Even the foundations of health economic theory have ethical underpinnings. Constantly we touch upon the boundaries between economics and medical ethics, since the Hippocratic basis often interferes with the utilitarian ethics. This section briefly draws attention to some ethical considerations in relation to economics and the consequences of this for health care. For a comprehensive review, see Mooney and McGuire (1988).

The application of medical ethics centres on the individual, requiring the doctor or pharmacist to give full attention to their individual patient or customer. Health professionals are not required to treat only those who would benefit from it, but the one in the greatest need. The need for health care is determined by the professional – not the patient, nor the treatment result.

Utilitarian ethics, on the other hand, takes a broader and more public perspective. It is claimed that resources should be used as efficiently as possible. The objective of resource allocation is to maximise the greatest benefit for the greatest number of people. The pharmacist has to pay attention not only to the customer in front of him/her, but also to the other customers waiting for service. It then follows that the society has to choose between the different possible alternatives in which the resources could be utilised, to achieve the best possible total result in terms of utility. The concept of choice also implies that the concept of cost has to be treated in a special way. The opportunity cost recognises the value of the resources used in relation to the benefits missed as a result of not using resources in the best alternative way. This principle underpins what is often referred to as 'evidence-based medicine'.

The two ethical systems place health professionals, including pharmacists, in a dilemma. They traditionally pay full attention to the patient in front of them and use resources for this patient even if the chance of treatment success is low and a waiting patient has greater need for the pharmacist's services than the current one. The painful dilemma arising from the two ethical systems can be reduced to some degree by good leadership and clear professional rules at the pharmacy level, or higher.

CONCLUSION

Health economics can be an important tool for pharmacists, to encompass the complex and multidimensional nature of high technology pharmaceutical care. From the health economic perspective, pharmaceuticals are valued in their proper environment, not only in a limited financial sense, but in a broad social and humanistic framework. They are scrutinised to extract the best available treatments. Their therapeutic effects are related to the costs of the treatment and to other treatment options.

The predominant health economic activity is the evaluation of new or existing treatments, from a social viewpoint. The sound application of health economic theory into practical assessment techniques is crucial for the understanding and fair comparison of treatment options. To that end, a small, but important number of conventions and guidelines are applied, and increasingly required in the publishing of scientific results. Pharmacists involved in clinical efficiency studies will benefit from recognising the importance of these.

Finally, this chapter has highlighted the political and ethical implications of health economics in the potential conflict between the professional and the ethical systems. Evaluation techniques are not ethically neutral, and depending on what technique is used, the social implications will differ and hence, health economic evaluations should not be applied mechanically.

FURTHER READING

Mooney, G. and McGuire, A. (Eds.) (1988) *Medical Ethics and Economics in Health Care*, Oxford Medical Publications, Oxford.

REFERENCES

Arrow, K.J. (1963) Uncertainty and the welfare economics of medical care. *American Economic Review*, **53**, 941–973.

Drummond, M.F., O'Brien B., Stoddart G.L. and Torrance G.W. (1989) *Methods for the Economic Evaluation of Health Care Programmes* (2nd Edn.) Oxford Medical Publications, Oxford.

Evans, R.G. (1984) *Strained Mercy*. Butterworths, Toronto.

Mooney, G. and McGuire, A. (Eds.) (1988) *Medical Ethics and Economics in Health Care*. Oxford Medical Publications, Oxford.

Parkin, M. (1997) *Economics* (5th Edn.) Addison Wesley, Harlow.

SELF-ASSESSMENT QUESTIONS

Question 1: Often the efficiency of health care is said to increase with increased competition (i.e. more '*of market*' mechanisms). Indicate the areas in pharmacy where this may be true or false.

Question 2: Why is the time perspective so important in health economic evaluations?

Question 3: Why should the medical staff costs be included in the calculation of marginal cost, but not the staff employed to garden the hospital grounds?

KEY POINTS FOR ANSWERS

Question 1: More *'of market'* mechanisms are suitable where the three intrinsic health care characteristics are small or not present. For instance, normal dispensing, without questions, simple self-medication without involvement of other people and frequent purchase of self-paid medication with few side-effects. All these areas could be suitable for supermarket sales. Areas where such mechanisms are unsuitable might include complex medication schemes and public health aspects.

Question 2: Consider the equation for discounting and notice that time appears as an exponent. That means that the value of future health effects lose their importance rather quickly. Fifteen years ahead, the effects have lost more than half their values at a discount rate of 5% (check it).

Question 3: Medical staff can be released from treatment, if the treatment strategy is changed, and reinstalled in other treatment activities. The gardening staff will probably not be affected at all as treatments are changed. The former are part of the *'variable cost'*, the latter are part of the *'fixed cost'*, and fixed cost elements should be excluded from calculations of marginal cost.

PART SEVEN

Research Methods

24 Measurements of Health and Illness

Sally-Anne Francis

INTRODUCTION	412
THE CONCEPT OF HEALTH	413
Why measure health?	414
APPROACHES TO MEASURING HEALTH AND ILLNESS	414
Types of measure	414
Mortality data	415
Morbidity and service-use data	415
Subjective health measures	416
Health-related quality of life	418
THE SCIENCE OF HEALTH STATUS MEASUREMENT	419
Choice of an instrument: generic, condition-specific or patient-specific?	419
Characteristics of instruments	421
Administration method	421
Scoring method	422
Psychometric properties of standardised instruments	423
Conceptual and measurement models	423
Reliability	424
Validity	425
Responsiveness	426
Interpretation	426
Burden	426
Alternative forms of instrument	426
Cultural and language adaptations	427
CONCLUSION	427
FURTHER READING	427
WEBSITES	428
REFERENCES	428
SELF-ASSESSMENT QUESTIONS	430
KEY POINTS FOR ANSWERS	431

INTRODUCTION

Health care comprises preventive care, public health strategies, health promotion and the medical and surgical treatment of established disease and illness (Barlow 1999). One of the most significant challenges of the 21st century is the international aim *'to increase healthy life expectancy for all'* (World Health Organisation 1999). This does not mean to sustain life, despite people's physical, psychological and social functioning, but to increase both the quantity and quality of life experienced by the world's population. Inherent to this aim is the need to achieve a more equitable distribution of health care resources among the world's population. So what strategies have been recommended to enhance quality of life worldwide? (Box 24.1).

Box 24.1 Strategies for enhancing quality of life worldwide (World Health Organisation 1999)

- Health systems should focus on delivering a limited number of interventions that have the greatest impact in reducing the excessive burden of disease
- Health systems should be pro-active in counteracting potential health problems as a result of economic crises, unhealthy environments or risky behaviour (e.g. tobacco addiction)
- Health systems should be developed so that, at the point of delivery, there is universal access to services with no, or minimum fees
- Health systems should be encouraged to invest in expanding the knowledge base and so continue health gains into the 21st century

Each of these recommendations demonstrates the need for effective development of current health care systems, the consequences of which must be evaluated in terms of the impact on the health of the population, i.e. the health outcome.

Traditionally, health care practitioners have used objective criteria such as signs of disease, laboratory data and radiological examination to inform the diagnosis of disease and its management. Measures of morbidity and mortality have been used to evaluate the consequences of medical treatment. However, in recent years, broader measures of health outcomes have been added that include both objective and subjective indicators, such as functional ability, self-reported health status and positive concepts of health such as quality of life. Increasingly, social and economic approaches to measuring health outcomes are employed alongside traditional methods, and the patient's viewpoint has become central to the monitoring and evaluation of health care interventions.

This chapter will review current approaches to the measurement of health and illness. Traditional approaches such as morbidity and mortality data will be described, followed by broader measures, such as subjective health indicators and health-related quality of life. The choice of approach is dependent on the definition of health adopted (i.e. the conceptual model) and the purpose for which health is being measured. Therefore, the chapter begins with a brief discussion of the concept of health.

THE CONCEPT OF HEALTH

A dictionary definition of disease is: *'an abnormal condition of the body with a complex of physical signs, symptoms and effects that can be attributed to a cause (known or unknown)'* (Youngson 1992). Illness is a subjective state resulting from a perceived change in functioning where disease may or may not be present. Sickness is endorsed behaviour that signifies illness, despite the presence of disease or illness (See Chapter 7).

Health is less easily defined. For example, the health of a population may be said to have improved if the life expectancy of that population has increased. Similarly, if a person who is diagnosed with schizophrenia receives a novel drug therapy that is effective at reducing the symptoms of illness and has an improved side-effect profile compared with previous drug therapy, then it may be said that the health of that individual has improved. Each of these perspectives can claim to be defining an aspect of 'health' (Hunt 1988).

Health may be defined in negative terms such as the absence of disease, illness and sickness. However, the widely acknowledged World Health Organisation's definition of health goes beyond the absence of disease, to: *'a state of complete physical, mental and social well-being'* (World Health Organisation 1948). A number of limitations have been identified with this definition, e.g. its lack of clarity, its exclusion of physiological states and its lack of guidance on which health-states are preferable to others and the boundaries of social well-being in relation to health (Patrick and Erickson 1993). A more recent definition of health (Ware 1995) compounds the criticism that health is often unrealistically represented as an ideal state: *'Health also connotes completeness – nothing is missing from the person – and proper function – all is working efficiently.'*

Absolute definitions such as these are often unhelpful in providing a conceptual base to guide the measurement of the concept, i.e. to serve as an operational definition. By developing measures without a firm conceptual base, confusion arises when interpreting the results of studies and making comparisons between studies. Consequently, the measurement of health is often represented by health indicators due to the lack of a consensus on the concept of health. For example, the number of times a person consults with their general medical practitioner may be considered a health indicator. However, it is unlikely that one indicator alone, such as general practitioner consultation rates, could reliably measure the multidimensional concept of health; more frequently a number of indicators are employed. For example, the health status of a patient after a hip replacement operation may be determined by the results of radiological examination, range of movement compared with the pre-operative state, experience of pain and the use of analgesia, and functional ability, e.g. ability to carry out activities of daily living (such as climbing stairs).

Why measure health?

Current health systems are concerned with the most effective treatment strategies, while considering the best use of their finite resources for a given population. In clinical settings, health status measurement may be concerned with determining the choice and effectiveness of interventions for an individual patient or comparing the outcomes of different treatment approaches between patient groups.

Population-based health outcome measurement can provide a baseline against which to measure future medical and public health practices, and any consequent social and economic legislation. For example, what would be the health consequences to the public if pharmacists supplied emergency hormonal contraception under direct supply as an over the counter medicine according to a group prescribing protocol compared to sale as a Pharmacy Medicine? Also, examination of the relationships between health status and the environment provides evidence for the aetiology of disease and informs the control of infectious diseases.

Life expectancy has improved worldwide. In the developed world, this has been largely due to preventive care and health promotion strategies, in conjunction with effective treatments for major causes of mortality. Consequently, demands on health care services continue to grow due to the increased prevalence, and presentation, of chronic, noncommunicable disease. This has shifted the objective of many treatments to reducing morbidity rather than curing or prolonging life. In addition, advances in health technology have raised society's expectations of health care interventions. There is a drive to increase the involvement of consumers of treatments in decisions concerning the risks and benefits of different treatment options. Therefore, the measurement of health outcomes has become increasingly important in allocating scarce resources, informing clinical decision-making and facilitating patients' autonomy.

APPROACHES TO MEASURING HEALTH AND ILLNESS

Types of measure

Mortality, morbidity and service-use data have traditionally been used as measures of health outcome. Such indices are based on the 'disease model', i.e. where health is expressed as the absence of disease. For example, in cancer studies, outcome measures may be represented by markers of disease such as radiological and pathological examination, tumour response to treatment and the effects of chemotherapeutic agents.

Mortality data

Mortality data provide population-based information on the patterns of disease and causes of death. The crude death rate is calculated by dividing the number of deaths in a given population by the total number of people in that population. This permits the comparison of death rates between populations and over time. However, the composition of a population can influence its death rate (e.g. the proportion of elderly people, the proportion of men or women). Therefore, 'standardised' values are often calculated to take into account factors such as the age and gender structure of a given population. Expressed as standardised rates, mortality data are important indicators of public health and may be used to estimate the size and distribution of health problems. For diseases where treatment is likely to have an impact on length of life, survival time is frequently used as a primary endpoint in the evaluation of new drug therapies.

The application of mortality statistics as a global indicator of health status has limitations. For example, patterns of mortality in the developed world have changed, i.e. death from disease is now more commonly age-related. Also, it is an insensitive health outcome measure for assessing the impact of most health care interventions. It is essential that health outcome measures can identify the impact and consequences of alternative treatment options, even if there is no effect on survival.

The advantages of using mortality data as a measure of health are twofold:

- Mortality data are often routinely collected by age, gender, cause of death and geographical area;
- Data are inherently reliable indicators since death is definitive.

However, there are also two notes of caution:

- The extreme nature of the endpoint makes mortality data insensitive to identifying important changes within people's continuum of health and illness experiences;
- Cause of death information has limited value regarding patterns of disease over time due to the continued refinements made to the classification systems of disease.

Morbidity and service-use data

Morbidity data aim to capture information about the experience of disease and illness. In health care evaluation, frequently used morbidity data include biological endpoints such as blood pressure, condition-specific markers such as symptom lists, or performance-related indicators such as number of days absent from work through illness. However, external factors such as environmental conditions and advances in diagnostic criteria can influence patterns of disease. In particular, performance-related indicators have a number of limitations. For example, in recent years, changes in employment patterns and society's attitude to work and sickness suggest that 'days absent from work through illness' has severe disadvantages as an indicator of health. It may represent information on a range of other factors such as age, economic and social opportunities, and the provision of health care resources. Also, it is only providing information on the proportion of the population who are in the workforce, thereby excluding children, full-time students, the unemployed, the retired, those looking after a home and full-time carers.

Service-use data (e.g. the number of people discharged from hospitals over a given period of time, hospital readmission statistics and general practitioner consultation rates) are frequently used as indicators of health status but can obscure the true picture of health or disease in society. Access and availability of services and the illness behaviour patterns of a population will affect the use of health services.

Morbidity and service-use data are often collected through service-based audits and surveys. For example, the Office for National Statistics, the Royal College of General Practitioners and the Department of Health in Great Britain carried out the fourth national study of morbidity in England and Wales for the years 1991–92 (Office for National Statistics 1995). This survey (which has been repeated at approximately 10-year intervals) provides information on the reasons, as perceived by the doctor or practice nurse, that people consult their general practitioner (as an indicator of the general health of the population) and prevalence trends in sickness (to help inform health service practitioners and planners).

The main limitation associated with morbidity and service-use data is whether patterns of change can be attributed to a change in health status or whether it is identifying change in some external factor. Other limitations include the lack of information about the impact of treatment on the patient's life and the difficulties associated with making comparisons across different groups or populations. Comparisons between international data can often reflect the influence of different cultural values and health care systems as well as identifying differences in the health of the populations being studied.

Subjective health measures

Mortality, morbidity and service-use data focus on disease, illness and access to health care services. However, determinants of the effects of treatment go beyond symptom alleviation and biological and physiological functioning to include patients' outcome criteria such as role performance (e.g. the ability to go to work, ability to fulfil household duties), levels of interest and energy, and the ability to enjoy oneself (Hunt and McKenna 1993). Therefore, subjective measures of health such as functional ability, self-reported health status and health-related quality of life are broader outcome measures that focus on the impact of disease and treatment on the lives of individuals.

Subjective health measures are important approaches to health outcome measurement since they reflect a comprehensive range of factors known to influence a patient's health outcome such as motivation, psychological well-being, adherence to treatment, social support networks and an individual's value system (Bowling 1997). Also, directly involving patients in the assessment of health outcome has been identified as the best approach to determining whether a treatment or medical intervention facilitates a patient to meet their needs or expectations (Ware 1995).

In Great Britain, government-sponsored surveys are carried out to collect subjective data about the nation's health and use of health services. For example, the General Household Survey (GHS), which has been running since 1971, is carried out with a sample of the general population resident in private households in Great Britain over a 12-month period and includes five core topics: population and family information, housing, health, employment and education. The GHS also permits the inclusion of additional topics, e.g. household burglary and questions on health behaviour such as smoking, alcohol and contraception. By understanding the health behaviour of populations, appropriate interventions can be designed that aim to increase both the quantity and quality of life.

For many disease states, future drug therapies and surgical procedures are likely to have marginal effects on quantity of life. This has shifted the awareness of health care practitioners and researchers to incorporate broader, patient-led measures such as functional status, health status and quality of life into the assessment of health outcome.

Functional measures focus on the impact of the disease and its treatment on activities of daily functioning. Interruption of usual activities and roles are often important outcome indicators for the individual. This approach also permits comparison of the burden of disease between different disease states. One of the oldest measures of functioning is the index of Activities of Daily Living (ADL) (Katz et al. 1963; 1970). This was developed for use with elderly people where an observer rates the degree of independence/dependence associated with the completion of activities such as bathing, dressing, mobility, continence and feeding. As with any standardised instrument, the judgement is limited to functioning in those areas included within the content of the instrument. Therefore, functioning in relation to other activities that may be important to individuals is not considered.

Health status measurement can encompass functional status, physiological measures (e.g. signs, symptoms, clinical data) and measures of subjective well-being: thereby permitting the identification of differences in the clinical condition and functional capacity of people with the same 'disease'. There are two approaches to measuring health status: the first focuses on an individual's subjective perception of their health and the second comprises symptom checklists (Bowling 1997) Health status measures can provide valid assessments of the health of individuals or populations and the positive and negative outcomes of health care interventions. Health status measurement may be presented as a single global index or a profile. These approaches to measurement are discussed later.

Health-related quality of life has multiple components and considers the impact of disease and its treatment on aspects of life such as functional ability, health status and life satisfaction. It should be noted that health-related quality of life is a narrower concept than quality of life, *per se*. The concept of quality of life is more than those aspects of life affected by disease and its treatment, and includes life areas such as the environment, standard of living and financial status. While the World Health Organisation's (1948) definition of health may be criticised for its idealistic stance, its commitment to a positive concept of health and related concepts such as quality of life, must be acknowledged.

'Quality of life is defined as an individual's perception of their position in life in the context of culture and value systems in which they live and in relation to their goals, expectations, standards and concerns. It is a broad ranging concept affected in a complex way by the person's physical health, psychological state, level of independence, social relationships, and their relationship to salient features of their environment' (World Health Organization Quality of Life Group 1993).

Health-related quality of life

Health-related quality of life is an important endpoint for those diseases where treatment is likely to have a limited impact on survival. The importance of including measures of health-related quality of life is of particular significance where the benefits of treatment are weighed against potential impaired functioning due to disabling adverse effects. With the increased prevalence of chronic disease due to increased life expectancy in the developed world, the primary outcome measure must focus on the well-being of those being treated.

The importance of pharmacists' understanding of concepts and measurement of health-related quality of life is shown in Box 24.2.

Increasingly, the economic analysis of competing treatment options has an important role in health care evaluation (see Chapter 23). One approach that has received much attention is the Quality Adjusted Life Years (QALYs). This method assesses the benefit associated with a treatment option through calculating the expected gains in both quantity and quality of life. QALYs have been used to compare different treatment options for the same group of patients, and more contentiously, different programmes of care for different patient groups (Spiegelhalter *et al.* 1992).

Box 24.2 Reasons pharmacists need to understand the concept and measurement of health-related quality of life (MacKeigan and Pathak 1992)

THE SCIENCE OF HEALTH STATUS MEASUREMENT

With increasing emphasis placed on measuring the outcome associated with health care interventions, it is essential that scientific methods are adopted to measure subjective indicators of health in a reproducible and valid way. Superior data are collected when using a standardised, well-tested instrument with robust psychometric properties (Bowling 1995).

Choice of an instrument: generic, condition-specific or patient-specific?

Standardised instruments have been developed for use as generic or condition-specific measures. Generic health measures focus on functional status and well being. They assess health concepts that are relevant to basic human values. Generic measures have a limited number of core health concepts that are sensitive to the impact of a wide range of diseases (e.g. physical and social functioning, role performance and mental health). As such, they should be administered in studies where one wishes to draw conclusions about general health outcomes. The advantage of generic methods is that the breadth of areas of life (domains) covered by the instrument maximises the opportunity for detecting unexpected or iatrogenic effects. However, the disadvantage is that by including such a wide range of domains, responsiveness to the measurement of outcomes of health care can diminish. Generic measures are more suited to measurements across populations for estimating the burden of disease, and can provide useful information for comparing alternative treatments.

The choice of generic measure is extremely important, when comparing the outcome of different diseases or alternative treatment programmes, to avoid confounding (see Chapter 22). Preferably, one must ensure that the items included in the measure do not favour the symptoms of a particular disease or the adverse effects of a particular treatment (Ware 1995).

Condition-specific measures are developed with a detailed knowledge of the disease, the treatments and interventions used in the management of that disease, e.g. cancers, respiratory conditions, cardiovascular diseases (see Bowling 1995 for a comprehensive review of condition-specific measures). Therefore, condition-specific measures are more likely to detect subtle changes resulting from treatment within a particular patient group (MacKeigan and Pathak 1992). Administering both generic and condition-specific instruments concomitantly can capture the burden of disease and treatment effects in specific terms as well according to general health outcome indicators.

Using standardised instruments has been criticised for reducing the individual to Mr and Mrs Average (Hunt, 1997). Alternative, patient-specific measures have been developed in response to the question of the relevance of standardised instruments when an external value system is imposed on respondents, e.g. Schedule for the Evaluation of Individual Quality of Life (SEIQoL) (O'Boyle 1994). This approach to outcome assessment permits the respondent to nominate the areas of life that determine their quality of life and the relative importance of each of these life areas.

Some authors have recommended the use of a patient-specific approach in clinical trials, since measurement of items nominated by respondents has an increased sensitivity to change that allows a smaller sample size to be employed compared with standardised instruments (Tugwell et al. 1990; Chambers 1993). Similarly, a risk-benefit analysis of treatment, weighing the positive effects of the medication (in terms of treating the disease) against the toxicity of the treatment, is an individual judgement and levels of acceptable toxicity are likely to vary between individuals (Fayers 1992). Individuals have different coping abilities and will make different adjustments to their lives in response to various health states (Hunt 1997).

By adopting a patient-specific approach, cross-sectional data will vary between individuals, but the responsiveness of individual measurement is likely to be greater, when considering the effects of different interventions and detecting unexpected or iatrogenic effects. A disadvantage of the patient-specific approach is that items reported at a follow-up interview may not be related to those items reported at the baseline. On such occasions, respondents could be asked to re-prioritise baseline items also.

The argument against the use of individual measurement of quality of life and condition-specific measurement is that such measurement cannot inform resource allocation decisions because there is limited potential for comparison between individuals, groups, or societies with different diseases (Cairns 1996).

Characteristics of instruments

Administration method

The most common method of collecting subjective data is by questionnaire, self-administered or administered by an interviewer. Measurement strategy depends on the purpose of the study, financial resources and the characteristics of the respondents.

Self-report instruments are the most popular methods since they access subjective assessments of health and its related domains, such as functional status and well-being. Self-report measures may be single item measures, a battery or scale. The usefulness of a single item method is limited, since it is unlikely to provide comprehensive information about a given concept. Scales are the preferred method of measurement because they contain a large number of items, and the summed and weighted scores are more able to withstand statistical analysis.

Interviewer-administered instruments introduce the potential of rater-bias into the assessment process. However, depending on the target population, interviewers may be essential in studies of patients with reading or cognitive difficulties that preclude use of some self-administered instruments. Bowling (1995) advises the use of trained interviewers to reduce bias in health-related quality of life studies. Interviewers must be as objective as possible and it is preferred that they are not staff responsible for the health or social care of the respondents. This can help guard against respondents wishing to give desirable answers. Interviewer-administered instruments also have the potential advantages of boosting response numbers, giving participants the opportunity to clarify issues or ambiguous questions, helping motivate respondents to complete the interview, and if sufficient rapport is developed, can lead to increased reliability in the reporting.

The length of an instrument is another important factor in choice of administration method. Shorter instruments are more akin with self-completion, although they are likely to be less sensitive. Longer instruments may be preferable. However they are more expensive to administer (especially if interviewer-administered) and more time consuming to analyse (See also Chapter 25). Given that respondents may perceive health-related quality of life as an abstract concept, another issue of importance is the perceived need by respondents to answer such questions. One study that has considered these issues concluded that patients enjoyed completing the questionnaires and thought the information relevant for their doctor to know (Nelson and Berwick 1989).

Scoring method

Three alternative methods used for scoring measurement instruments are the health profile, health battery and the health index, Box 24.3

- The *health profile* is derived from a single instrument that scores a number of individual dimensions separately (e.g. physical functioning, psychological well-being, social functioning). This method does not attempt to aggregate the component scores into a single summary score
- The *health battery* comprises a series of questions, or independent instruments, that each measure a separate dimension of the same concept. Each dimension is scored separately
- The *health index* is a single instrument whose dimension scores are aggregated to form one summary score. It is not usually recommended to simply sum the components; each dimension should be weighted before totalling

Health profiles and health batteries provide comprehensive information pertaining to impairments in those dimensions of life measured (e.g. physical functioning, role performance, psychological well-being). However, limited information can be achieved with these methods in comparative studies unless measurement is higher in all dimensions for one comparator. Some health indexes provide dimensions' scores, as well as an overall score, which are useful for their descriptive detail. Other health indexes simply provide the summary score which cannot be disaggregated and are therefore less sensitive. Health indexes have the advantage of being easier to analyse and to inform decisions, particularly for economic analyses.

Weighting reflects the preferences and priorities of certain items/ domains within a given scale. Values (which may be represented by the number of items proportional to significance) are often assigned to constructs during the testing of the instrument. However, Joyce (1994) questioned how likely the weightings developed during testing would be identical to those an *individual* may set with whom the scale may be used. Najman and Levine (1981) also drew attention to the arbitrary nature with which weightings and priorities are given to any life area. They believe that the values and perceptions of the respondents should be understood to be able to interpret the ratings. Critics may want to consider the year and place of testing of the instrument, the sample characteristics used to derive the weightings, and whether these reflect the sample and study conditions for which the instrument is to be employed. Joyce (1994) recommended that, ideally, to assess an individual's quality of life, weights should be allocated to each item (or at least the dimension) for each individual on each test occasion. Two examples of patient-specific measures where authors have adopted this method successfully are the McMaster Health Index Questionnaire (Chambers 1993) and the Schedule for the Evaluation of Individual Quality of Life (SEIQoL) (O'Boyle 1994).

Other approaches do not examine the preferences of the respondents, but assume equal weighting amongst items. Häyry (1991) suggested that it is contrary to common sense to suppose that all items in a given scale have equal importance and equally unrealistic to assume that all individuals would have the same preferences and priorities. Methods where the values comprise a single score, and then groups of patients are aggregated to form a single mean score, have been criticised since they lose any aspect of an individual's preferences and values (Rosenberg 1995; Hunt 1997).

Psychometric properties of standardised instruments

The selection of an instrument to measure health or illness should be influenced by its psychometric properties. The Medical Outcomes Trust (1997) recommended eight attributes by which to evaluate an instrument (Box 24.4). The relative importance of each criterion depends on the instrument's intended use and application. For example, if the instrument is intended for discriminative or evaluative purposes between individuals or populations, or if the instrument is intended for research or clinical practice settings, the criteria should be assessed accordingly. The context of use is an essential factor that influences the properties of an instrument and therefore, evidence should be presented for each of the instrument's intended applications. A clear description of the sample size, characteristics of the sample, testing conditions and study design methods should be detailed for any work undertaken to test or adapt a new instrument. Bowling (1995) has also listed a review of the important criteria to consider when generally selecting and administering a scale.

Box 24.4 Criteria by which to evaluate a measure's strengths and weaknesses (Medical Outcomes Trust 1997)

- Conceptual and measurement model
- Reliability
- Validity
- Responsiveness
- Interpretation
- Alternative forms
- Burden
- Conceptual and linguistic equivalence

Conceptual and measurement models

A conceptual model is the justification for, and description of, the concept(s) that the instrument claims to measure and the relationship between those concepts. A measurement model represents the structure and scoring methods of the instrument's scale and sub-scales. The scale should also demonstrate adequate variability in domain scores relative to its intended use (i.e. the avoidance of *'floor'* or *'ceiling'* effects). The level of measurement (e.g. ordinal, interval or ratio scales) and the rationale for the chosen scoring methods (e.g. use of raw scores, standardisation or weighting) should be stated.

Reliability

The reliability of an instrument is a measure of the degree of freedom from random error and may be judged using a number of methods: test-retest reliability, inter-rater reliability or intra-rater reliability. Reliability can be expressed as *'a ratio of the variability between individuals to the total variability in the scores'* and is represented by a number between zero (indicative of no reliability) to one (perfect reliability) (Streiner and Norman 1989).

For instruments used on two or more occasions with the same group of participants, a *test-retest reliability* (also known as reproducibility or external reliability) attribute may be tested, i.e. on repeated administrations of the same instrument, to what extent are similar results obtained when conditions have remained stable. However, the influence of the first administration may affect the responses collected on the second administration causing reliability to be overestimated. This is known as a *repeat-effect*. Conversely, reliability may be underestimated due to the detection of true variations. Careful consideration should be given to the time permitted between measurements and the nature of the underlying concept, i.e. is the concept likely to change in given circumstances?

If more than one interviewer is involved in administering an interview and coding the data, *inter-rater reliability* may be measured, i.e. the degree of agreement between two interviewers. The reliability of measurements made by the same interviewer on two separate occasions may also be determined: *intra-rater reliability*.

The *internal consistency* of an instrument considers the relationship between multiple items of a scale. It is an estimate of the reliability based on all possible correlations between two sets of items within the test on a single administration of the instrument. Is the group of items consistently measuring different aspects of the same underlying construct? One of the most frequently used statistics for estimating internal consistency is Cronbach's alpha (Cronbach 1951).

An explicit decision must be made concerning the acceptable level of variation in measurement. Acceptable levels of the reliability coefficients differ according to whether comparisons are being made between groups (0.70) or between individuals where the standard is much higher (0.90 or above) (Nunally 1978). Cronbach (1951) reported that a value greater than 0.50 was an acceptable level of good internal consistency, as well as test-retest reliability. Other authors are more conservative and expect values of greater than 0.8 for internal consistency and greater than 0.5 for external reliability (Streiner and Norman, 1989; Bryman and Cramer 1997).

Validity

While reliability data indicate the random error associated with measurement of an attribute, it does not mean that the correct attribute is being measured. The validity of an instrument is concerned with the extent to which a measure assesses the underlying attribute. Evidence of validity may be gained through observation, expert and lay judgement, and empirical enquiry.

Face validity is a measure of whether the items included in the scale make sense, are unambiguous and could reasonably measure the underlying concept. Face validity is an estimate of the meaning and relevance of the items (Bowling 1997). *Content validity* is a judgement of the standard of clarity, comprehensiveness, and redundancy of items and scales of an instrument, relative to its intended use and name. A definition or conceptual framework is required, as a standard, against which content validity may be evaluated. All items should be relevant to the content areas (domains) of the instrument. Items should be reviewed for their relevance to the instrument's objectives, and similarly, the instrument's objectives should be reviewed for comprehensiveness. The number of items per domain should reflect the relative importance of that domain to the instrument construct. Lay groups have been suggested as the best source for determining the content validity of measures of subjective health status (Hunt *et al.* 1986). It is important that due consideration is given to the items and domains of instruments in light of the specific condition under study. This is of particular significance, when the data from the questionnaire are reduced to a single index and so mask the items and domains tested by the instrument.

Construct validity is concerned with *hypothetical* instrument attributes that cannot be directly measured. Testing of the instrument involves developing theories about the relationship between the instrument attribute and other measures. Testing is undertaken to confirm or dispel these theories. Problems arise when the hypothesis is disproved since it is not clear whether the hypothesised theory was wrong or if there is a problem with the instrument. Construct validity may be subdivided into *convergent* and *discriminant validity*. Assessment of the relationships between the new instrument and other variables, and also other constructs to which it should be related are tested. Correlations provide evidence of the extent of these relationships. If the correlation coefficient is too high, the new instrument may be measuring the same concept. Convergent validity requires the new instrument to correlate moderately with measures of the same construct (0.4–0.8) (Streiner and Norman 1989). Discriminant validity requires the instrument to have no associations with dissimilar variables. It has been suggested that a low or zero-correlation is more informative, since it clearly shows that instruments are measuring different concepts.

Criterion validity refers to the ability of an instrument to correlate with other widely accepted validated measures of the construct under test. It is difficult to perform tests of criterion validity with health outcome measures due to the lack of widely accepted measures of health and related concepts such as quality of life. Criterion validity may be sub divided into *concurrent* and *predictive validity*. Concurrent validity involves administering the new instrument and the criterion instrument simultaneously to establish if the new measure may be a suitable substitute for the criterion measure. Predictive validity considers the ability of the new instrument to predict future differences. For this test the criterion is available at a future endpoint.

Responsiveness

Responsiveness (i.e. the extent to which scores change when the concept under study improves or deteriorates) is a particularly important criterion for studies that occur over a period of time. Sufficient sample sizes and variability of scores are required to detect a real change. When evaluating the impact of a health care intervention, it is vital that instruments can detect change, both clinically and that which is important to patients.

Interpretation

The degree to which qualitative meaning may be assigned to the quantitative scores of an instrument is an important aspect of interpreting the scores of that instrument. For example, if the instrument is scored so that it provides a summary score, it is important that this number has meaning.

Burden

During the administration of an instrument, demands may be placed on those participating in the study and those conducting the study. Consideration must be given to the abilities of the participants and the feasibility of the study. Missing data (questions not answered by participants) and refusal rates should be made explicit, as measures of acceptability of the instrument to the target population.

Alternative forms of instrument

The above properties should be reported during the development of any instrument in combination with the form of the instrument (e.g. telephone-administered, interviewer-administered, self-administered, observer-rated, proxy reports etc.). All instrument criteria and information relating to its use must be demonstrated with the alternative forms of the instrument. It is unacceptable practice to use an interviewer-administered instrument for a postal survey by assuming that the psychometric properties of the instrument will be stable.

Cultural and language adaptations

Of concern to many health providers and researchers is the need to include the views of participants that are representative of local populations. However, this can cause problems when using standardised instruments for measuring health and illness with respondents who have a variety of cultural backgrounds and speak different languages. The reliability and validity properties of instruments developed in a particular language or culture must be reassessed if translated into a different language or adopted for use in a new culture.

The main concerns are of *conceptual equivalence* (i.e. what are the relevance and meaning of concepts across different languages and cultures?) and *linguistic equivalence* (i.e. are the wording and meaning of questions in all aspects of the instrument shared across different languages?). Conceptual and linguistic equivalence equally apply to the use of American measures in the UK and other European settings and vice versa.

CONCLUSION

From the range of approaches to measuring health, it is evident that there is not a single best method. The choice of approach is determined by the conceptual model and the purpose for which health is being measured. Multiple approaches offer the most comprehensive method for measuring health. All health care professionals should be interested in determining the impact of disease and treatment from the patient's perspective and using this information alongside clinical variables to optimise the health care of their patients.

It is essential that considerable thought is given to the choice of instrument for measuring health and illness. Uncritical use of instruments can influence decision-making in an inappropriate manner. The relative strengths and weaknesses of instruments influence their appropriateness for measuring change in certain illnesses, and consequently data can give inaccurate pictures of the impact of interventions.

FURTHER READING

Aggleton, P. (1990) *Health*, Routledge, New York and London.

Armstrong, D. (1994) Measuring Health and Illness. In: D. Armstrong (Ed.) *Outline of Sociology as Applied to Medicine* (4th Edn.) Butterworth-Heinemann, Cambridge.

Bowling, A. (1995) *Measuring Disease: A Review of Disease-Specific Quality of Life Measurement Scales*, Open University Press, Milton Keynes.

Bowling, A. (1997) *Measuring Health: A Review of Quality of Life Measurement Scales* (2nd Edn.) Open University Press, Milton Keynes.

Coggon, D., Rose, G. and Barker, D.J.P. (1993) *Epidemiology for the Uninitiated* (3rd Edn.) British Medical Journal Publishing Group, London.

WEBSITES

Department of Health, Great Britain – http://www.doh.gov.uk

World Health Organisation – http://www.who.int

REFERENCES

Barlow, P. (1999) Health care is not a human right. *British Medical Journal* **319**, 321.

Bowling, A. (1995) *Measuring Disease: A Review of Disease-specific Quality of Life Measurement Scales*, Open University Press, Milton Keynes.

Bowling, A. (1997) *Measuring Health: A Review of Quality of Life Measurement Scales* (2nd Edn.) Open University Press, Milton Keynes.

Bryman, A. and Cramer, D. (1997) *Quantitative Data Analysis with SPSS for Windows. A Guide for Social Scientists*, Routledge, London, New York.

Cairns, J. (1996) Measuring health outcomes. Condition specific and patient specific measures are of limited use when allocating resources. *British Medical Journal*, **313**, 6.

Chambers, L.W. (1993) The McMaster Health Index Questionnaire: an update. In: S.R. Walker and R. Rosser (Eds.) *Quality of Life Assessment: Key Issues in the 1990s*, Kluwer Academic Publishers, London, pp. 131–149.

Cronbach, L.J. (1951) Coefficient alpha and the internal structure of tests. *Psychometrika*, **22**, 293–296.

Fayers, P. (1992) Untitled contribution to the discussion on Cox D. et al. Quality-of-life assessment: can we keep it simple? *Journal of the Royal Statistical Society*, **155**, 382.

Häyry, M. (1991) Measuring the quality of life: why, how and what? *Theoretical Medicine*, **12**, 97–116.

Hunt, S.M. (1997) The problem of quality of life. *Quality of Life Research*, **6**, 205–212.

Hunt, S.M. (1988) Measuring health in clinical care and clinical trials. In: G. Teeling Smith (Ed.) *Measuring Health: A Practical Approach*, John Wiley and Sons, Chichester.

Hunt, S., McEwan, P. and McKenna, S. (1986) *Measuring Health Status*. Croom Helm, London.

Hunt, S.M. and McKenna, S.P. (1993) Measuring quality of life in psychiatry. In: S.R. Walker and R.M. Rosser (Eds.) *Quality of Life Assessment. Key Issues in the 1990s*, Kluwer Academic Press, London.

Joyce, C.R.B. (1994) Requirements for the assessment of individual quality of life. In: H.M. McGee and C. Bradley (Eds.) *Quality of Life Following Renal Failure. Psychosocial Challenges Accompanying High Technology Medicine*, Harwood Academic Publishers, Amsterdam, pp. 43–54.

Katz, S., Downs, T.D., Cash, H.R. and Grotz, R.C. (1970) Progress in development of the index of ADL. *Gerontologist*, **10**, 20–30.

Katz, S., Ford, A.B., Moskowitz, R.W., Jackson, B.A. and Jaffe, M.W. (1963) Studies of illness in the aged. The index of ADL: a standardized measure of biological and psychosocial function. *Journal of the American Medical Association*, **185**, 914–919.

MacKeigan, L.D. and Pathak, D.S. (1992) Overview of health-related quality of life measures. *American Journal of Hospital Pharmacy*, **49**, 2236–2245.

Medical Outcomes Trust. (1997) *Source Pages. A Resource Directory for the Health Outcomes Field*, Medical Outcomes Trust, Boston.

Najman, J.M. and Levine, S. (1981) Evaluating the impact of medical care and technologies on the quality of life: a review and critique. *Social Science and Medicine*, **15F**, 107–115.

Nelson, E.C. and Berwick, D.M. (1989) The measurement of health status in clinical practice. *Medical Care*, **27**(Suppl. 3), S77–S90.

Nunnally, J.C. (1978) *Psychometric Theory* (2nd Edn.) McGraw-Hill, New York.

O'Boyle, C.A. (1994) The Schedule for the Evaluation of Individual Quality of Life (SEIQoL). *International Journal of Mental Health*, **23**, 3–23.

Office for National Statistics. (1995) *Morbidity Statistics From General Practice – Fourth National Study 1991–92*, HMSO, London.

Patrick, D.L. and Erickson, P. (1993) *Health Status and Health Policy. Quality of Life in Health Care Evaluation and Resource Allocation*, Oxford University Press, New York.

Rosenberg, R. (1995) Health-related quality of life between naturalism and hermeneutics. *Social Science and Medicine*, **41**, 1411–1415.

Spiegelhalter, D.J., Gore, S.M., Fitzpatrick, R., Fletcher, A.E., Jones, D.R. and Cox, D.R. (1992) Quality of life measures in health care. III: resource allocation. *British Medical Journal*, **305**, 1205–1209.

Streiner, D.L. and Norman, G.R. (1989) *Health Measurement Scales. A Practical Guide to Their Development and Use*, Oxford University Press, Oxford.

Tugwell, P., Bombardier, C., Buchanan, W., Goldsmith, C., Grace, E., Bennett, K.J., Williams, H.J., Egger, M., Alarcon, G.S., Guttadauria, M., Yarboro, C., Polisson, R.P., Szydlo, L., Luggen, M.E., Billingsley, L.M., Ward, J.R. and Marks, C. (1990) Methotrexate in rheumatoid arthritis: impact on quality of life assessed by traditional standard item and individualised patient preference health status questionnaires. *Archives of Internal Medicine*, **150**, 59–62.

Ware, J.E. (1995) The status of health assessment 1994. *Annual Review of Public Health*, **16**, 327–354.

World Health Organisation (1948) *Official Records of the World Health Organisation*, No. 2, World Health Organization, Geneva, p. 100.

World Health Organization Quality of Life Group (1993) *Measuring Quality of Life: The Development of the World Health Organization Quality of Life Instrument (WHOQOL)*. World Health Organization, Geneva.

World Health Organisation (1999) *The World Health Report 1999: Making a Difference*. World Health Organization, Geneva.

Youngson, R.M. (1992) *Collins Dictionary of Medicine*, Harper Collins Publishers, Glasgow.

SELF-ASSESSMENT QUESTIONS

Question 1: What is meant by positive and negative definitions of health?

Question 2: What are the limitations of simply counting the number of deaths in a given population as an indicator of the health of that population, and comparing this with other populations?

Question 3: What are the differences between generic, condition-specific and patient-specific approaches to assessing the health outcome of a population?

Question 4: What is the difference between the reliability and validity of a measurement instrument?

Question 1:   Negative definitions of health are based on the absence of disease, illness or sickness. Positive definitions of health include the wider concepts of physical, mental and social well-being.

Question 2:   In the first instance, the number of deaths needs to be presented as a fraction where number of deaths is the numerator, and the total population at risk of dying is the denominator. The population may be defined within geographical boundaries. Secondly, depending on the make-up of that population, factors that affect death rates such as the number of elderly people or the number of the very young should be taken into account when comparing crude mortality rates between populations.

Question 3:   Generic approaches to health outcome measurement are broad measures that include core health concepts such as physical, social and mental health. Condition-specific measures have been developed according to a detailed knowledge of that condition and its management. Each of these approaches has a standardised content. Patient-specific approaches allow the preferences and priorities of the respondents to be represented in the instrument and therefore, this approach is claimed to have greater sensitivity for detecting change.

Question 4:   Reliability is concerned with the accuracy of measurement on repeated applications of the instrument. Validity is concerned with the concepts being measured by the instrument and if they reflect the intended purpose of the instrument.

Survey Methods

Jill Jesson and Rob Pocock

INTRODUCTION	434
PERSPECTIVES ON RESEARCH AND SCIENCE	434
MODELS OF HEALTH, ILLNESS AND DISEASE	435
Bio-medical model	435
Social model	436
HISTORICAL DEVELOPMENT OF SURVEY METHODS IN PHARMACY PRACTICE RESEARCH	437
PARADIGMS AND THE PRACTICALITIES OF CONDUCTING RESEARCH	437
CRITERIA FOR APPRAISING SURVEY RESEARCH	438
Scientific rigour	438
Validity	438
Reliability and replicability	439
Values	439
Ethics	439
Stages of research which require ethical considerations	440
Deciding to do the survey	440
Sampling	440
Generation of the data	440
Contents of the questionnaire	440
Data processing	441
Presentation of the results	441
Fraud	441
PLANNING AND DESIGNING A SURVEY	441
Selecting appropriate survey methods	441
Secondary data	442
Referencing	442
Surveys	442
CHOICE OF METHOD	443
Project planning and scheduling	444
Samples and sampling frames	445
Grouping and categorising samples	446
QUESTIONNAIRE DESIGN, ADMINISTRATION AND RESPONSE	447
Self-completion questionnaire surveys	447
Construction and layout	447
Question design	448
Piloting	448
Administration of the survey	449
Letter content	449
Self-completion, non-postal surveys	450
Processing replies	450
Face to face interviews	451
Telephone interviews	452
Response rates	453
CONCLUSION	454
FURTHER READING	454
REFERENCES	454
SELF-ASSESSMENT QUESTIONS	455
KEY POINTS FOR ANSWERS	455

INTRODUCTION

Along with health care professionals, such as nurses, physiotherapists and other professions allied to medicine, one of the biggest hurdles pharmacists researching pharmacy practice encounter is the introduction of *'alien'* thought patterns for which their academic training has often left them ill-prepared. The pharmacy degree is based on the *'positivist'* philosophical approach to science and the natural world, but to understand the social world, a social scientific approach is necessary. Some social scientists would argue that all knowledge is socially constructed i.e. scientific procedures and conclusions are, in fact, not neutral, objective enterprises but are *'cultural products'*. Empirically based scientific *'facts'* then, are not simply determined by the nature of the observable physical world – they are also dependent upon socially derived assumptions.

Scientific *'facts'* are inseparable from the assumptions, traditions and relations of people at a particular time and place. These assumptions and traditions are motivated by, and in themselves motivate, conceptual modes of thought. Similarly, each professional group develops its own way of knowing. Pharmacists, doctors, lawyers, social scientists are all socialised into the culture, language and methods of their respective disciplines. Consequently they each make sense of the world in different ways, and investigate the world according to their own rules and perspective.

PERSPECTIVES ON RESEARCH AND SCIENCE

The social sciences are not constructed on the same principles as the natural sciences. Human actions, unlike the observed effects of molecules when heated, have meaning for both the observer and the observed and involve a process of interpretation. To explore social actions a different range of methods is used. In the social sciences it is accepted that there is not one, but several ways of looking at the world. These ways of looking at the world are known as *paradigms* or *perspectives*. Each may have its own internally valid *'truths'* but accepting the valid existence of several different paradigms means accepting the reality of several possible conflicting truths instead of one single universal truth. *'Paradigm shift'* describes the development of new ideas. A classic clinical paradigm shift in beliefs centres on the cause of peptic ulcer. In the past it was believed genetic factors, a faulty diet, or stress caused the condition. Now, with the emergence of bacteriological infection as a primary cause, as Lefanu (1999) observes *'helicobacter has provoked another paradigm shift in changing scientific understanding, not only of the diseases with which it is directly associated but of all disease.'*

MODELS OF HEALTH, ILLNESS AND DISEASE

In pharmacy practice research and health care research two paradigms come into conflict, the biomedical and the social model of health, illness and disease.

Biomedical model

The dominant model of disease worldwide, the biomedical model, is based on the Cartesian philosophy (after the philosopher, Descartes) of the body as a machine. Underlying this perspective is the concept that if a body system malfunctions it can be repaired or replaced. Thus, the biomedical model is concerned with the treatment of dysfunction. By contrast, illness is the subjective experience of dysfunction. The medical model is based on notions of scientific rationality, with an emphasis on objective, numerical measurement. In this model health is conceptualised merely as the absence of disease.

The theoretical framework underpinning the biomedical model is termed *Positivism*, an approach to knowledge based on quantitative measurement. This is a view of the world which suggests that phenomena which convey knowledge and meaning are those which are observable and measurable. Positivist researchers are those who believe that by careful observation, it is possible to identify the relationship between observable and measurable things. It could then be argued that events that cannot be measured cannot be understood. The key relationships of interest are those of *'causality'* in which the state of one variable can be said to *'cause'* the state of another one – the *'cause and effect'* relationship. This is the principle underlying all physical *'laws'*.

In the natural sciences, positivists begin with a tentative idea or hypothesis about relationships between variables and then repeatedly test these ideas against the available evidence. This process leads to validation of theory based on the results of observation. Positivism holds that social aspects of human life can be measured objectively and analysed following the principles of the scientific method, i.e. it can be explained in the same way as the natural sciences and other natural phenomena. Such an approach implies we can predict and explain behaviour. We can produce a set of *'true'*, *'precise'* and *'universal laws'*, from which we can generalise about the population as a whole.

The gold standard research method for positivists is the Randomised Controlled Trial (RCT) carried out in a controlled setting such as the clinical laboratory or hospital, often with a drug therapy or surgical intervention-based treatment of the *'subject'*. The principle is a simple experiment where the allocation of remedy to patients is unknown to the physician. Comparing the outcome in patients given a remedy with the outcome of a similar group (the control) who are not, provides a test for the efficacy of the remedy. If there is a measurable improvement it can be *presumed* that the remedy has had a beneficial effect.

Social model

The subject matter in the social model is *social action*. Social scientists have a range of paradigms they draw on in order to understand the world. Pharmacy practice research frequently draws on a *'realist'* paradigm. One way of understanding this is to distinguish between the medical model concept of disease and the subjective feelings and perceptions of *disease*, usually called *illness* or *sickness* by non-health professionals. Illness is not always detectable by biochemical indicators, a person can be diseased without feeling ill, for example, they may have undiagnosed cancer, or feel ill without any obvious biological cause, e.g. *myalgic encephalomyelitis* (ME). The social model's definition of *'health'* can best be described as: *'not merely the absence of disease but a state of complete physical, psychological and social well-being.'*

The varied range of methods used in social science (Box 25.1) includes: surveys, secondary source data analysis, ethnography, observation and interviews. The social science methodologies are often regarded to be a product of the 1960s. However their origins go back over a century. For instance, William Henry Duncan, the first Medical Officer of Health in England and Liverpool, conducted a survey of housing conditions in Liverpool in the 1830s. His findings were used by Edwin Chadwick, a 19th century pioneer of the public health movement in the UK, to argue for public health measures to deal with the social causes of the high rate of mortality in Liverpool.

Quantitative methods

- Randomised controlled clinical trial (RCT)
- Experiments: usually laboratory-based
- Surveys: using postal questionnaires or interview schedules. The method can be self-completion or face to face interviewer administered
- E-mail and faxback offer new choices and samples of respondent

Qualitative methods

- Ethnography
- Participant observation and interview
- Focus group discussions

Other methods

- Documentary – secondary data
- Life history, narratives
- Diary completion
- Historical or comparative perspective
- Nominal group technique
- Case study
- Critical incident analysis

Evaluation

- Uses all methods

Box 25.1 The range of research methods

HISTORICAL DEVELOPMENT OF SURVEY METHODS IN PHARMACY PRACTICE RESEARCH

Pharmacy practice has only recently emerged as an internationally recognised discipline. The first international workshop on social pharmacy was held in Helsinki in 1980. The first volume of the English language international *Journal of Social and Administrative Pharmacy* describes the historical development of the subject in the USA and Europe (Wertheimer *et al.* 1983). This journal remains one of the best sources of published international pharmacy practice research papers. The range of different nations involved is extensive, papers have been published from many nations, including European nations, with the Nordic countries playing a leading role; the United States of America, Canada, Africa, Australia and New Zealand.

The Royal Pharmaceutical Society of Great Britain's Director of Pharmacy Practice Research established a Research Task Force in 1997, which published its strategy for the future development of pharmacy practice research. The strategy comprised four key goals (Box 25.2).

Box 25.2 Four key goals for the development of pharmacy practice research (Mays 1997)

- A clear focus to ensure that the research asks and answers critical questions and produces results that inform not only the profession but also the wider health and social care policy agenda
- High quality, to ensure that the research produces scientifically rigorous results that enable it to be a persuasive and effective force for change
- Raised awareness, to ensure that the results from research are routinely used to improve the effectiveness, efficiency, appropriateness and quality of practice and services provided, as well as to inform professional and policy development in pharmacy
- Sound funding, to secure the future of pharmacy practice research with adequate investment that is targeted and used to maximum effect

PARADIGMS AND THE PRACTICALITIES OF CONDUCTING RESEARCH

The description of the medical and social models of health, together with positivist and realist paradigms (Table 25.1), is a polarised view, used here to illustrate the conceptual framework that researchers (often unquestioningly) carry with them. However, research often requires a more pragmatic approach. The most effective pharmacy practice research often draws from a range of paradigms with associated methodologies relevant to the research question. Thus researchers may use three different methods (triangulation) to explore different aspects of the same phenomenon.

Positivist	Realist
Phenomena can only be termed real if their existence can be demonstrated through quantifying empirical evidence	Studying individuals and organisations is different from studying the physical world. Social reality is the product of social interaction
Positivist research begins with experimental design, based on hypotheses and involves the investigation and discovery of cause and effect relationships	Naturalistic inquiry questions the value of preconceived hypotheses and objectification and emphasises qualitative research, which describes and explains human behaviour
Positivist research is based on measurement and deductive statistical analysis of large number data sets. Emphasis on treatment and control group, dependent and independent variables	Small numbers or case studies of examples are valid. Narratives, descriptions, comments can help to give meaning to inductive analysis
Positive researchers are objective, unbiased, apolitical. They remain aloof from the research objects	Researchers admit subjective influences and use the practice of reflexivity to discuss the interpretation of results

Table 25.1 Key features of Positivist and Realist research paradigms

CRITERIA FOR APPRAISING SURVEY RESEARCH

Pharmacy practice research in its infancy was characterised by lack of rigour and inadequate reference to the hallmarks of high quality survey research.

Scientific rigour

All research should be conducted rigorously in relation to the scientific paradigm. The essence of science, that applies equally to the social sciences, is the commitment to the 'rules' governing the line of enquiry – the means by which knowledge ('science' as in Latin scio = I know) is acquired. Positivists emphasise validity and reliability; realists will also look for a statement of context and values in the methodological writing.

Validity

There are two forms of validity: internal and external validity. Internal validity applies to the study setting and concerns whether or not the empirical evidence properly describes the concepts under investigation. In other words: 'Am I measuring what I think I am measuring?'. External validity is the extent to which findings can be generalised beyond the immediate study setting. Replication can confirm findings, and may also uncover '*trimming*' – the selection of data which fit hypotheses; '*cooking*' – manipulation of the data to make them look better, and '*forging*' – a complete fabrication of data. Validation requires you to consider, for example, if you study one pharmacy in one area, to what extent can you generalise the findings to all pharmacies, and to all areas? In other words, how artificial or atypical is the setting and has this constrained the findings such that they are particular to one setting and do not represent a valid general model?

Reliability and replicability

Reliability is extremely important in laboratory-based research. Reliability is less easy to ensure in social scientific studies because we cannot, for both ethical and practical reasons, create precise social conditions and interactions in an experimental setting. Reliability and replicability are often confused with each other. Replicability is about the consistency of results, i.e. the extent to which the research findings are replicable and reproducible using a comparable sample, design and conditions.

Values

The notion that researchers are '*value free*' is questionable. In the realist paradigm we can question to what extent the researcher imposes their own values on the study. Values, as illustrated by the example in Box 25.3 can be subjective. This subjectivity is expressed through the choice of problem or subject, the theoretical framework underpinning the study, its concepts, indicators and question design, the choice of research methods, the analysis and report writing.

Ethics

In the UK, all research involving patients has to be approved by a Local Research Ethics Committee (LREC). Ethical issues to be considered are listed in Box 25.4.

A question in a self-completion postal questionnaire to general practitioners (GPs) asked:

'*Would you support your medical practice funding a GP Pharmacist?*'
❒ Yes   ❒ No

50% said yes, 50 % said no.
The researcher analysed this as a negative, disappointing result and wrote in the report: '*only 50% of GPs were prepared to pay for a GP pharmacist*'. This statement caused some concern at the medical practice because it was perceived to be negative. The report was changed, the word '*only*' removed (Jesson *et al.* 1998a).

Box 25.3 An example of subject value placed on data

Box 25.4 Ethical issues in research

Stages of research which require ethical considerations

Deciding to do the survey

Deciding whether a survey can answer the research question is a technical matter, but to undertake a survey which cannot answer the question is unethical if you are aware of it and incompetent if you are not.

Sampling

There are no ethical problems about the use of public records such as electoral registers or postcode lists, but patient medical records will need ethics committee approval.

Generation of the data

This applies equally to interview or postal surveys. A respondent has the right to know:

- Who you are;
- Why the study is being done;
- How their name and address was obtained;
- How the person was chosen;
- What is to be done with the information.

It is best for the researcher to avoid assuming the dual role of both practitioner and researcher, as the patient may feel compromised and under an obligation to participate. Confidentiality also requires that information is not supplied to anyone outside the research team. Finally, prior to commencing the study, a researcher should plan the action to be taken if a respondent asks for advice, or appears to need medical or psychological help.

Contents of the questionnaire

Consider whether is it reasonable to ask people about certain subjects which they may find embarrassing or painful. Particular care must be taken for some marginalised groups or where sensitive issues are involved, such as terminal illness or sexual health.

Data processing

Ensure that data recorded on computer cannot be related to individuals, without reference to other lists or records correlating names with serial numbers. Researchers should also be aware of any legislation governing the storage of survey data.

Presentation of the results

In presenting qualitative data, quotations may be used to illustrate concepts, ideas, or other activity. These will usually need an identifier code, e.g. Pharm.24 would mean pharmacist interview 24. There is a question as to what extent you should camouflage the identity of places, organisations or respondents. Sometimes it may be difficult if the work is commissioned. Finally, there may be a dilemma over the suppression of data. Some funding bodies may wish to suppress unfavourable findings, as illustrated in Box 25.5, which is an extract from a review of Local Authority Social Services Departments.

Box 25.5 An example of sensitivity to the subjects of research

> *'Almost by definition, research on complaints procedures is going to involve issues that are sensitive for the authorities concerned. The research has in-built bias. It deals only with situations where something, at some stage, has gone wrong; it does not even begin to look at the things the Department got right. Not surprisingly, they (the Departments) wish to remain anonymous'* (Simons 1995).

Fraud

It is clearly unethical to fabricate data. Some researchers have been caught out when other researchers have tried to replicate the study. Many research organisations now have Research Guidelines or Research Codes which members are expected to uphold (Kimmel 1996; British Medical Journal 1998). The Market Research Society has a code of conduct requiring that a proportion of those interviewed are re-contacted by a supervisor to check that the interview has actually been carried out, as well as conformity with codes of etiquette and courtesy.

PLANNING AND DESIGNING A SURVEY

Selecting appropriate survey methods

Early in an investigation, it is necessary to decide what means of enquiry is best suited to meeting the objectives of the study. There is no one best approach to research methodology, but there is a need to select the approach which is going to be most effective for addressing the research question(s). Before embarking on a survey, researchers should identify what they are seeking to find out. Perhaps there is already a set of someone else's data (secondary data) that will suffice?

Secondary data

The research process involves a review of current knowledge. This may vary from a cursory consideration of everyday knowledge, to a full-scale systematic literature review. Online computer search data bases are a valuable source of information, but they should be supplemented with a manual search of journals and books.

Readily available secondary sources of data include routinely collected census data and government statistics. Before deciding to produce your own survey data, consider whether they have already been collected by another agency. There is a standard format to all research, beginning with a secondary data review and critical analysis, shown in Box 25.6. Selecting the appropriate method takes place at a much later stage.

1. Critical review of the literature (secondary data stage)
2. Develop the aims, objectives and hypothesis of the research, specify concepts and theories
3. Clarification of independent and dependent variables
4. Consider research ethics
5. Selection and design of the methods of research and the measurement instruments
6. Data assembly, either secondary sources or through fieldwork and implementation
7. Analysis
8. Report and dissemination of findings

Box 25.6 Basic steps in carrying out a research project

Referencing

It is important at the commencement of a project to note all your sources of information systematically as you proceed. Record every source; write the source on photocopies, journal or news articles because you may not find the original again. Begin a card index or computer file. There are two referencing systems: Harvard and Vancouver. Some studies prescribe the format to be used but in general it does not matter which you use, so long as you consistently use one style.

Surveys

Having decided that a survey is appropriate, it is necessary to work through the associated parts of the process described in the remainder of this section. A survey is a quantitative method (although qualitative data may be obtained through free text using 'open-ended' questions) In the main however, it deals with quantities of data and relationships between variables, involving the generation and analysis of highly structured data in the positivist tradition. Generally the technique involves the systematic, structured questioning of a large (statistically

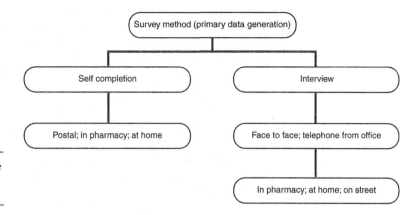

Figure 25.1 The range of options within the survey method

valid) sample of people. The structured questioning can be undertaken by self-completion or by interview. Figure 25.1 shows the range of options available within the survey method. An interviewer completes interviews; they can be face to face in the pharmacy, the surgery, at home, on the street, or by telephone. A new and less well developed option is to distribute the questionnaire through IT based World Wide Web or email, if a suitable database of respondents is available (Murray and Sixsmith 1998).

The survey is one method of collecting information from a sample of the population of interest – but not necessarily the whole population. Surveys are suitable in situations where there is sufficient pre-existing knowledge, which can be incorporated into a standard structured *'research instrument'* as the questionnaire is often termed. There are many textbooks that describe the survey method in greater detail than is possible here. A comprehensive review of UK pharmacy practice surveys was undertaken by Smith (1997a; 1997b). For a critical review of health service surveys see Cartwright (1988).

CHOICE OF METHOD

All too often, researchers decide on the method before being clear on the information they need. The availability of resources, of time, money, sample of participants or pharmacies often determines options and choices. Although the remainder of this chapter is mainly about quantitative surveys, we look briefly at the full range of options. Box 25.7 illustrates that if you need insight and understanding of rationales for people's beliefs and attitudes, you need a qualitative method such as a focus group (see also Chapter 27) or depth interview (see also Chapter 26). If you want baseline population data on behaviour patterns (e.g. what percentage of people are loyal to one pharmacy) a quantitative technique such as a self-completion questionnaire form will be appropriate.

Box 25.7 Is a survey appropriate?

The method by which the survey will be administered is a key early decision. The presentation of the questionnaire or interview schedule, and format of the questions is determined by the method of accessing respondents, i.e. is it to be postal, face to face or telephone? At an early stage in learning about research, it is easy to start writing a questionnaire without first thinking about how it will be administered. The words and expressions used will vary considerably, just as written and spoken English is very different.

The design of the research instrument will thus depend on the target audience and the strategy to access them. Before writing the questionnaire, it is important to think through what you want to achieve from your survey. How much time have you got? What research questions do you want to answer? If you are testing a hypothesis, which statistical test will you be using, what size of response will you need? Who is going to respond to your survey and how will you identify them?

Project planning and scheduling

Project management is rarely mentioned in research methods textbooks but it is crucially important. Keep records of everything that you do on the project; set up a systematic filing system; retain a copy of all correspondence; make a note of all telephone calls and purchase or invoicing orders. There should be a file of all design drafts of research instruments. You can never be sure that computer held files will not be deleted or lost. This documentation package will be an integral record of the research process, and may be important when you write up the methods section of reports or papers. The bigger the survey, and the longer the project, the more important a robust data organisation system becomes.

The best way to manage day to day activities is by using the so-called GANTT project management method. By drawing up a '*GANTT Chart*' project time plan at the outset you can see whether the work is feasible

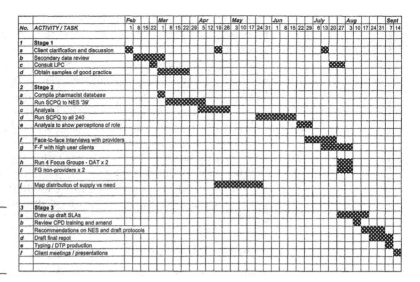

Figure 25.2 GANTT plan of community pharmacy and drug abuse study

within the time allowed, and which activities are dependent on another. For more complex or commissioned work it is the means of identifying resource costs, whether staff, materials or funding.

Figure 25.2 shows a GANTT chart for a survey of pharmacists and their views about services to drug misusers, such as needle exchange schemes and supervised methadone consumption. The project consisted of a number of different methods. The project plan shows a two-tier system of organisation – firstly dividing the project into three stages, and then within each stage, itemising the activities to be undertaken. Stage and activity are the building blocks of project management. Some activities depend on others having been done first, and these 'dependencies' set demands and constraints on the resulting schedule. Working out the dependencies is vital in helping you decide in what order to do the various tasks.

Samples and sampling frames

The type and availability of the sample often determine the choice of survey method. Before you can begin to decide on the choice of research instrument, decide who the respondent sample will be and how you are going to elicit the information you need. What sort of information do you want? If you want to measure 'how many', such a question can easily be answered by a tick box closed option, thus a self-completion postal survey, or telephone survey could be the choice. If you want more detail, in depth and to understand 'why' or 'how', then a face to face interview will be needed (see also Chapter 26).

Who will respond to your inquiry? Think through the availability of your respondents. Can you realistically access your sample? Will you need a gatekeeper or can you access them directly? Do pharmaceutical

bodies, or the electoral register hold an established database, such as
the membership lists, or will you need to be more creative in finding
respondents?

Surveying customers in a pharmacy might appear easy, but what if
you need subjects to meet specific criteria, such as people with coeliac
disease, or substance misusers, or homeless people? If the target audience is small and difficult to access by post or telephone, or you want
in-depth information and to understand a social process, then a face to
face interview will be a more appropriate technique.

Table 25.2 shows the key terms, and the range of sampling
options commonly encountered in pharmacy practice research. As
you move down the list the sampling method becomes necessarily
more opportunistic in order to access the more difficult to reach
samples.

Grouping and categorising samples

Often, pharmacy practice researchers want to survey pharmacies.
Surveys can cover a whole health authority, a random sample of
registered pharmacy owners, or all pharmacists as the sample frame.
Yet, if differing types of pharmacy are sought, how are they to be
categorised? Traditionally, pharmacies have been categorised by ownership or by location, because that is the easiest variable to identify
from existing databases. The competitive nature of pharmacy as a
business means that it is extremely difficult to categorise pharmacies

Sample	The research population
Sampling frame	List of population from which sample is drawn (contains everyone)
Sampling units	Can be pharmacies, general practitioners, Health Authorities, employees in a firm, or residents on an electoral register, or customers, patients at home, in the street or attending a clinic
Types of sampling	Simple random sample – each element has same chance of being selected, use random sample tables
Systematic sampling	More even spread of sample across a list
Sampling interval	When total N is known (1 in 10) n = sampling interval
Stratified sampling	Identify key characteristics, sex, age, social class
Cluster sample	When geographically distributed, e.g. towns in a national survey
Quota sampling	Use Census to match proportions in population (market research)
Snowball or network	People recommend someone they know
Convenience sampling	Anyone you can get
Purposive sampling	A setting chosen for its features
Illustrative sample	A small number of case studies, which describe concepts or behaviours

Table 25.2 Key
concepts in sampling

Chapter Twenty-five

by physical size, prescription level, or income, yet these may be much more meaningful criteria for understanding the contribution of pharmacy to health care.

There is another important consideration in surveying pharmacies. Researchers often make the mistake of not defining clearly whether it is the pharmacy or the pharmacist they are trying to study. These two entities are intrinsically intertwined, but from the research perspective they should be distinguished. Surveying practising pharmacists is in one sense a simple task because the individual is the single entity under study. Pharmacies as businesses are much more complex. Business data such as prescription volumes, financial returns from prescriptions, over the counter (OTC) and non-medical sales may be seen as highly sensitive and confidential. Then there is the problem of *'chains'*. A small chain is often seen in business terms as a single entity or sample. Financial and operational data (such as counter staff employment) may only be held in aggregate form for the chain. The large multiples often have corporate protocols prohibiting individual pharmacists from responding as individuals – the chain providing a single group response.

In such cases, questions need to be phrased and expressed having regard to the *'corporate'* respondent. Similarly, research concepts such as the *'response rate'* are less meaningful and expectations should be geared to the *'norms'* of business surveys (where responses of over 15% are acceptable) rather than for surveys of individuals or professionals, where such a response would be seen as unacceptable.

QUESTIONNAIRE DESIGN, ADMINISTRATION AND RESPONSE

Self-completion questionnaire surveys

Construction and layout

The questionnaire format and question construction are two separate issues, but there are a few key rules that can be quickly used for reference purposes. Box 25.8 shows the complete instrument design for the

1. Think about what you want to ask, what are your aims and objectives
2. Begin design
3. Check for clear unambiguous questions
3. Check layout and visual aspects
4. Beware of the length
5. Order Freepost envelopes
6. Set up database of sample for logging replies and follow-up
7. Design letter
8. Pilot or pre-test, redesign, pilot again if necessary
9. Print
10. Stuff envelopes and post (select Thursday or Friday, check time of year, holidays)

Box 25.8 Standard postal survey design process

postal self-completion survey process. Most self-completion questionnaires are sent by post, but this is not always the case. In a pharmacy, customers can be asked to fill in questionnaires while waiting for the prescriptions to be dispensed. The same can be done at a general practitioner's surgery, or at relevant locations for target groups such as young parents at play groups, older people at day care centres and so on.

With postal, self-completion questionnaires the layout and design should encourage the recipient to respond. The first thing is to have a title, and an introductory sentence explaining the reason you are asking for the information. Then number each question Q1, Q2, Q3, and provide instructions for each question, e.g. *please tick box* or *write in your own words, rate on a scale 1 to 5 where 1 is low and 5 is high* and so on. Questions should be written in a clear typeface that looks attractive. The use of arrows, boxes, and italics, bold and underline can draw attention to key words or instructions.

The visual impact of the instrument is important. Use A4 size paper and a strong staple to hold pages together. An alternative might be A3 paper folded into a booklet form; this makes it easier to turn the pages and it is less likely that the back page will be lost. Questions should not be split across two pages. You do not have to say *'please'* in every question. Aim for not more than 50 questions, or 10 pages, printed back to back. In a lengthy questionnaire it is important to print on both sides of the page as this has a positive psychological effect on the recipient who may not reply to a thick document.

Finally, don't forget to include a reminder about the Freepost address, stamped addressed envelope or fax number on the last page. In order to track replies it is usual to stamp a code or ID number on the back page. This is important when following up non-responders.

Remember, self-completion and postal survey questionnaires are limited in the range of information that can be obtained. In a self-completion questionnaire you can only measure: *Attitudes, Beliefs, Behaviour, Knowledge, Attributes or Demographics.*

Question design

The way in which questions are designed depends on the survey technique. Do not formulate specific questions until you have thought through the research question. Keep asking yourself: *Why do I want to know this? What will I do with the answer?* – the *'So-what?'* question. Box 25.9 has some tips on question design that are applicable to all survey types, not just self-completion surveys.

Piloting

Every survey instrument should be piloted before it is ready to be printed. Test it on colleagues, edit and revise; test on other

Box 25.9 Tips for good question design

people of the same respondent group by post and by sitting down with them and asking what they are thinking as they read each question.

Check that the instructions are clear, the design is professional and looks acceptable to the recipient, that language is easy to understand and questions are clear and unambiguous. Are the pre-coded options comprehensive, are the skips (instructions to complete only appropriate questions) correct and question numbers sequence accurate, is there sufficient space to write an answer to open ended questions? Finally, check how long it takes to complete. It is then ready for printing.

Administration of the survey

Ideally a self-completion questionnaire is limited to 50 questions that take about ten minutes to complete. It should be printed on attractive paper, with a balance of words and space, easy to complete and handle, and well stapled. From the research management side, it needs to be easy to record responses in an appropriate manner for statistical analysis (*coding*), and to identify. A survey needs a covering letter to motivate completion. It is important to get the letter right, to maximise the number of completed questionnaires returned (*the response rate*). The covering letter must answer all the recipients questions, the who, what, why and when explanations. It should look attractive, be no longer than a page, each sentence short and purposeful. Even the heading on the letter can influence completion.

Letter content

- Explain the purpose of the study
- Attempt to convince the reader that they are being useful and have valued information/opinions
- Ensure confidentiality and anonymity if relevant
- Do not forget to mention a contact name and number and the Freepost or stamped addressed envelope

The advantage of a postal questionnaire is usually cost. Postal surveys can cost only a third as much as interviews because there are lower organisational costs per respondent (e.g. stamps are cheaper than the equivalent interviewer fees). It is also easier to have a random geographical sample in a postal survey than in an interview model. You can reach working people, those who are rarely at home at 'normal' times and sparsely populated country areas or 'unsafe' housing estates. Self-completion helps to eliminate interviewer bias and personal or embarrassing questions may be answered more frankly. The respondent has more control of the instrument and has time to reflect on their answers before posting at their convenience. Finally, there is a degree of anonymity, which may encourage completion.

The disadvantages of a postal questionnaire are linked to the limitations of the instrument and the completion process. In this method it is not possible to use lead questions to get at a sub-set of issues; questions have to be simple, short and straightforward. Thus, they lack qualitative depth and are inflexible.

Once the instrument has been posted there is no control over the sequence of reading or completing and answers cannot be probed or checked. Loss of control over the process means that it is not always possible to determine who is a non-responder, or reasons for non-response. Returned forms may be incomplete or inaccurate because the person misunderstood or did not read the instructions. One can never be sure who filled the questionnaire in – whether it was the target person or a group effort. There is only the letter to motivate response. Thus, the main disadvantage is the risk of poor response rates and a biased skew to the sample.

Self-completion, non-postal surveys

Some self-completion surveys are completed by the respondent in the pharmacy or a general practitioner surgery. The non-postal instrument lacks a target respondent unless someone agrees to hand questionnaires out on your behalf. Quite often they are left lying around, or on the counter, waiting to be noticed.

In one survey, self-completion questionnaires were to be handed out to all patients attending a surgery over two weeks, the anticipated target had been calculated on attendance numbers to be 500. The reality was that since no-one had responsibility for the distribution it actually took six weeks to achieve 289 replies. The following year a repeat survey was managed differently and that produced a return of 257 after two weeks (Jesson et al. 1998b).

Processing replies

Once you are ready for distribution, here are some tips to help. With postal surveys, you should print two and a half times the number in the sample, to allow for two follow-up reminders. Buy self-sealing envelopes to make the *'stuffing'* process quicker. Post towards the end of the week to arrive for completion at the weekend. The whole mailing process can take up to nine weeks.

You can expect:

- 30% returned from the first mailing after 3 weeks
- 20% returned from the second mailing after 3 weeks
- 10% returned from the third mailing after 2 weeks

If the sample is small an alternative option is to telephone and ask whether the respondent has returned the survey instrument. This way you can find out something about the non-responders attitudes. Sometimes subjects will be prepared to respond over the phone (i.e. you fill in a spare copy of the survey form while they give you the answers).

Each questionnaire needs a code number before distribution, so you can tag the replies as they come in ready for the follow-up mailings. Set up the questionnaire database and code the replies for entering into a database.

Face to face interviews

Face to face interviews can be held with patients in their own home, or in the street. It is important to remember in face to face interviews that this is social interaction between an interviewer and respondent, so the dynamics of information exchange are different from that obtained in self-completion surveys. There are two types of interview: the structured interview, which produces quantitative data, and the exploratory depth interview, which produces qualitative data (see also Chapter 26). The choice of interview model depends on the purpose of the research, the stage of the research (development or testing), the time available for interview and the skill of the interviewer.

In a structured face to face interview, as in a self-completion survey, the questions are standardised. This method is most commonly used in market research surveys, for public opinion polls and in government surveys. The interviewer uses a standard technique, following the format rigorously so that every interview should be the same. In quantitative, structured interviews the questions are fixed by the designer before the interview, exact wording is prescribed for each respondent and the sequence is always the same. The interviewer should attempt to be unbiased and objective. However, there is a debate about the extent to which this is possible and whether there should be matched interviewer and respondent, in terms of age, sex and ethnicity. The large sample size means that the data should be valid, replicable and reliable, drawn from a representative sample, which then allows generalisation.

The advantage of structured, quantitative interviews is that interviewers can reach a large proportion of the sample. Standardisation of the instrument makes comparison and statistical analysis easier. The quantitative interview allows more scope for creativity through the use of prompts and show or shuffle cards, especially when it takes place indoors. House interviews can take up to an hour, or longer, and have the advantage of building up rapport with the respondent. Quicker, on-street surveys take about five minutes.

The disadvantage of this method can be the unavailability of respondents. It can be a frustrating experience standing outside a pharmacy, in the cold, trying to catch the attention of customers, and it may take some time to reach the desired sample size. If you want to interview a pharmacist, this method is problematic for interviewing them in the pharmacy. In addition to the demands of dispensing there is rarely a suitable place to sit. You may also have to offer to pay a locum fee to cover work time. Recruiting and training good interviewers can also be time consuming and expensive.

Time and the cost of interviewers will influence the sampling strategy. Every pharmacy is different. Sometimes quotas are used, but more often than not it is likely that an interviewer will approach every other pharmacy customer. Problems arise when the pharmacy is a very busy one, because it is difficult for one person to approach every other customer. Conversely in quiet pharmacies there may be a lot of '*down time*' because of lack of customers.

Telephone interviews

Telephone interviews are increasingly used in survey work and may be more suitable for interviewing pharmacists. A telephone interview needs to be fairly short, taking about 10 minutes at most. It will need a different construction and format from a face to face interview schedule, with more attention needed for spoken explanations.

The main advantages are convenience, the capability of rapid data collection, lower cost than face to face, better access, adaptability and greater interviewer control plus lower costs in term of time, effort and money. Telephone interviews share many of the advantages of a face to face interview: a high response rate, the potential for correction of obvious misunderstandings and the potential to use probes and prompts. They are also safer for interviewers, who do not have to enter unknown homes. The disadvantage is the limitations on scope and complexity of questions that can be asked. A typical call will last up to 10 minutes. The lack of visual cues may cause some problems in interpretation of answers.

The sampling frame is usually telephone and business directories. This too, can have a bias based on gender and social class. Further, new subscribers are not listed; more and more people are now ex-directory, use a mobile phone or subscribe to one of a range of telecommunication companies. Similarly, the telephone number of pharmacies may not be held centrally by the profession's registering body. For more random sample surveys, the technique of random digit dialling is used, which involves the local part of a telephone number being generated randomly using a table or a computer.

The response rate to a telephone survey can be higher than the postal method because the immediacy of the approach give respondents less time to refuse, or they have the option of calling back at a convenient time. Telephoning pharmacies may not produce the anticipated response rate, especially if it has a busy dispensary and the pharmacist is constantly interrupted or called away from the telephone. Halfpenny *et al.* (1998) describe the experience of a telephone survey of small companies, with a 33% refusal rate. The companies in question had developed resistance to telemarketing because they were deluged with telephone calls that were unproductive for them, because the callers want something other than goods or services sold by the companies. It wastes their time, and prevents customers getting through.

In a face to face or telephone interview the time scale can be much shorter than in the postal survey, depending on the size of the sample. You print exactly the sample number of schedules. No reminders are needed. There are no envelopes, Freepost inserts or postage costs. Instead you will need to set up interviewer claim forms, travel cost payments and so on.

Response rates

Response rates to survey questionnaires vary tremendously according to the sample, the method (postal, interview, telephone), design, the topic of interest and the time of year when they are sent out. Smith (1997a) describes a range of methods for increasing survey response rates. Her review of surveys involving community pharmacists found a range of rates from 30%–90%, with patients the range was 34%–88%. The best results for postal surveys can be obtained by sending at least three mailings. The response rate should be described in the report, so that readers are able to understand the scientific validity of the results.

There is no consensus on acceptable response rates. Many research textbooks base their estimates on clinical or medical studies and assert that anything less than a 70% response is not good enough, because there is a potential bias in the data. Bowling (1997) mentions 40% as common in postal surveys.

In addition to the usual reluctance to answer survey questionnaires, the response rate for pharmacy surveys in the UK is associated with competition and competitive advantage. This is because, as stated previously, a pharmacy survey is often analogous to a *'business survey'*. Although the pattern of pharmacy ownership varies with every health authority, so that in the West Midlands two multiples dominate; whilst in the south of England there are more multiples, competitive advantage limits the amount and type of information that can be obtained. When undertaking a survey that includes the multiples, the Superintendent Pharmacist should be contacted in advance of posting the questionnaire. The instrument may require amendment, but if support is given the response rate will be higher.

Conclusion

Surveys are a popular way of generating data in pharmacy practice research. They can be easy to do, or extremely difficult. The complexity varies with the study. In this chapter we have not set out to review the work of published surveys. Instead we have described the philosophical basis of survey methods as applied to pharmacy practice research, and shown the need to bring into pharmacy practice the social or *'realist'* paradigms of social survey research. This chapter has demonstrated three basic model options within the survey model, and has described in practical detail the key stages in undertaking a survey using these methods.

It should be borne in mind that survey research is, in itself, a learning process and has to adapt to a dynamic social and technological environment (people are increasingly reluctant to take part in surveys but on the other hand technology is opening up new ways of accessing people). There is no definitive text on the subject nor have we attempted to provide one, because the state of the art is still rapidly developing. Rather, we hope to have stimulated reflective thinking on the subject in order to raise the overall standards of survey research.

Further reading

Edwards, A. and Talbot, R. (1999) *Hard Pressed Researcher* (2nd Edn. Longman, London.

Kumar, R (1999) *Research Methodology. A Step by Step Guide for Beginners*, Sage, London.

Shipman, M. (1997) *The Limitations of Social Research* (4th Edn. Longman, London.

References

British Medical Journal (1988) The Randomised Control Trial at 50 *British Medical Journal*, **317**, 1217–1246.

Bowling, A. (1997) *Research Methods in Health*, Open University Press Buckingham.

Cartwright, A. (1988) *Health Surveys in Practice and Potential: A Review of Scope and Method*, King's Fund, London.

Halfpenny, P., Hudson, S. and Jones, J. (1998) Researching small companies' charitable giving through telephone interviews. *International Journal of Social Research Methodology*, 1, 65–74.

Jesson, J., Lacey, F. and Wilson, K.A. (1998a) *Second Year Evaluation of the North Birmingham Total Purchasing Pilot Pharmacy Project*. A Report to the TPP, Aston University, Birmingham.

Jesson, J. and Wilson, K. (1998b) An *evaluation study for the Isle of Wight Health Authority*. Newport Pharmacy Service Survey, Aston University, Birmingham.

Kimmel, A.J. (1996) *Ethical Issues in Behavioural Research*, Blackwell, Oxford.

Lefanu, J. (1999) *The Rise and Fall of Modern Medicine*, Little Brown, London.

Mays, N. (1997) *A New Age for Pharmacy Practice Research. Promoting Evidence Based Practice in Pharmacy. The Report of the Pharmacy Practice R&D Task Force*. Royal Pharmaceutical Society Great Britain, London.

Murray, C. and Sixsmith, J. (1998) E-mail: a qualitative research medium for interviewing? *International Journal Social Research Methodology*, 1, 103–121.

Simons, K. (1995) *I'm Not Complaining But ... Complaints Procedures in Social Services Departments*, Joseph Rowntree Foundation, York.

Smith, F. (1997a) Survey research: *(1)* Design, samples and response. *International Journal of Pharmacy Practice*, 5, 152–166.

Smith, F. (1997b) Survey research: (2) Survey instrument, reliability and validity. *International Journal of Pharmacy Practice*, 5, 216–226.

Wertheimer, A., Claesson, C. and Londen, H.H. (1983) The development of the discipline of social pharmacy. *Journal of Social and Administrative* Pharmacy, 1, 113–115.

SELF-ASSESSMENT QUESTIONS

Question 1: What can you do to increase the potential response rate in a postal self-completion survey?

Question 2: What are the key limitations of doing research in pharmacies?

Question 3: Should a questionnaire be written from the viewpoint of the researcher or the respondent?

KEY POINTS FOR ANSWERS

Question 1:

- Make sure the mailing list is up to date
- Enclose a covering letter with a motivational message and a '*P.S.*'
- Use Freepost reply envelopes
- Use one or preferably two reminders
- Make sure the questionnaire and letter are in '*plain English*'

Question 2:

- Gaining access to multiples
- Gaining approval of independents
- Finding space to speak to customers
- Lack of record of users
- People who will only spend three to five minutes in the shop
- Finding sufficient time with the pharmacist to be interviewed

Question 3:

- The respondent is the one who has to use it so it should be written from the '*user perspective*', i.e. use language, concepts and expressions familiar to respondents
- This often means translating professional or academic concepts and expressions
- However, the questionnaires must also be written with a view to how the results will be analysed and written up
- Try doing a checklist table when designing a questionnaire – lay each page of questions on the left hand side and a blank page next to it on the right. Read each question, imagine a result, then on the blank page write down what the question tells you and how it contributes to the research question.

26 Interviews

Madeleine Gantley

INTRODUCTION	458
APPROPRIATE RESEARCH QUESTIONS	458
SAMPLING STRATEGIES IN QUALITATIVE RESEARCH	458
INTERVIEWS VERSUS FOCUS GROUPS VERSUS OBSERVATION	459
PREPARATIONS	461
MAKING THE FAMILIAR STRANGE	461
PREPARING AN INTERVIEW TOPIC GUIDE	462
TYPES OF INTERVIEW QUESTION	463
GETTING IN: NEGOTIATING ACCESS AND RECRUITMENT	463
Introducing yourself	464
Ethical issues	464
GETTING ALONG	465
Interviewing colleagues	466
Keeping on track	466
RECORDING THE DATA	466
Taking notes	467
Tape recording	467
DATA ANALYSIS	467
VALIDITY AND RELIABILITY IN QUALITATIVE RESEARCH	468
CONCLUSION	468
FURTHER READING	469
REFERENCES	470
SELF-ASSESSMENT QUESTIONS	471
KEY POINTS FOR ANSWERS	471

INTRODUCTION

This chapter addresses interviewing as one means of collecting research data. In some ways, pharmacists use informal, brief interviews as an integral part of their work. However, the shift to research interviewing requires an acknowledgement of the distinction between routine conversations with the aim of extracting information in order to make a particular decision, and the semi-structured interview designed to encourage research respondents to talk at some length about a particular phenomenon.

The choice of data collection methods is made within the broader choice of research methods appropriate to answer a particular research question (see Chapter 25). Interviews may be formal or informal, structured or unstructured. The formal, structured interview, often centred around the administration of a questionnaire, falls within the quantitative framework in which researchers focus on the collection of large structured data sets. The informal, semi-structured interview, in contrast, is one of the key methods of data collection within qualitative research, which is designed to produce detailed data from a relatively small number of research respondents with experience of a particular phenomenon.

APPROPRIATE RESEARCH QUESTIONS

Qualitative research is essentially exploratory, and the choice of qualitative methods is made in order to maximise the amount of data generated. If the research question focuses on how many people at risk of heart disease take aspirin regularly, the appropriate method is a large survey, using a standard data collection tool. If, on the other hand, the question is why people with heart disease do not take aspirin regularly, then a relatively small number of in-depth interviews will provide appropriately detailed information to help the researcher understand their concerns. An example of a qualitative study is illustrated in Box 26.1.

SAMPLING STRATEGIES IN QUALITATIVE RESEARCH

Bearing in mind the nature of qualitative research, sampling concentrates on maximising either the range or depth of explanations and reasoning. Sampling is described as purposive, and is subdivided into a number of different strategies. The most frequent include maximum variety, intensity, typical and dissonant case. These are summarised in Box 26.2.

Sampling *strategy* is of more importance than sample size, but qualitative studies tend to draw on 30–40 hours of data collection. For

Box 26.1 A qualitative study of ideas about medicines

a review of sample sizes in qualitative research, see Denzin and Lincoln 1994.

INTERVIEWS VERSUS FOCUS GROUPS VERSUS OBSERVATION

Face-to-face interviews, of course, are not the only way of collecting data for qualitative research. Many qualitative studies use a mixture

Box 26.2 Sampling strategies (Patton, 1990)

of interviews and focus groups, and some also draw on observation. It is important to be clear about the strengths and weaknesses of each method (Table 26.1), and to choose the most appropriate. Each method is a balance between gathering appropriately detailed data, and ensuring that such data are relevant for the research question. Interviews have maximum potential for obtaining such data, allowing the interviewer to follow the respondents' own priorities, and to encourage discussions at some depth. Focus groups (see Chapter 27) are a relatively rapid method for generating a range of topics, but may be more difficult for the facilitator to control. Thus, the data may lack both relevance and depth. Observation may be either direct or participant, depending on the nature and relevance of the researcher's involvement in the research site, and entails prolonged exposure to the research setting. It may be used to supplement information collected by interviews, or may comprise the principal method of data collection as with ethnographic studies. Observation is very time consuming, but has the advantage that the observer sees what people do, rather than collecting data on what they say they do. However, there is no guarantee that data are relevant and the researcher has minimal control over the research setting. Bear in mind that for each method, the researcher has an impact on the research setting. For a comparative discussion of methods of data collection see Fitzpatrick and Boulton 1994.

Advantages	Disadvantages
INTERVIEWS	
Depth	Skilled interviewer essential
Opportunity to explore ideas	Sampling strategy essential
Context rich	Expensive
Data collected in *'natural setting'*	
FOCUS GROUPS	
Generate breadth of ideas	Skilled facilitator essential
Document development of ideas	Tape recording more difficult
Spin off among participants	May be hard to control
	May be dominated by vociferous participants
Relatively rapid data generation	Expensive
	May tend to consensus
OBSERVATION	
Seeing people in *'natural setting'*	Skilled observer essential
Observing process	No control over setting
Context rich	Time consuming
Can be used to complement interviews	Lack of focus
Sensitising researcher to research setting	

Table 26.1
Advantages and disadvantages of qualitative methods

PREPARATIONS

The first step in conducting a qualitative study is the preparation of a topic guide. This involves a critical assessment of relevant literature and reflection on your own beliefs and assumptions about the research question. In conducting the literature review, ensure that you search across different disciplinary fields, including sociology, anthropology and psychology, as well as pharmacy and other relevant fields such as primary care. Reflecting on your own assumptions is rather more difficult. This is sometimes known as *'bracketing'*. Ahern, in a recent paper for Qualitative Health Research, provided ten *'tips for reflexive bracketing'* (Box 26.3).

MAKING THE FAMILIAR STRANGE

Another technique for promoting reflection on your own assumptions is that of *'making the familiar strange'*.

Imagine you are on holiday in France. Your companion twists a knee and needs to buy painkillers and a knee bandage. You go into the local pharmacy. Here is my brief account of what happened last year in a small town to the east of Paris!

'My immediate impression was that I had entered a clinical environment. White coats, bright lights, a slightly antiseptic smell. The assistant was immediately at hand, behind a glass-topped counter. She offered anti-inflammatories, insisted on my companion sitting down, while she measured the painful knee in order to fit a support bandage. She then offered an array of walking sticks of varying heights and strengths. Two other people entered the pharmacy while we were being attended to, and joined in the provision of advice and help.'

This kind of observation is useful in encouraging us to reflect on what is familiar to us in our own cultures. It is what anthropologists call *'making the familiar strange'*, or recognising what we take for granted in our own cultures. The short account above identifies the notion of the clinical environment, the focus on serving the customer rather than self-service, and a consultation involving inspection and tailoring of care to the individual concerned. I remember each of these aspects precisely because of the contrast with my own perceptions of visiting a pharmacy in the UK.

Beware, however, of the apparently simple observation: *'Don't they do things differently here!'* This has been characterised as *'the trap of tourism'* by David Silverman (1993), and carries the inherent danger of focusing on what is different while ignoring those features that are common to both settings.

1. Identify some of the interests that you, as a researcher, might take for granted in undertaking this research, for instance the assumption that you will be able to gain access to your professional peers to conduct research, or broader assumptions associated with power, gender, skin colour, socioeconomic status and so on.
2. Clarify your personal value systems and acknowledge areas in which you know you are subjective. This is important in recognising the assumptions that you bring to the analysis of the data, and developing a critical perspective throughout the research process.
3. Identify possible areas of role conflict, and your responses to particular types of situations. How would you respond, for instance, to being interviewed about your own professional practice? How is this likely to influence recruitment of research respondents, and the data collection process?
4. 'Gatekeepers' are people with whom you need to negotiate in order to recruit research respondents. For instance, the pharmacist may be the gatekeeper to his or her customers; or the Local Pharmaceutical Committee may be the gatekeeper (or one of them) to pharmacists in a particular area. Try to identify gatekeepers' interests and consider their enthusiasm, or lack of it, towards your research.
5. Identify and recognise feelings that could indicate a lack of neutrality on your part. This could include, for instance, your feelings towards injecting drug users, or female colleagues combining professional practice with parenthood. How will you deal with these feelings in conducting the research?
6. Is anything new emerging from the data collection or analysis? This may be an indication of 'saturation' or a lack of critical reflection. This is the time to talk to colleagues, ideally drawn from a variety of academic and professional backgrounds, to increase your capacity for reflection.
7. Learn to recognise 'blocks' in the research process and to reframe them. Think laterally, review the methodology, is additional data collection needed, or an alternative method?
8. As you complete the analysis, reflect on the presentation of the data. Are you citing one person more than another? Why? Are you citing the articulate professional, rather than the quiet layperson?
9. Review the literature that you have cited. Does it too bring a critical perspective to the findings of the research, or have you selected the literature in order to reinforce your own research question or findings?
10. Become aware of potential 'analytical blindness', that is ignoring data that does not support your conclusions. Again, draw on multi-disciplinary discussion of data analysis to reflect on your own assumptions about the data.

Box 26.3 Ten tips for reflexive bracketing (Ahern 1999)

PREPARING AN INTERVIEW TOPIC GUIDE

The next step is the preparation of the interview topic guide. This is a list of topics to be covered in each interview (see also Chapter 27). Topics may be addressed in any order, and the list may be added to throughout the research collection period. An example of a topic guide for use in a pharmacy setting is shown in Box 26.4.

Box 26.4 Example of an interview topic guide

The topic guide may then be developed into a semi-structured interview guide, with specific open questions, followed by more exploratory, probing questions. An example is shown in Box 26.5. Some researchers find it easier to work with a topic guide, and some with a semi-structured interview guide. It may also be that at an early stage of the research process a topic guide is appropriate, and as the research develops, a semi-structured interview guide becomes more useful.

Box 26.5 Example of a semi-structured interview guide

TYPES OF INTERVIEW QUESTION

As can be seen from the interview guide in Box 26.5, there are a number of different types of question that can be used. Box 26.6 summarises the range of approaches that may be helpful.

GETTING IN: NEGOTIATING ACCESS AND RECRUITMENT

Having identified your sampling strategy, the next step is recruitment. How will you identify and reach appropriate respondents? How will you present the research to potential participants? How will you ensure that respondents' confidentiality is maintained, and that they understand the nature and potential use of the research data?

> **Introducing questions**: opening questions designed to yield spontaneous, rich descriptions where respondents provide what they experience as the main dimensions of the phenomena under investigation. May include *'can you tell me about'*, or *'do you remember an occasion when'*.
>
> **Follow up questions**: The interviewer adopts a curious attitude, inviting the respondent to explain through a further question, a nod, non-vocal encouragement, or repeating significant words.
>
> **Probing questions**: Asking the respondent to explain, or provide an example of a particular phenomenon. Recognising areas of concern to the respondent, finding alternative ways of addressing such areas.
>
> **Specifying questions**: Invite the respondent to provide more detail, often specific to their own experience rather than general beliefs: *'What did you do then?'*, *'How did you react?'*
>
> **Direct questions**: Used only later in the interview, after opening exploratory questions.
>
> **Indirect questions**: Invite the respondent to comment on how other people might feel or react; useful in conjunction with direct and specifying questions.
>
> **Structuring questions**: sometimes called *'signposts'* and used to indicate to the respondent the sequence of questions to be used, or the stage of the interview that has been reached.
>
> **Interpreting questions**: A variety of follow-up questions, allowing the interviewer to check that their understanding or interpretation matches that of the respondent.
>
> **Silence**: Don't be afraid to pause, to leave the respondent to break a silence. Sometimes people need time to think, some respondents speak less, or more slowly, than others. Allow the respondents to pace the interview, and to use (short) silences for reflection.

Box 26.6 Interview questions (Kvale 1996)

Introducing yourself

Make sure people know who you are, what role you are in (particularly important if respondents know you either as a professional colleague, or as a local pharmacist), the purpose of the research, what will happen to their interview (e.g. transcribed anonymously, data analysed, extracts may be used in a final research report, and in publications for academic journals), offer to let them see a copy and to comment on it. Assure them that they may withdraw from the research at any time, and it will have no impact on their care/service. Offer a prepared information sheet, to be left with respondents, to provide information to them, to reassure them of your own identity, and to allow them to contact you if they have comments to add.

Ethical issues

What sort of ethical issues are raised? If your respondents are also pharmacists, or other health professionals, are specific professional or ethical issues raised? If your respondents are clients, what sort of professional and ethical dilemmas might be raised?

Kvale (1996) suggested a number of ethical questions that should be addressed at the start of an interview study (Box 26.7).

Box 26.7 Ethical questions which should be asked at the start of an interview study (Kvale 1996)

GETTING ALONG

Having prepared a topic guide, managed recruitment of research participants, and negotiated access, you are now in a position to start talking. The aim of the interview is to be respondent-centred, to establish the respondent as the expert, and to place them in a position to explain to you their views of a particular topic. It is the researcher's role to guide, to establish an atmosphere in which the respondent feels comfortable to talk in depth, and to ask questions that allow the respondent to think and reflect on their particular experiences. Thus, it is important to emphasise that there are no '*right*' answers. The point of the exercise is a '*guided conversation*' rather than a series of questions and answers. It is important to recognise that, particularly in research of this kind, the knowledge generated is a social product, that is to say that it is the result of the interaction between you as interviewer, and the interviewee.

As a research interviewer you will be expected to strike a balance between the needs of the research, and creating a guided conversation using the topic guide or interview guide that makes sense to your respondent. For this reason, the sequencing of questions is important, from the general to the specific, and from the relatively easy to the more complex topics. One strategy is to start with the '*grand tour*' question, to ask respondents an initial open question that allows them to talk at some length. To return to the example of aspirin, an opening grand tour could be '*could you start by telling me about your general feelings about taking medicines*'.

Another useful strategy is to use '*signposts*' to let your respondent know the broad direction of the interview, when you are changing topics or focus, and when you are getting close to the end of the interview. Phrases such as: '*I'd like to start by asking you to tell me about.*', '*I'd like to move on now*' can be used. A signpost such as '*the final thing I would like to ask you about is …*' tells your respondent that the end is in sight, and may prompt them to relax and speak more discursively. It is always worth finishing with '*any other comments you would like to make about this?*'

Interviewing colleagues

There are particular issues in interviewing colleagues, sometimes encapsulated as the '*you know what it's like*' syndrome. If this happens, have probe questions at your disposal to encourage respondents to make their views explicit; these may be phrases such *as 'if you were describing this to a new colleague, how would you do so?*', or '*imagine you were explaining this to a colleague from abroad, how would you start?*'

There are both advantages and disadvantages to interviewing colleagues. On the one hand, it is likely to be relatively easy to gain access to professional peers, and on the other hand you may simply reinforce each other's beliefs, and not create an environment in which respondents can think critically and question their own professional beliefs and assumptions. It may be that it is less easy to give a glib, publicly acceptable answer to an outsider than to a pharmacist colleague. For instance, if you were asked to be interviewed for a study of the role of community pharmacists in Primary Care Groups, you may say very different things to a pharmacist than to a non-pharmacist; and as an interviewer in this particular scenario, you are well placed to ask the probing follow-up question.

Keeping on track

While it is important to encourage respondents to be discursive it is equally important to keep them on track. Strategies such as '*could I bring you back to?* '*You mentioned …*' or '*some people have mentioned*' are subtle ways of steering an interview, while remaining informant-centred and working with your own agenda as a researcher.

RECORDING THE DATA

There are two important aspects to recording data, note taking and tape recording.

Taking notes

Taking brief notes during each interview, and expanding them immediately afterwards, allows you to record your own observations of the interview, to note wording that either did or did not work well, to identify new topics or opinions that were generated during the interview, and to identify additional topics for future interviews. In short, it is the beginning of the work of data analysis, of generating an analytical framework from the data.

Tape recording

The second way of recording data is through the use of a tape recorder. Use as high-quality a machine as possible, ideally with a separate microphone. Don't try to use a dictaphone. Frequent changes of short tapes interrupt your concentration and the flow of the interview. Make sure you have spare batteries; make sure the pause button is not on; don't use *'voice activation'*; use 60-minute tapes. In short, take every care to avoid losing data and to allow you to concentrate on the interview, not on problems with recording. Tapes then need to be passed to a transcriber (who will need a special transcribing machine). Tapes should be anonymised and numbered before being passed to the transcriber. In costing for research of this kind, ensure you budget for a tape recorder, tapes, transcriber, and transcribing time of approximately five hours for each hour of interview time.

Remember that if the transcription is not going to be undertaken by the researcher, it may take several weeks for transcripts to be produced. During this time you will be carrying on with data collection. Again, notes taken after each interview allow you to keep track of the data collection process, and of new topics emerging from interviews, and of ways of addressing particular topics. Ensure that notes are numbered in sequence in the same way as interviews, in order to allow you to link the notes with their original interview, and to establish their place in the sequence of data collection.

DATA ANALYSIS

Much contemporary health services research adopts an approach to knowledge that could be described as *'common sense'*, accepting a physical world that is both knowable and researchable. Such an approach relies on a positivist definition of the world (see Chapter 25), in which what is being researched may be reduced to its constituent parts, understood and reassembled, either physically or metaphorically. Such an approach is appropriate in certain circumstances, for instance the assessment of the physical impact of a particular drug. However, in addressing more complex questions, which relate to the social world, or to the way in which we attempt to explain or make sense of particular phenomena, a more complex consideration of knowledge allows the development of a more subtle and complex analysis. Qualitative research is used appropriately in little understood areas, and its methods are embedded in disciplines such as anthropology and sociology, which provide scope for a more theoretical analysis (see Chapter 27). The choice of the depth of analysis lies in the nature of the research question.

There are a number of methods that are used in qualitative research, from '*framework*' analysis (at the most empiricist end of the spectrum), through thematic analysis, conversation, discourse and narrative analysis, to grounded theory. The general principle of qualitative analysis is that the analytical framework is generated from the data, rather than being predetermined by the researcher. Data analysis commences at the same time as data collection, and new data are used by the researchers to review their sampling strategy and data collection methods. The analytical framework is developed throughout the data collection period, with new data being used to question or refine the analysis. For further reading see Strauss and Corbin 1990; Ritchie and Spencer 1994; Gantley *et al.* 1999.

VALIDITY AND RELIABILITY IN QUALITATIVE RESEARCH

The British Medical Journal criteria for assessing the rigour of qualitative research are largely methodological, but emphasise that the methods need to be discussed within their theoretical framework. This is particularly important given that the research process is essentially inductive, which is to say that the analytical framework is derived directly from the data, and therefore reflects both the theoretical and practical concerns of the researcher and the researched. It is therefore essential to make explicit your own theoretical and practical starting points as outlined above in the discussion of bracketing and reflexivity. There is no absolute expectation that any two researchers will analyse data in precisely the same way; the question to be asked is *why* conflicting analyses are different. Is it a feature of the researcher's theoretical background in a particular discipline, or a result of assumptions based on experience and beliefs? Consequently, there are a number of pertinent questions one should ask when presented with a qualitative study (Box 26.8).

CONCLUSION

The research interview is one powerful method for the collection of qualitative data. Choosing both to conduct a qualitative study, and to use interviews within the study, has a number of specific implications for the conduct of the research. While all qualitative studies entail careful sampling strategies and the collection and

Box 26.8 Questions to ask of a qualitative study (Mays and Pope 1995)

management of detailed data, interview studies require particular reflection on the ways in which the interviewer affects the data collected and the data analysis. When the interviewer is also known in a professional capacity, and is interviewing either fellow professionals or clients, a number of specific strategies need to be adopted in order to protect the confidentiality of research informants and the integrity of the data.

FURTHER READING

Britten, N. (1995) Qualitative interviews in medical research. *British Medical Journal*, **311**, 251–253.

Crabtree, B. and Miller, W. (1992) *Doing Qualitative Research*, Sage, Newbury Park.

Gantley, M., Harding, G., Kumar, S. and Tissier, J. (1999) *An Introduction to Qualitative Methods for Health Professionals*, Royal College of General Practitioners, London.

Glaser, B. and Strauss, A. (1967) *The Discovery of Grounded Theory*, Aldine, CA.

Hoddinott, P. and Pill, R. (1997) A review of recently published qualitative research in general practice. More methodological questions than answers? *Family Practice*, **14**, 313–319.

Kirk, J. and Miller, M. (1986) *Reliability and Validity in Qualitative Research*, Sage, London.

Kitzinger, J. (1995) Introducing focus groups. *British Medical Journal*, **311**, 299–302.

Mays, N and Pope, C. (1995) Observational methods in health care settings. *British Medical Journal*, **311**, 182–184.

Mays, N. and Pope, C. (1995) Rigour and qualitative research. *British Medical Journal*, **311**, 109–112.

Murphy, E. and Mattson, B. (1992) Qualitative research and family practice: a marriage made in heaven? *Family Practice*, **9**, 85–91.

Patton, M.Q. (1990) *Qualitative Evaluation and Research Methods*, Sage, Newbury Park.

Riessman, C. (1993) *Narrative Analysis*, Sage, London.

Ritchie, J. and Spencer, L. (1994) Qualitative data analysis for applied policy research. In: A. Bryman and R. Burgess (Eds.) *Analyzing Qualitative Data*, Routledge, London.

Silverman, D. (2000) *Doing Qualitative Research: A Practical Handbook*, Sage, Thousand Oaks, London and New Delhi.

Strauss, A. and Corbin, J. (1990) *Basics of Qualitative Research*, Sage, London.

Tesch, R. (1991) *Qualitative Research: Analysis Types and Software Tools*, Falmer Press, London and Philadelphia.

REFERENCES

Ahern, K.A. (1999) Ten tips for reflexive bracketing. *Qualitative Health Research*, **9**, 407–411.

Britten, N. (1994) Patients' ideas about medicines: a qualitative study in a general practice population. *British Journal of General Practice* **44**, 465–468.

Denzin, N. and Lincoln, Y. (1994) *Handbook of Qualitative Research*, Sage, Thousand Oaks, London and New Delhi.

Fitzpatrick, R. and Boulton, M. (1994) Qualitative methods for assessing health care. *Quality in Health Care*, **3**, 107–113.

Gantley, M., Harding, G., Kumar, S. and Tissier, J. (1999) *An Introduction to Qualitative Methods for Health Professionals*, Royal College of General Practitioners, London.

Kitzinger, J. (1995) Introducing focus groups. *British Medical Journal*, **311**, 299–302.

Kvale, S. (1996) *Interviews*, Sage, Thousand Oaks, London and New Delhi.

Mays, N. and Pope, C. (1995) Rigour and qualitative research. *British Medical Journal* **311**, 109–112.

Patton, M.Q. (1990) *Qualitative Evaluation and Research Methods*, Sage, Newbury Park.

Ritchie, J. and Spencer, L. (1994) Qualitative data analysis for applied policy research. In A. Bryman and R. Burgess (Eds.) *Analyzing Qualitative Data*, Routledge, London.

Silverman, D. (1993) *Interpreting Qualitative Data: Methods for Analysing Talk, Text and Interaction*, Sage, London.

Strauss, A. and Corbin, J. (1990) *Basics of Qualitative Research*, Sage, London.

SELF-ASSESSMENT QUESTIONS

Question 1: What features of a research question would make it appropriate for qualitative methods?

Question 2: How would you ensure that you maximised the rigour of the research?

Question 3: Map out the research process adopted with qualitative methods. Show the key stages and how they interact with each other.

KEY POINTS FOR ANSWERS

Question 1: Appropriate questions for qualitative research should:

- Be exploratory, often '*how*' or '*why*' questions, not amenable to questionnaire-based research
- Require in-depth data for which informal interviewing is essential
- Address process, change over a period of time
- Be those in which the researcher gives precedence to the priorities and perceptions of the researched

Question 2: Maximise rigour by:

- Ensuring that data collection and analysis is reviewed by a multidisciplinary panel, in order to avoid the analysis simply reflecting the researcher's views
- Ensuring that the researcher has sought out views that apparently contradict those of other participants, and ensuring that the analysis can incorporate such views
- Adopting a range of different data collection methods
- Using constant comparison of data
- Ensuring that transcripts and data analysis are accessible and retrievable, in order to demonstrate transparent links between data and analysis

Question 3:   Mapping the research process

The key elements are shown in Figure 26.1.

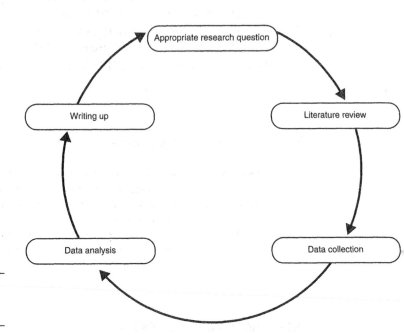

Figure 26.1 Key elements of the research process

Note the arrows! The process is circular or iterative, rather than linear. Each stage of the process entails a review of each of the other elements: thus the literature review will inform the data collection, but new data may take you back to other areas of literature. Similarly, the data provides the bases for the analytical framework, but as the analysis proceeds new questions may be generated which in turn will affect the decisions made about sampling and data collection.

27 Focus Groups

Felicity Smith

INTRODUCTION	474
ABOUT GROUPS	474
RESEARCH OBJECTIVES FOR WHICH FOCUS GROUPS MAY BE APPROPRIATE	475
SAMPLING: SELECTION OF THE GROUPS AND/OR THE PARTICIPANTS	476
GROUP SIZE	478
VENUE AND ENVIRONMENT	479
ROLE OF FACILITATOR AND CO-FACILITATOR	479
THE INTERVIEW TOPIC GUIDE	480
DATA ANALYSIS	480
ETHICAL CONSIDERATIONS	480
CONCLUSION	481
FURTHER READING	482
REFERENCES	482
SELF-ASSESSMENT QUESTIONS	483
KEY POINTS FOR ANSWERS	483

INTRODUCTION

Focus groups (group interviews) are an increasingly popular technique in health services and pharmacy practice research. They are a qualitative method used to explore issues from the perspective of particular population groups in the context of their experiences, views, priorities and concerns.

Focus groups are often seen as an alternative means of data collection to face to face interviews. Interaction between group members is the essential feature that distinguishes focus groups from one to one interviews (see Chapter 26). Researchers generally opt to conduct a group rather than individual interviews when they believe that the group interaction will have a positive effect on the effectiveness of the data collection process and the quality of the data.

Group interviews are believed to confer a number of advantages over individual interviews (Kitzinger 1994; Kreuger 1994; Barbour 1995). They may for instance, uncover more wide-ranging thoughts and ideas as the participants may stimulate each other. Listening to the views and arguments of other group members may assist individuals in developing and clarifying their own thoughts. Should differences of opinion be expressed, the researcher has the opportunity to explore the reasoning behind them. Usually, group members will share some common background or experience. Thus, from the group discussion the researcher will be able to gain some insights into the concerns of particular population groups.

ABOUT GROUPS

Interaction between people is part of everyday life. Thus, in some respects, focus group research simulates a natural interactive process in which people express and modify their views and opinions. As with all qualitative research, the aim of the researcher is to explore issues from the perspective of people's lives, experiences and concerns and is thus context-specific.

When individuals come together in a group, each brings their own personal history, views and perspectives which contribute to the character of the group. Consequently, all groups will be unique. All members then share the experience of being part of the group and in the production of data.

Many researchers and authors, in particular in the sociology and psychology literature, have examined and reviewed aspects of group behaviour. However, although in focus group research, interaction between group participants is seen as an important feature (often the reason the approach is selected) the implications of group dynamics for the analysis and interpretation of data have received only limited attention (Carey 1994; Kitzinger 1994).

Group polarisation is widely acknowledged. This is defined as: '*a group-produced enhancement of members' pre-existing tendencies*' (Myers 1993). Researchers have observed that group discussion has the effect of strengthening the average or dominant view within the group, rather than resulting in a split within it. Thus, a group of people with a tendency to take risks, following a group discussion, would be expected to assert enhanced risk-taking tendencies, whilst a group of people naturally more prudent would tend to more cautious views. A number of explanations are given for this. For example, in a group discussion a high proportion of contributions from the group would favour the dominant view, whilst minority viewpoints, if expressed, may not receive the corresponding attention. Participants may be unaware of the extent to which alternative or competing views are considered. People are also more likely to be persuaded by the arguments of individuals with whom they identify. In the context of focus group research, the participants in a group will generally share some background and/or experiences.

Thus, as well as being specific to the lives and perspectives of the group participants, group interview data is also a product of the group interaction process in which it was derived. The data should be analysed and interpreted with this context-specificity in mind.

RESEARCH OBJECTIVES FOR WHICH FOCUS GROUPS MAY BE APPROPRIATE

The aim of the researcher is to explore issues from the perspective of the group members. This may be to gain insights into people's understanding and perceptions of issues, and to explore how these relate to people's experiences, priorities and concerns. In general, qualitative methods are used to explore the research questions '*how?*' and '*why?*' rather than to quantify frequency of events and statistical relationships between variables. They are used to generate hypotheses and facilitate the development of theory to explain phenomena rather than to provide conclusions based on quantitative assessments.

Focus groups are commonly employed in the early stages of a research project to assist researchers in developing their research agendas. They may be used to inform the development of a quantitative study (e.g. a survey instrument) ensuring its content validity, i.e. by identifying the issues of importance to the population of interest and ensuring that these issues are covered and that closed questions include an appropriate range of responses (Jepson *et al.* 1991). Focus groups have also been used by researchers subsequent to quantitative work, to explore in greater depth, topics of interest arising from previous work, or in combination with one to one qualitative interviews, as an alternative method of data collection. In a study of older women's perceptions of control, health and ageing, data was collected in three group interviews and ten one to one interviews. The researcher found that more in-depth discussions were achieved in the individual interviews than in the groups (Mitchell 1996). Thus, depending on the research objectives, either group or one to one interviews may be more effective. The generation of a comprehensive range of issues in a group interview may be at the expense of detailed discussion of particular issues of greatest concern to individual participants. In the light of the objectives of the study, and preliminary fieldwork, the researcher must decide the most effective method of gathering the data required.

SAMPLING: SELECTION OF THE GROUPS AND/OR THE PARTICIPANTS

Focus group research has been conducted in both established community groups and those convened by the research team for the purpose. Each approach has its own advantages and disadvantages.

Research among established community groups enables the researcher to gather data in the context of a *'real life'* situation. Qualitative studies, in particular ethnographic work, aim to examine people's views, priorities and concerns in the context of their daily lives and experiences. The groups people join are natural settings in which they will discuss issues, hear views and form and modify their thoughts and ideas. Thus, research among these pre-existing groups enables the researcher to follow some principles of ethnographic research, collecting data in a natural social context rather than in an artificially created research environment.

Group interviews with established community groups will often be conducted as part of a regular meeting of the group. If people are interested in the research, then willingness to participate may be high. The meeting may be held at a group's usual venue which minimises both the costs (e.g. room hire) and the administrative tasks associated with organising the meeting.

However, there may be important disadvantages. In attending the meetings of established community groups, the researcher has only limited control over who attends and the suitability of the venue. The quality of the data and the extent to which research objectives are met may be severely compromised if, for instance, the number of participants is too large, or the room is unsuitable. In arranging the meeting, researchers must ensure that their minimal requirements (determined in advance) can be met.

Convening groups specially for the purpose of the research, generally involves more administration than arranging to meet with established groups and attending one of their regular meetings. Costs may also be greater, for example financial incentives may be required to elicit cooperation from individuals. However, subject to response rates, the researcher retains control over the group size, who attends the group and can ensure the suitability of the venue.

Inevitably, interaction and relationships between group members will have an impact on the data collected. This applies to both established community groups and those specially convened for the study. Participants in established groups will often know each other well, are likely to be friends, and may be more likely to be supportive of each other, rather than unfriendly or antagonistic. They may also be less shy and more willing to participate in discussion, and natural '*leaders*' may have emerged. Groups which are convened for the purpose of the study, may or may not include individuals known to each other. Members of the group are generally selected on the basis of sharing some experience or characteristics. They may include health professionals from a particular geographical area, or people who have been involved in a particular initiative. It is not necessarily possible or desirable to ensure group members are unknown to each other.

Decisions regarding sampling procedures relate to both the groups and the individual members of the groups. The researcher will often have limited control over the individuals attending established community groups. However, they do make decisions regarding the selection of the groups themselves and similar considerations will apply.

Appropriate procedures will depend on the objectives of the study. In the selection of individuals into groups convened for a study, the researcher may wish to ensure that group members are broadly representative of the population of interest. Where a sampling frame (a list of all members of a population) is available (e.g. of community pharmacies, pharmacy students, people attending a surgery or clinic) the researcher can randomly select individuals and invite them to participate. In many cases, a sampling frame may not be available and the researcher may have to resort to less rigorous methods of achieving some degree of representativeness in the groups. Quota sampling involves the selection of individuals with particular characteristics, e.g. ensuring representation from people in particular age-groups. Although not randomly selected, the group will include representatives of people with particular characteristics. In preliminary fieldwork, convenience samples (individuals accessible and willing to participate) may be acceptable to the researcher. Some studies require the participation of individuals who share some common experience, have taken part in particular programmes or possess other characteristics. Individuals may be '*purposively*' selected for these studies. See Chapter 26 for further discussion of sampling strategies.

In discussion, groups in which the individuals are from varied backgrounds may raise a wider range of issues than groups of like-minded individuals. However, groups in which the individuals share background characteristics and experiences may provide the researcher with an opportunity to explore in some depth issues of concern to them. Thus, there may be some trade-off between the variety of issues raised for discussion and the depth of discussion achieved surrounding each of these issues.

In selecting or convening groups, the researcher must decide the extent to which their study objectives are best served by either groups whose members share many common features or those more heterogeneous in nature. The number of groups required will be determined by the objectives of the study. If the aim of the researcher is to include issues important to individuals' to inform a more structured instrument, sufficient groups should be consulted so that the researcher is confident that all important perspectives are identified. A technique that can be employed is to meet with successive groups until no new issues emerge. In some studies, with a very specific focus or among a limited population group, all major issues may emerge from just one or two meetings.

GROUP SIZE

The groups should be small enough to allow all participants to contribute to the discussion. If the group is too large there may also be a tendency for:

- The group to fragment
- Inaudible comments made to neighbours (lost to the data set)
- Several people attempting to speak at once
- The contributions of some individuals relevant to the discussion not being voiced

In a large group, the task of the facilitator in maintaining a single 'floor' for the discussion and participation of all individuals is more difficult. A wide range of viewpoints may be shared but this may be at the expense of more detailed exploration of specific issues.

Bales *et al.* (1951) found that as group size increased, larger proportions of participants contributed less than their fair share, that there was greater differentiation between the most active people and others and that the involvement of the group leader increased. Participation in relation to group size was also analysed in a series of focus groups held with community groups to discuss views of reclassification of medicines from prescription-only to non-prescription (Smith 1999) Group size ranged from four to ten. Irrespective of group size, the proportionate contributions of the most active members were similar Increasing the group size beyond about six participants had the effect of increasing the number of participants who made a minima contribution.

Krueger (1994) in discussing developments in focus group methodology points out that the numbers considered as optimal have decreased. Five to seven participants are now generally preferred, as opposed to previous norms of 10–12.

Venue and environment

The venue and environment must be conducive to a group discussion. The surroundings should be comfortable and the layout of the room such that all participants feel equally part of the group and able to take part in the discussion with similar ease. Prior to the start of the meeting, the researchers should prepare the room to ensure that these needs are met.

The usual procedure (as in all qualitative interviews) is for the meeting to be audio-taped (see Chapter 26). The microphone should be situated where contributions from all group members will be picked up.

Role of facilitator and co-facilitator

Focus groups are conducted by a facilitator and co-facilitator. The facilitator has responsibility for steering the group discussion. He or she will endeavour to encourage participation by all members of the group. In welcoming people to the group and explaining its purpose, group members should be informed of the importance of sharing their views, that individual group members may have different perspectives, experiences and concerns regarding the issues to be discussed and that all are important. The facilitator should encourage participants to express differences of opinion when these arise, enabling the researcher to obtain a more accurate picture of the range of views and explore the rationale behind them.

In accordance with the interview guide (see below), the facilitator will introduce topics for discussion and follow up responses and contributions from group members to obtain further details or contextual information, rationale for particular viewpoints, alternative perspectives and reasoning behind these, and experiences and feelings of other group members relating to the issues raised.

The co-facilitator's role is to ensure the smooth organisation of the group meeting, including operating the audio-recording equipment so a high quality recording is obtained and noting contextual information to aid the interpretation of the transcript (e.g. interruptions or late arrivals, nonverbal behaviours etc.). The co-facilitator should be seated close to recording apparatus (and mains electricity if used) so he or she can easily check all contributions are being recorded and turn or change the tape or disc when necessary. He or she also needs to be able to see all participants and identify who is speaking. As the discussion proceeds the co-facilitator should maintain a record so that contributions of different group members can be identified and attributed in the transcript. A diagram of the seating plan should be made, including the position of the facilitator, co-facilitator, all groups members, the tape-recorder and any other relevant features that may be useful.

Meetings are generally followed by a '*debriefing*' session between the facilitator and co-facilitator in which relevant observations or thoughts can be noted, for example, features of the interactions between group members that may be important and not apparent from the audiotape.

THE INTERVIEW TOPIC GUIDE

Following an introduction to the meeting, the group discussion will be based around an interview topic guide (see also Chapter 26). The interview guide will generally comprise a series of predominantly open questions on topics relevant to the subject area of the research. Open questions allow group members to respond with issues which are important to them. They give participants an opportunity to express their views, experiences and concerns in their own words.

The interview guide may also include a range of prompts and probing questions to assist the facilitator in achieving an in-depth discussion of the issues raised in response to the open questions. For example:

- Would you say more about ...?
- Why do you think ...?
- What do you think are the reasons for ...?
- Has anyone else had a similar experience?
- Does anyone have a different view?
- What others issues are important regarding ...?

As is common in all qualitative interviews, the issues raised and discussed are determined by the respondents, rather than following the agenda and perspectives of the researcher.

DATA ANALYSIS

In analysis of focus group data, the principles of one to one qualitative interviews are generally followed (see Chapter 26). However, the data from focus groups has the added complexity in that the group process will have an impact on the data obtained. The analysis and interpretation of the data should be undertaken bearing in mind the context in which they were derived.

ETHICAL CONSIDERATIONS

All research raises ethical issues. Some of these are common to many types of study, whilst other considerations are pertinent to particular methodologies or procedures. Maintaining the confidentiality of data must be addressed in all research. Researchers generally remove individual (and possibly group) identifiers from transcripts of focus group discussions prior to analysis.

Focus group discussions are generally audio-taped. Verbatim transcripts are seen as important to ensure that detailed and comprehensive data required for qualitative analytical procedures are obtained. In individual interviews, respondents will be informed of the researcher's wish to audiotape the interview and their consent will be requested. A similar procedure is adopted when working with groups. An objection by any member of the group must be respected. If the reasons for the need to audiotape are stated (i.e. that it is important that everyone's views and thoughts are documented), permission is generally granted. However, a single objector may feel unable to speak out. Researchers who require a verbatim transcript, should also respect the rights of individuals to feel able to voice their concern.

Researchers frequently choose to conduct focus groups rather than individual interviews, because they believe that they will be more effective in identifying a wide range of issues, considering alternative viewpoints and securing an in-depth discussion. This will be the case only if group members are willing to share their thoughts and experiences with others. If relevant issues are not raised in the discussion this will impact on the validity of the data. In groups that include people who know each other, individuals may have had experiences that they have shared with another group member, but that they would not wish to be raised for open discussion in the context of the research study. Circumstances could arise in the course of the discussion that leave individuals feeling vulnerable and uncomfortable.

There are examples in the literature of focus group research that has been conducted over the telephone. This enables the participants to remain anonymous, when discussing a 'sensitive' topic whilst retaining the advantages of interaction between individuals in the production of the data (White and Thomson 1995). An attempt has also been made to conduct focus groups via the Internet (Murray 1997).

CONCLUSION

Focus groups are a valuable tool, increasingly used in health services and pharmacy practice research (Smith 1998). Often viewed as an alternative to one to one interviews for data collection, they possess important distinguishing features that should be observed in data processing and analytical procedures.

FURTHER READING

Barbour, R.S. (1995) Using focus groups. *Family Practice,* **12,** 328–334.

Krueger, R.A. (1994) *Focus Groups: a Practical Guide to Applied Research,* Sage Publications, London.

Morgan, D.L. (1988) *Focus Groups As Qualitative Research,* Sage, London.

Smith, F.J. (1998) Health services research methods in pharmacy: focus groups and observation studies. *International Journal of Pharmacy Practice,* **6,** 229–242.

REFERENCES

Bales, R.F, Strodtbeck, F.L, Mills, T.M and Roseborough, M.E. (1951) Distribution of participation as function of group size. *American Sociological Review,* **16,** 461–468.

Barbour, R.S. (1995) Using focus groups. *Family Practice,* **12,** 328–334.

Carey, M.A. (1994) *Group Effect in Focus Groups. Critical Issues in Qualitative Research Methods,* Sage, London.

Jepson, M., Jesson, J., Pocock, R. and Kendall, H. (1991) *Consumer Expectations of Community Pharmaceutical Services. A Report for the Department of Health,* Aston University/MEL Research Birmingham.

Kitzinger, J. (1994) The methodology of focus groups: the importance of interaction between research participants. *Sociology of Health and Illness,* **16,** 103–121.

Krueger, R.A. (1994) *Focus Groups: A Practical Guide to Applied Research* Sage Publications, London.

Mitchell, G. (1996) A qualitative study of older women's perceptions of control, health and ageing. *Health Education Journal,* **55** 267–274.

Murray, P.J. (1997) Using virtual focus groups in qualitative research. *Qualitative Health Research,* **7,** 542–549.

Myers, D.G. (1993) *Social Psychology* (4th Edn.) McGraw-Hill, London.

Smith, F.J. (1998) Health services research methods in pharmacy: focus groups and observation studies. *International Journal of Pharmacy Practice,* **6,** 229–242.

Smith, F.J. (1999) Analysis of data from focus groups: group interaction – the added dimension. *International Journal of Pharmacy Practice,* **7** 192–196.

White, G.E and Thomson, A.N. (1995) Anonymised focus groups as a research tool for health professionals. *Qualitative Health Research,* **5** 256–261.

SELF-ASSESSMENT QUESTIONS

Question 1: When are focus groups an appropriate research method?

Question 2: List the main stages of planning a research study where data are collected using focus groups.

Question 3: When facilitating a focus group, what types of question would you include in an interview guide?

KEY POINTS FOR ANSWERS

Question 1: Focus groups are a qualitative method used to explore issues from the perspective of particular population groups in the context of their experiences, views, priorities and concerns; especially when the researchers believe group interaction may uncover wide-ranging thoughts, as participants may stimulate each other.

Question 2: In planning a study:

- Decisions have to be made about the appropriateness of group interviews to achieve the study's objectives
- Identification or convening of groups
- Number of groups and participants in each
- Ensuring a suitable venue and environment
- Develop and test the interview guide to ensure that relevant and comprehensive data are obtained

Question 3: As in all qualitative interviews, predominantly open questions on issues relevant to the study objectives, with probing questions or prompts to elicit more detailed discussion, reasoning behind particular views, additional comments from other participants and to encourage expression of alternative viewpoints.

28 Analysing Qualitative Data

Geoffrey Harding, Madeleine Gantley and Kevin Taylor

INTRODUCTION	486
THEORY-ORIENTED VERSUS PROBLEM-ORIENTED QUALITATIVE	
RESEARCH	486
AN EMERGENT COMMON GROUND	488
TREATING 'COMMON SENSE' AS A TOPIC FOR ANALYSIS	489
INTRODUCING A THEORETICAL PERSPECTIVE: AN EXAMPLE	489
CONCLUSION	490
ACKNOWLEDGEMENT	490
FURTHER READING	490
REFERENCES	491
SELF-ASSESSMENT QUESTIONS	491
KEY POINTS FOR ANSWERS	491

INTRODUCTION

Quantitative methods, and social surveys in particular, have long comprised the methodological bedrock of pharmacy practice research (Chapter 25). More recently qualitative methods, such as depth interviews (Chapter 26) and group interviews (Chapter 27), have gained in popularity, as investigators explore the broader context of pharmacy, e.g. the behaviours and attitudes of users and providers of pharmaceutical services. The use of qualitative methods in pharmacy practice research, as in much health services research, produces analytical insights from recounted experiences, beliefs and views.

Using qualitative methods in pharmacy practice research without an understanding of the theory that informs the types of questions asked, and the data generated from these methods, can result in their being used merely as a technique for collecting or organising data. Qualitative research is frequently a *'catch all'* term used variously to describe the type of data to be collected (e.g. documents, transcripts of interviews); the method of data collection (e.g. participant observation); methods of data analysis, or the particular theoretical perspective adopted (e.g. interpretative).

THEORY-ORIENTED VERSUS PROBLEM-ORIENTED QUALITATIVE RESEARCH

The *'theory-oriented'* and *'problem-oriented'* distinction in research reflects researchers' contrasting epistemological stances, that is to say differing assumptions about what constitutes legitimate knowledge. Theory-oriented research is essentially exploratory and theory-generating. Thus, the nature and significance of empirical inquiry are fully meaningful only within the context of social science theories. On the other hand problem-oriented research is embedded within an epistemology in which *'facts'* do not require theoretical interpretation but are readily observable and describable.

Published qualitative studies in pharmacy practice, based on depth interviews, are frequently characterised by a similar presentational format, with raw data (i.e. selected quotes) grouped together and listed along identified themes to generate an account of individuals' actions. Such qualitative studies are then little more than a reiteration of what subjects reported when interviewed. Typically these publications comprise little more than a stream of selective quotes whose significance is assumed to be self evident in relation to the conclusion of the research.

'Applied' research, as exemplified by health services and pharmacy practice research, is generally less theoretically driven than *'pure'* social science research, which has many theoretical assumptions. Pharmacy practice research has a clear end objective defined in terms of outcomes, centred on the efficient and effective delivery of pharma

ceutical services. However, without an appreciation of the theoretical framework that underpins such research methodologies, investigators run the risk of conducting 'shallow' analyses yielding apparent insights which differ little from common sense or which are invalidated by the misapplication of a particular method.

Qualitative methods in the theoretical disciplines comprising the social sciences require interpretation of data from a theoretical perspective. At the core of such interpretation lies the assumption that what people say and do can be analysed as a particular form of behaviour – that is – *social action*. Behaviour is therefore not self-evident, but requires interpreting within a wider social and cultural environment. The interplay with this environment both shapes, and is shaped by, social action. Thus, principles of social theory, (for example, ethnomethodology or symbolic interactionism, which regard social interaction as comprising meaningful communicative activity between people) essentially define the nature of a sociological research problem, how it is to be explored, and the interpretation of the qualitative data collected. In contrast to 'theory-oriented' social science research however, pharmacy practice research has largely utilised 'common sense' rather than 'theory', derived from a discipline, as a basis for analysis. Theory in qualitative analysis becomes secondary to assembling 'facts' and descriptions in order to answer predefined research questions, such as how to contain prescribing costs or how to identify the constituent elements of 'best practice'. The scope of problem-oriented qualitative research questions and the chosen method of analysis becomes defined then, by practical rather than theoretical considerations. Transcripts and notes recounting experiences, views, and beliefs are taken at face value. Problem-oriented qualitative research thus becomes little more than a set of simple techniques or practices as in 'content analysis' which involves identifying and cataloguing themes from transcripts.

It is arguable whether pharmacy practice researchers should (and equally important could) adopt the social scientist's approach to qualitative analysis. In short, is qualitative data interpreted within say a sociological epistemology, valid and relevant to the objectives of pharmacy practice research? Correspondingly, should qualitative methods in pharmacy practice research be informed by, and interpreted within a social theory frame of reference? When used as a managerial tool for planning and rationing services, where the role of problem-oriented research is to provide information to bring about organisational change, pharmacy practice research which draws on social theory is neither tenable nor necessary. However, to avoid too simplistic an application of qualitative methods, and to enhance the quality of qualitative analysis in pharmacy practice research, a theoretically-informed approach is vital. Qualitative pharmacy practice research should develop beyond such a 'cookbook approach', i.e. simply following a recipe for data collection and interpretation (Figure 28.1). Rather, the potential contribution of theoretical frameworks from within the social

Figure 28.1 Problem-oriented research

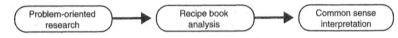

sciences, particularly sociology, social psychology and social anthropology should be considered, in framing research questions and informing subsequent analysis (Figure 28.2).

Figure 28.2 Theory-informed research

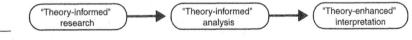

AN EMERGENT COMMON GROUND

The problem-oriented approach of pharmacy practice and health services research, and the preeminence of theory in social scientific research might seem irreconcilable. However, common ground is emerging, as funding for theoretically-oriented research is diminishing, relative to funding available for health services research. This has led social scientists to increasingly temper their emphasis on analytical or exploratory research with pragmatism, researching social rather than sociological concerns. Likewise, pharmacy practice and health services researchers can develop a theoretical foundation by framing research questions within a broad theoretical perspective (Figure 28.3). Thus, the theory-oriented/problem-oriented dichotomy is less defensible and less relevant in the current economic climate.

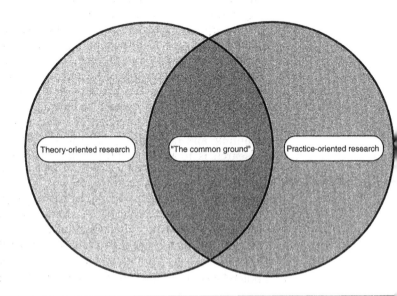

Figure 28.3 The common ground

However, while arguing against pharmacy practice research simply applying qualitative methods, divorced from a theoretical context, it should nevertheless draw on social theory only to the extent of building up its own theoretical foundation, which in turn would be subject to a continual process of refinement through hypothesis testing. A first step would be for practice researchers to eschew qualitative analyses founded on the principles of what has been termed *'abstracted empiricism'*, i.e. treating what people say and do as self-evident, leading in turn to the discrete accumulation of empirical data – thus stultifying the development of theoretical insights, however limited. Qualitative analysis should extend beyond ordering the content of individuals' responses along identified themes. The question becomes, not simply what pattern can be discerned from people's responses, but also, why this pattern and not others? A central assumption of a theoretically-informed qualitative analysis in pharmacy practice research then, may be that the authenticity of people's experiences are not necessarily to be taken at face value.

TREATING 'COMMON SENSE' AS A TOPIC FOR ANALYSIS

In the absence of theory, it is not possible for pharmacy practice researchers to produce a detailed analysis of the processes whereby meanings are attached to behaviour. Theoretical structures are needed in which to analyse the common sense assumptions of both the researcher and the subjects of research to lend meaning to behaviour. A leading figure in sociological qualitative analysis, David Silverman (1993), notes the philosopher, Wittgenstein's observation that *'The aspects of things that are most important for us are hidden because of their simplicity and familiarity'*. Silverman suggests this applies equally to the social sciences as to philosophy. Introducing a theoretical perspective from the social sciences thus seeks to make common-sense knowledge of the way in which the world (and indeed pharmacy) is organised *the* topic of analysis because once perspectives enter the category of *'common sense'* they cease to be examined or questioned.

INTRODUCING A THEORETICAL PERSPECTIVE: AN EXAMPLE

A pharmacy-based example of theory-informed practice research might be a study of the relationships between pharmacists and other health professionals. Typical questions to pharmacists and general practitioners might include: *'how would you describe your relationship with your colleagues? Do you participate in joint decision making? How would you describe good inter-professional communication?'* In the absence of a theoretical underpinning, responses to such questions would not inform the researcher about the broader social processes which have formed that response. A research methodology and an analysis of the data informed by social theory, for example the application of theoretical concepts of *'proletarianization'* and *'bureaucratization'* of professions, would however, enable searching questions to be posed to explore the extent to which inter-professional collaboration is influenced by the various professions' susceptibility to these processes and their impact on collaboration. Such questions might include: *'how do you make professional judgements? To what extent can your judgements be challenged by other professions?'* The answers to such questions will then provide insights into the dynamics of the relationship between occupational groups, each staking claims to making professional judgements in health care.

CONCLUSION

By paying attention to the unremarkable, and to seemingly uneventful descriptions and events, as well as the strikingly different, qualitative pharmacy practice research, informed by social scientific theories, has the potential to contribute to our understanding both of social processes and how they may be modified in the pursuit of desired ends. While using a recipe book approach to research methods may produce practical solutions to specific problems, it does not provide researchers with the broader concepts in which to place contemporary and/or immediate problems. Theory is *'good to think with ...'* (Levi-Strauss 1964) and provides researchers with new insights, and a broader context for the development of a theoretical foundation for pharmacy practice research.

ACKNOWLEDGEMENT

This chapter is a modified version of a paper published in Family Practice (1997) 15, 576–579 and is reproduced by permission of Oxford University Press.

FURTHER READING

Britten, N. (1995) Qualitative interviews in medical research. *British Medical Journal*, **311**, 251–253.

Bryman, A. and Burgess, R. (1994) *Analysing Qualitative Data* Routledge, London.

Fitzpatrick, R. and Boulton, M. (1994) Qualitative methods for assessing health care. *Quality in Health Care*, **3**, 107–113.

Harding, G. and Gantley, M. (1998) Qualitative methods: beyond the cookbook. *Family Practice*, **15**, 76–79.

Kitzinger, J. (1995) Introducing focus groups. *British Medical Journal*, **311**, 299–302.

Mays, N. and Pope, C. (1995) Rigour and qualitative research. *British Medical Journal*, **311**, 109–112.

Mays, N. and Pope, C. (1995) Observational methods in health care settings. *British Medical Journal*, **311**, 182–184.

Silverman, D. (1993) *Interpreting Qualitative Data: Methods for Analysing Talk, Text and Interaction*, Sage, London.

Silverman, D. (2000) *Doing Qualitative Research: A Practical Handbook*, Sage, London.

REFERENCES

Levi-Strauss, C. (1964) *Totemism*, Merlin Press, London.

Silverman, D. (1993) *Interpreting Qualitative Data: Methods for Analysing Talk, Text and Interaction*, Sage, London.

SELF-ASSESSMENT QUESTIONS

Question 1: What are the key hazards of conducting qualitative research divorced from appropriate social theory?

Question 2: With reference to Chapter 12, how might an understanding of professionalisation as a social process inform the interpretation of pharmacists' willingness to participate in health promotion strategies?

KEY POINTS FOR ANSWERS

Question 1:

- Anecdotal accounts
- Lack of social context
- Failure to consider social processes

Question 2:

A pharmacist's apparent willingness or unwillingness to participate in a health promotion scheme may in fact reflect not solely their personal viewpoint but should be considered in the context of the following processes:

- Autonomy
- Conflict of commercialism and professionalism
- Consumer expectations
- Mystique
- Promotion of indeterminate knowledge and professional judgement

How each of these processes impact on the pharmacist's willingness to participate can be explored by appropriate analytical questioning.

29

Statistical Tests

Nick Barber

INTRODUCTION	494
LEVELS OF MEASUREMENT	494
Nominal	494
Ordinal	495
Interval and ratio	495
HYPOTHESIS TESTING	496
SIGNIFICANCE	499
CONFIDENCE INTERVALS	500
TESTS COMPARING GROUPS	500
ANALYSIS OF VARIANCE	503
REGRESSION	504
CONCLUSION	505
FURTHER READING	505
SELF-ASSESSMENT QUESTIONS	506
KEY POINTS FOR ANSWERS	506

INTRODUCTION

Imagine a lecture theatre of 100 students. I give half of them tea and the other half coffee; the 50 who receive coffee all die. Which statistical test should I use to determine whether the coffee was poisoned? The answer is none, as the answer is obvious. But what if I decided to try and improve my teaching, as 10% of students fell asleep in my statistics lectures? I revise my notes, slides, jokes, etc. and find 6% fall asleep during my next lecture. Is my new lecture better? I don't think the answer to this question is obvious – the variation (a reduction from 10% to 6%) may be due to chance or it may be caused by the new teaching methods. We are uncertain – I say it's my brilliant new lecture, you say its chance – how can we decide? It is here that statistical tests come to the rescue.

Statistical tests quantify uncertainty. They do not, contrary to popular belief, reveal what is true. Statistical tests are part of the experimental process; what is tested is an idea, a hypothesis, about reality. Statistics is part of the scientific process, which tries to establish the truth about reality.

This chapter focusses on the choice and interpretation of statistical tests, rather than the detail of how to execute them. The reason for this is that computers generally perform tests nowadays; the art is in the choice and interpretation of the findings.

Over the last half-century, around half of the papers in leading medical journals used the wrong statistical test. Most of these would have used the correct test if they had followed the simple principles outlined in this chapter. Most students who are taught statistics focus on calculations at the cost of the principles, but this is the wrong way round. There are many computer programmes that can do the calculation. The key to choosing a test is to understand the principles. We start by learning an enormously powerful principle that unlocks the choice of statistical tests – three simple levels of measurement.

LEVELS OF MEASUREMENT

We are so used to measuring things that we forget that there are different 'strengths' of measurement. An understanding of these is the key to understanding the choice of statistical tests. Measurement can be divided into three levels – nominal (based on name), ordinal (based on order) and interval/ratio (based on a known interval between measurements). Interval/ratio is really two separate levels, but they can be treated in the same way for most statistical purposes.

Nominal

Nominal measurement is the simplest, and is so much a part of life we may not recognise it. It involves putting experimental findings into named categories (it is also called a '*categorical*' level of measurement by some authors) – common examples are alive/dead, correct/incorrect, male/female, pass/fail, tablet/capsule/injection. Each new measurement is allocated to its appropriate category; at the end of the study the number in each category is counted. This data is therefore usually a form of frequency data. The categories must be mutually exclusive and at this level of measurement it is assumed that all members of the same category are equal (e.g. no one patient is more dead than another). For each new reading the decision to be made is whether it is equal or not equal to the other members in each category – if it is equal, count it as another member of that category (e.g. another male subject). No one category is higher or better than another.

Ordinal

Ordinal measurement is at a higher level as it allows categories to be put in some order. Examples are socio-economic group; pain scores on a scale of 1–5; palatability of formulations on a scale of +, ++, +++; or measuring sedation as the distance from the right of a 100 mm visual analogue scale marked '*wide awake*' at one end and '*nearly asleep*' at the other. Not only can this information be categorised, as with the previous level of measurement, but the categories can now be related by putting them in order. This level of measurement is sometimes called a ranking scale. Although we can put the categories in order, we cannot precisely define the distance between them. For example, we cannot say that an increase in a pain score from 1 to 2 is the same '*aliquot of pain*' as would raise the score from 4 to 5; nor can we say that someone with a score of 4 is in twice as much pain as someone with a score of 2. Any subjective measurement scale, where people rate themselves or others, must produce ordinal data. Expressed mathematically, in this scale the decisions made about a reading are whether it is equal, not equal, greater than or less than others.

Interval and ratio

Interval/ratio data is that on which scientists are raised. The data are continuous (not in categories), and the intervals between reading are the same. Examples include: height, weight, volume, temperature, concentration, pressure and time. Much more can be done with this data as it has precise relationships. Four kg is exactly twice as heavy as 2 kg; two 1-kg weights added together weigh 2 kg. Mathematically it cannot only describe whether readings are equal to or greater than each other, but also allows them to be added, subtracted, multiplied and divided.

HYPOTHESIS TESTING

Science is based on people coming up with ideas (hypotheses) and then testing them by trying to prove them wrong (called falsification) – only the strong survive. We determine whether a hypothesis is true or false by experiment. First of all two hypotheses need to be formulated. Then we conduct an experiment, which forces us at the end to accept one or the other. It is a close parallel to a legal trial, in which evidence is collected and leads to a decision of either innocence or guilt.

Let us say, for example, that we have a hypothesis that community pharmacists can improve patient adherence by phoning up the patient a week after they receive the prescription and giving advice. We call this the *alternative hypothesis* (H_1). We must have a different hypothesis to test it against, and this is called the *null hypothesis* (H_0; null = zero). The null hypothesis is that the new service has no effect on adherence.

Our experiment would consist of taking a representative sample of pharmacies and randomly allocating the service to half of them. We would assess the adherence of patients, perhaps two weeks after receiving their prescription. We would then choose an appropriate statistical test to test which of the hypotheses appears to be supported.

Note that technically we are interested in populations, yet study samples. The uncertainty in statistical tests comes from this fact – if we measured whole populations we would *know* if they were different. In the above example we would hypothesise that, if we introduced the new service into all pharmacies in Britain, adherence would increase. In real life this would be ridiculously expensive to study, so it is more *cost-effective* to take representative samples for the intervention and control group. Statistical tests then estimate, from the sample, the range of values that the population may have (it is a range as we cannot precisely predict a population from a sample). If both samples could have come from the same population we accept H_0; otherwise we accept H_1.

Statistical testing leads to a probability value, yet a dismally small proportion of researchers understand what this means. First the basics. *Probability* is denoted by the letter *p*, for example:

$$p = 1: \quad \text{certainty}$$
$$p = 0.5: \quad \text{a 1 in 2 probability}$$
$$p = 0.05: \quad \text{a 1 in 20 probability}$$
$$p = 0.01: \quad \text{a 1 in 100 probability}$$

When tossing a coin, the chance of it coming down '*heads*' could be expressed as $p = 0.5$. A p value is commonly quoted after testing an idea (hypothesis testing). Many people misinterpret the p value, so it is important to understand what it represents. When a hypothesis test has been applied (usually to determine if two groups were different in an experiment) and a conclusion reached, the conclusion may be correct, or one of two types of mistake could be made:

- It is decided that there is a real difference (choose H_1), when in reality there is not (H_0 is true)
- It is decided that there is no real difference (choose H_0), when in reality there is (H_1 is true)

The first of these (see Figure 29.1) is called a *Type 1 error*, the probability of it occurring is denoted by α, and it is the probability value (p value) usually quoted in experimental work. The experimenter should set a level for α (such as 0.05) before the study. The second type of error is rarely considered and yet is even more galling for the researcher – it occurs when H_1 is in fact true, but the results do not indicate that this is so. It is called a *Type 2* error. The probability of it occurring is β. Although these are called errors it does not mean we made a mistake in our experiment; it just reflects that our sample may not (by chance) be typical of its population.

A statement that one service is better than another (p = 0.05), means there is a one in 20 chance that the statement is wrong, in other words, that H_0 was true, there has been a Type 1 error, and there was no real difference between the two groups. It is good practice when coming across a p value, say x, in a research paper, to say to yourself '*there is a one in y chance that this statement is untrue, where y = 1/x*'. Considering the large number of published papers that make decisions at the

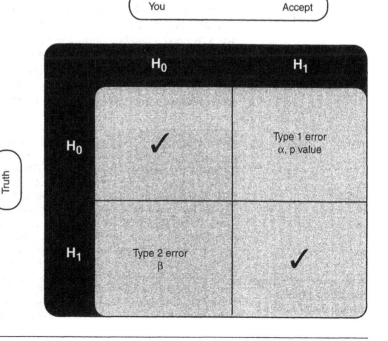

Figure 29.1 Errors in statistical testing. In an experiment you never know the truth (left hand side): whether H_0 or H_1 is true. All you can do is accept one of these hypotheses (top) from your findings. If what you accept is true (✓), then you have accepted the truth. If you accept a hypothesis that is not true, you have made one of two types of error. The probability of making that error is α (Type 1) or β (Type 2). α is the same as the p value (often 0.05), taken as critical in statistical testing.

p <0.05 level, it is inevitable that quite a number (somewhere between 1 in 20 and 1 in 100, as p <0.01 is the next level commonly reported) come to false conclusions. Remember that there is always some risk of a Type 1 error and rejecting H_0, when it is in fact true. A one in a million chance (p $= 0.000001$) will happen exactly 1 in a million times, even though you may be amazed that it has happened to you. This also illustrates that one experiment is never enough and can explain apparently contradictory findings in the literature.

How can these errors be reduced? The answer is to increase the sample size. Obviously, as our sample contains a greater proportion of the population we will be more certain of the population's characteristics. However, too large a sample is time consuming, expensive and often unethical. If it is too small, we are unlikely to discover a difference, even if it really exists.

There are several ways of calculating the correct sample size, but all depend on the same four factors:

- α
- β
- expected difference between groups
- variance

To calculate a sample size you first choose α and β. Although α is nearly always set at 0.05, β varies; 0.2 is commonly used, but if you wanted to show the value of a new pharmacy service, would you be happy that there was a 1 in 5 chance of missing it? A β of 0.1 or even 0.05 may be more suitable, although this will markedly increase the sample size. We also need some idea about the expected size of the difference between the groups. If we expect them to be widely different we will need a smaller sample size to demonstrate it. If a small difference is expected, a larger sample is needed. Finally, we need some idea of the variance within the sample (variance is a measure of spread – see Box 29.1). If the variance is large, we will need a large sample to reduce the confidence intervals and reveal a difference.

Box 29.1 n, standard deviation and variance

How can you describe your sample to other people? This is usually done by giving the number (n) in your sample, a 'typical' result (technically called a measure of central tendency) and a measure of spread (how wide the data is spread around the typical result). For Normally distributed interval/ratio data the 'typical' result is the mean, and spread is given by the Standard Deviation (SD). Have you ever thought how you could measure deviation from the mean? The simplest way would be to measure the deviation of each reading from the mean and add them together. Unfortunately they will add to zero, as half are negative. Statisticians get round this by squaring the deviations, so they all become positive, then adding them together. The size of this total will partly show the spread of the data, but will also increase as n increases. To counter this the number is divided by n to give the mean squared deviation (or variance). If the square root of this is taken we get the standard deviation.

It can be seen that calculating a sample size is not easy. It requires judgement and prior knowledge about the distributions and effect size. The prior knowledge may come from previous research papers or, more often, has to be established by a pilot study.

SIGNIFICANCE

There is a common and potentially misleading practice when describing results to refer to values of p <0.05 as 'significant' and those of p <0.01 as 'highly significant'. It is important to separate the p value – the objective probability of a Type 1 error – from the subjective decision that the results have significance. To illustrate the difference, suppose I asked you to play a game of squash with me, but told you that there was a 1 in 20 (p = 0.05) chance of you being knocked by my racket. Most people consider this probability insignificant. However, if you were a haemophiliac you would consider the same probability highly significant. The probability is the same, but the significance different.

There are two other consequences of linking significance and p values. The first is that the opposite of 'significant' is 'insignificant', so experimenters who find a p value of greater than 0.05 tend to think of the experiment as a failure and the results as uninteresting. This is clearly wrong for two reasons. First, it is as important to know that a hypothesis is likely to be untrue as to know that it likely to be true, however, there is a publication bias in the literature that leads to under-reporting of 'negative' findings. To illustrate the problem with an extreme example, if twenty experimenters conducted the same experiment for which H_0 was true, by chance we would expect one may get a result of p <0.05; this chance finding may be published and the others' papers may well be rejected or not submitted for publication. This also has implications for *meta-analysis* – the process by which studies, which meet minimum design criteria, are pooled and re-analysed to increase sample size and power. The second reason why the p = 0.05 watershed is inappropriate is that it focuses on one value, so that a result of p = 0.049 is treated differently to one of p = 0.051, yet the difference is only 2 in 1000.

The convention of using p <0.05 as a level at which to reject H_0 grew from early workers who were trying to balance the high costs of pursuing too many false hypotheses (which would happen if p was set at a higher level, such as 0.3) with the costs of conducting the large experiments needed in order to have a high level of certainty when rejecting H_0 and accepting H_1. However there is no statistical reason why p = 0.05 was chosen – early authors said it was 'convenient' and it stuck. Probabilities should be interpreted intelligently, according to the study.

Some statisticians think that there is an excessive use of hypothesis testing, as it is beset by the problems discussed above and because the acceptance or rejection of a hypothesis tells us nothing about the size of any difference; instead they prefer the use of confidence intervals, described below.

CONFIDENCE INTERVALS

A normal distribution is defined by its mean and SD. From this we can calculate the standard error of the mean (SEM): $SEM = SD/\sqrt{n}$. We know that for a normally distributed sample, 95% of the results are within $\pm 1.96 \times SD$ of the mean. Using SEM we can go further and extrapolate from the sample to the population. The population mean is 95% certain to be $\pm 1.96 \times SEM$ from the sample mean (i.e. there is a 1 in 20 chance, or $p = 0.05$, that the population mean is not in that range). As we are 95% confident, the mean ± 1.96 SEM are known as the 95% confidence intervals (CI). The importance of this is easy to see when you remember that hypothesis testing is based on testing whether or not groups come from the same population. If two groups' 95% CI overlap then they could share the same population mean (i.e. come from the same population, supporting H_0); if they do not overlap H_1 is supported at a level of certainty equivalent to $p < 0.05$.

To use an example, say two groups are treated with a potential antihypertensive or placebo. If the resulting diastolic pressures, shown as mmHg ($\pm$ 95% CI) were 95(3) and 91(2) we would accept H_0 as their CI overlap (92–98 and 89–93), so both could have come from the same population. Had the figures been 98(3) and 91(2) we would accept H_1, as the CI do not overlap (95–101 and 89–93) so we are 95% certain that they do not come from the same population.

Confidence intervals can also be used for other types of data, such as proportions. If we introduced a new ward drug distribution system to reduce medication administration errors and the incidence of errors fell from 6% $\pm$ 1 (mean $\pm$ 95% CI) to 3% $\pm$ 1, then as the CIs do not overlap we would accept H_1, that there was a significant reduction in error rate.

Many medical journals prefer mean $\pm$ CI rather than hypothesis testing alone, because it is thought that it stops readers focusing on statistically significant differences, when a closer look would show the difference between the two groups to be clinically irrelevant. The use of CI ensures both the difference between groups and hypothesis testing are presented together.

TESTS COMPARING GROUPS

Most pharmacists who ask about statistics are only interested in one thing – which test should they use for their data? This decision is relatively easy for most experiments as it depends on only three things:

- The level of measurement
- The number of groups being tested
- Whether the same subjects undergo each test condition

Once these three things are known they lead to an appropriate test. All tests are based on assumptions and the data should be checked to see that they have been met. Sometimes this is difficult to judge and statisticians may disagree over which test is correct. Note that proportions and percentages should be reduced to the original data or have special tests applied. Incidentally, a common mistake is to start thinking about choice of test once you have the data. Beware. You may find no test suitable. Always choose the test when designing your study.

Of the three factors that determine the choice of test, the level of measurement has been dealt with above. The number of groups being tested is important because tests designed for two groups should only be applied to two groups. If three or more groups are being studied, for example A, B and C, it is wrong to compare A with B, B with C and A with C using tests for two groups. If more than two groups are tested, a form of Analysis of Variance (often abbreviated to ANOVA) must be applied. The problem is that multiple testing of pairs of groups leads to '*false positives*'. P values are then misleading, as the true probability of a Type 1 error is much higher. The only exception to this is if the *Bonferroni correction* is applied. Sometimes only one group is tested, against population data for example.

The third factor in choosing a test – that '*paired*' studies, in which subjects undergo all experimental conditions (for example each of two treatments), should be treated differently to '*unpaired*' studies, in which a different group undergoes each treatment – is, unfortunately, sometimes ignored. It is to the experimenter's advantage to use the correct tests. Experiments on the same subjects (such as in crossover studies) have less variation; so more powerful tests can be applied to them.

Once these three elements can be distinguished it is easy to use the flow chart (Figure 29.2) to guide you to a suitable test. Other tests may also be suitable, and may be alternatives if your data does not meet the assumptions of the test shown. Now is a good time to test your learning by trying to answer the questions at the end of the chapter, using the flow chart. Some more detail about the tests is given below, together with alternative tests.

For all tests of nominal data, the *Chi squared* (X^2) test can be used, independent of the number of groups. It can even be used to test against an expected frequency distribution, for example that the number of prescribing errors are independent of the day of the week (i.e. do a seventh of all errors appear each day?). If the data forms a 2×2 table (for example two treatments and two outcomes) then the

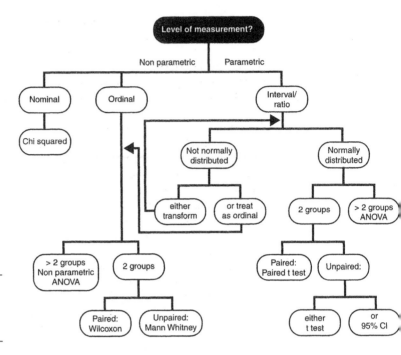

Figure 29.2 Flow chart for finding a suitable statistical test. Terms are described in the text.

X^2 test should have Yeates' correction applied. If the assumptions are not met for larger tables, it may be necessary to merge categories until they are met. An alternative 2×2 test, which may be used on small numbers if the conditions for X^2 are not met, is Fisher's exact test.

Ordinal data from two groups can be compared using the *Mann-Whitney test* for independent samples, and the *Wilcoxon test* for samples undergoing all conditions. In the Mann-Whitney test the results are pooled and put in rank order; special procedures should be followed if results in a group tie. An alternative to the Wilcoxon test is *the sign test.* These tests are powerful and easy to calculate.

The t test (its full name is *Student's t test*) is applied to two groups of small samples (n <30) of data at the interval/ratio level that is Normally distributed. If the samples are independent, then the *'unpaired'* t test is used; if the samples undergo all conditions, then the *'paired'* t test is used. If there are more than about 30 samples in each group, it is usual to test using the Normal distribution z statistic. This is sometimes called the z test. The t and z values become very close at this point and in practice many people use the t test for sample sizes larger than 30.

For interval/ratio data that does not follow the Normal distribution, the above non-parametric tests can be used or it may be possible to transform the results into a Normal distribution, for example by taking the logarithm of them, and then apply the t test.

ANALYSIS OF VARIANCE

This technique is used when more than two groups of observations are compared. Measurement at the ordinal level is analysed by non-parametric analysis of variance and at the interval/ratio level (provided it is Normally distributed, or can be transformed into a Normal distribution), by parametric analysis of variance. Analysis of variance if often shortened to ANOVA. The rest of this section deals with parametric ANOVA.

The nomenclature in ANOVA is often confusing and is based on the classes of variables used, for example testing drugs A, B and control would involve one class – the type of drug. Because the study has only been classified in one way, it is known as one way (written 1x) ANOVA; if a second class of variable, such as type of patient, had been introduced, it would be analysed by two way (2x) ANOVA. Non-parametric tests cannot go above 2x ANOVA, but parametric tests can go on to 3x, 4x or nx ANOVA, although such large studies are rarely performed.

The principle of ANOVA is explained in its name – it analyses variation in the results. As it is a hypothesis test we create H_0 and H_1. H_0 is that all the samples are taken from the same population and H_1 is that at least one sample is taken from a different population. Taking 1x ANOVA as the simplest case, using the example above, the type of drug would either have no effect (H_0) on the patient or would have an effect (H_1). First of all, the variation *within* each group is calculated. Then the variation *between* each group is calculated. A measurement called the mean square is used to give the extent of deviation – remember that mean squared deviations were used in calculating variance and standard deviation. If all samples have been taken from the same population the two mean squares will be similar. This is calculated by the *F test*.

$$F = \frac{\text{mean square between groups}}{\text{mean square within groups}}$$

The greater the value of F (i.e. the variance *between* groups is greater than that *within* groups), the less likely that it is that H_0 is true. Using tables of F produces a p value to support the alternative hypothesis. If there were only two groups, the p value would be the same as if the t test had been performed. Note that this test does not tell us where any differences lie, merely that all samples were not taken from the same population. Further testing is needed to find out where the differences lie (i.e. which groups are different from the control). Examples are the *Scheffé test*, the *t test with Bonferroni correction*, *Duncan's multiple range test* and the *Newman Keuls method*. The chances of finding a real effect are increased if there has been a good experimental design, which specifies a limited number of comparisons, rather than comparing everything with everything else in the hope of a significant result. Note that the results are only valid if the F test has first been shown to be significant – it is incorrect, and may lead to false conclusions, to perform the other tests without a prior F test.

Other assumptions important to ANOVA are that the sample size is the same in each group, as is the standard deviation. If these assumptions are not met then the data or calculations may have to be manipulated. In practice, equal sample sizes do not seem to be needed for 1x ANOVA, although they should not be too unequal. It is important for 2x ANOVA and above.

REGRESSION

Regression describes the relationship between two or more sets of data. One of its key features is that it lets us *predict* one variable when we have the value of the other one. We usually want to make these predictions because we can measure the predictor variable more accurately or more easily than the thing we are trying to predict. Examples could be predicting the concentration of a drug at t_0 from the concentrations at later times or predicting, from APACHE and other clinical scores, whether a patient on an intensive care unit is likely to live or die.

One of the hardest parts of regression is understanding the terminology:

The x-axis is called the *predictor* or *independent* variable
The y-axis is called the *outcome, response, yield* or *dependent* variable

The traditional names (independent and dependent) are being used less in modern texts because they are not particularly informative. I shall use *'predictor'* and *'outcome'*.

We shall first deal with the simplest case – linear regression between two variables. We have measured X and Y; in experimental settings we have chosen the values for X and measured Y at each of them.

After plotting the points for our two variables we want to fit a straight line. This is called a regression line and is calculated by a method called 'least squares'.

The straight line has the formula:

$$Y = a + bX$$

where Y is the outcome variable and X the predictor variable; a is the intercept on the Y-axis and b the gradient of the line. What does this tell us?

$$Y = 0.13 + 0.82X$$

means that when X increases by 1, Y increases by 0.82, and that when X is 0, Y will be 0.13.

Although it is helpful to know the equation of the line, we want to know other things as well, for example:

- Does the intercept or slope differ significantly from zero?
- What is the confidence interval of the line?
- What is the confidence interval around Y if I make a prediction for one patient from a value of X?

All of these are explained in more advanced statistics texts. There is another valuable calculation that can be made on regression lines, which is $100r^2$ (where r is the correlation coefficient). This figure tells us the percentage of variation in Y that can be explained by X. For example if $r = 1$, $100r^2 = 100\%$; so for a given value of X we could calculate Y precisely. If $r = 0.7$, then $100r^2 = 49\%$, so approximately half of the variability of Y can be accounted for by X, and our estimate of Y, given X, would be more uncertain.

In addition to simple linear regression there is multiple regression, in which there may be many predictor variables explaining the outcome variable. For example, the number of interventions made by hospital pharmacists to alter prescriptions on wards (Y), may be predicted by their grade (X_1) the type of ward they visit (X_2) and the time they spend on the ward (X_3). The technique is sometimes used the other way around to find out which of many variables predict an outcome – for example, 10 or 20 possible predictors may be fed into the regression model; all the significant predictors will emerge, together with an r^2 value. This is often used in epidemiological studies: Y may be a clinical condition such as blood cholesterol or having had a heart attack, and the X values could be dietary and lifestyle factors. If the outcome can be only one of two possibilities (e.g. alive or dead) then a special technique called logistic regression is used.

CONCLUSION

It has never been easier to perform statistical tests, and it has never been easier to misuse them. Statistical tests are there to test hypotheses. They depend on good experimental design and execution, careful exploration of the data, meeting the assumptions behind the test and intelligent interpretation of the findings. They do not reveal the truth, merely quantify uncertainty.

FURTHER READING

These books are in increasing levels of advancement, and will provide more information on the concepts described here, on the tests themselves, and on a variety of other tests.

Bowers, D. (1997) *Statistics Further from Scratch*, Wiley, Chichester.

Altman, D.G. (1991) *Practical Statistics for Medical Research*, Chapman & Hall/CRC, London.

Armitage, P. and Berry, G. (1994) *Statistical Methods in Medical Research*, Blackwell Science, Oxford.

SELF-ASSESSMENT QUESTIONS

For each of the studies below, identify the level of measurement and suggest an appropriate statistical test. Assume there are sufficient subjects in each group and any interval-ratio data has a Normal distribution.

Study 1. Excellitol, whisky or a placebo is given to 3 groups of volunteers with hangovers, who are asked to rate (on a scale of 1–5) the effect of the drug on their hangover after an hour.

Study 2. Comparison of Bugoff capsules and placebo in 2 groups of patients with urinary tract infections. Compare the percentages still infected at the end of a week's treatment.

Study 3. Comparison of 3 treatments post myocardial infarction Study survival in each group at 10 years.

Study 4. Which is most effective in lowering blood pressure – aspirin, atenolol or venesection of 2 pints of blood? Compare the fall in blood pressure in each of the 3 groups of patients.

Study 5. Effects of Grinalot versus placebo in a crossover study of patients with depression. Subjects ranked by a psychiatrist on the extent of their depression before and after treatment.

Study 6. A new drug is thought to have a hyponatraemic effect and is compared with placebo. Plasma sodium is measured before and after treatment. Patients undergo both treatments in a crossover design.

Study 7. Which causes more weight gain – 3 pints of beer a day or 1/2 lb chocolate a day? Use 2 groups of volunteers.

Study 8. The ethics committee has asked you to add a placebo group to the above study. Which test would you use?

KEY POINTS FOR ANSWERS

Study 1. Level of measurement is ordinal (it is a ranking scale) so the test would be a non-parametric ANOVA.

Study 2. Level of measurement is nominal as patients are either '*infected*' or '*not infected*'. Many people are confused by the percentage – remember this is just a proportion; you must look behind it to the actual data. The test would be Chi-squared.

Study 3. Level of measurement is nominal (alive or dead), so a Chi-squared would be appropriate.

Study 4. Level of measurement is interval/ratio; as there are 3 groups the test is parametric ANOVA.

Study 5. Level of measurement is ordinal (ranking scale). As it is a crossover study (each patient is his or her own control) the Wilcoxon test would be appropriate.

Study 6. Level of measurement is interval/ratio (concentration of sodium). The study has a crossover design, so a paired t test would be appropriate.

Study 7. Level of measurement is interval/ratio (weight). As there are two separate groups the test would be an unpaired t test.

Study 8. Level of measurement as above. The third group means that parametric ANOVA would be appropriate.

30

Evaluating Community Pharmacy Services

Felicity Smith

INTRODUCTION	510
WHAT IS EVALUATION?	510
FRAMEWORKS FOR EVALUATION	511
Efficacy, effectiveness and efficiency	511
Efficacy	511
Effectiveness	512
Efficiency	512
Appropriateness, acceptability and accessibility	513
What to evaluate?	513
Appropriateness	513
Acceptability	514
Satisfaction with services	514
Accessibility	515
Structure-process-outcome	515
STUDY DESIGN	516
Randomised controlled trials	516
Other study designs	517
Sampling	518
Response rates in evaluative studies	518
Data collection in the community pharmacy setting	519
CONCLUSION	521
FURTHER READING	521
REFERENCES	521
SELF-ASSESSMENT QUESTIONS	522
KEY POINTS FOR ANSWERS	522

INTRODUCTION

In response to changing health needs and expectations of populations, and the priorities and policies of governments and health authorities, health care professions are continually reappraising the services they offer. In many parts of the world, pharmacy's professional bodies, researchers and practitioners have been evaluating services to assist in the development of strategies for future provision.

Pharmacy practice and health service researchers have conducted many evaluations of existing services, professional developments and local initiatives (for a review see Smith 1999; 2000). For successful service development, it is essential that initiatives are demonstrated to be:

- Effective in achieving their objectives
- Deliverable in a wide range of pharmacy settings
- Appropriate to the needs and expectations of clients
- Cost-effective

Evaluation provides the pharmaceutical profession with an invaluable picture of the strengths and weaknesses of existing services and potential developments, as well as providing data to support its endeavours to secure health services resources.

The methodological principles of service evaluation are transferable across different branches of the health services. However, the application of different designs and methods in various settings, including community pharmacy, will present a unique set of considerations and challenges. In addition, because of the diversity within community pharmacies, procedures which are feasible and acceptable in one may be unworkable in another.

WHAT IS EVALUATION?

The World Health Organisation (WHO) has defined evaluation as: '*the systematic and scientific process of determining the extent to which an action or a set of actions was successful in the achievement of predetermined objectives*' (Shaw 1980). Within this definition, a number of components can be distinguished that must be addressed when evaluating health (including pharmacy) services. A scientific approach requires the use of an appropriate study design, with systematic data collection and analysis. Evaluation against predetermined objectives requires the selection of valid measures pertinent to the goals and purposes of the study.

Many studies evaluating aspects of pharmacy services are undertaken and/or commissioned by individual practitioners, professional bodies and health authorities who may have vested interests in demonstrating particular outcomes. It is important that the research is objective and can be seen to be free from prejudices and judgements of interested parties.

Evaluation of community pharmacy services frequently requires the involvement of a number of sites. The research process (including methods of data collection and measures) must be devised to ensure adherence to protocols and the systematic collection of comprehensive and reliable data, workable in different environments and conditions. The research design (e.g. randomised controlled trials, before-and-after studies and cohort studies) is an important determinant of the generalisability and validity of findings. All designs have their own advantages and disadvantages when employed in the evaluation of health services in community settings.

Researchers generally make a distinction between evaluation and audit. Audit consists of reviewing and monitoring current practice against agreed standards. As a cyclical process it includes evaluative procedures. It is often undertaken as an integral part of the normal provision and delivery of health services, as a means of maintaining and improving standards of care (see Chapter 32).

FRAMEWORKS FOR EVALUATION

Efficacy, effectiveness and efficiency

Evaluation may be considered in terms of efficacy, effectiveness and efficiency, which all relate to the extent that the objectives of a pharmacy intervention are met:

- Efficacy – can it work?
- Effectiveness – does it work?
- Efficiency – is it cost-effective?

Efficacy

Innovations in pharmacy frequently begin with individual practitioners who perceive a need in the population they serve. They may develop a service in response to this need and then evaluate it in terms of the extent to which specific objectives are achieved. Many local developments, prior to widespread implementation, are evaluated as pilot projects and may involve small numbers of pharmacies and pharmacists who are keen to participate.

It may be expected that in these special conditions (of self-selected settings and personnel) an innovative service may be more likely to succeed than in a wide range of more representative environments. Thus, the study may be seen as an *'efficacy study'* the question being *'can this work?'* If the service is unsuccessful in *'ideal'* conditions then it is unlikely to work in a more diverse range of settings.

These studies are also referred to as *'feasibility studies'*, that is, they focus on the assessment of specific features or objectives that would be deemed essential for success, prior to recommendations for more extensive implementation. For example, before offering a community pharmacy-based therapeutic drug monitoring service, researchers undertook a study to assess the extent to which community pharmacists could produce reliable biochemical results. This was seen as an essential requirement for the programme to be successful when subsequently offered to patients (Hawksworth and Chrystyn 1995a; 1995b).

Randomised controlled trials frequently share many features of efficacy studies in that they commonly have narrow eligibility criteria (restricted to people from specific population groups), are confined to a small number of settings, and data are collected on a limited number of outcomes.

Effectiveness

Having demonstrated that a particular service development can work, in terms of achieving specific objectives in selected settings, the next question may be '*does it work*' when implemented more extensively? That an innovation can work in a particular setting, does not necessarily mean that it will work when delivered more widely. The effectiveness of any new intervention should be assessed in a range of environments and conditions that reflect the diversity of the settings in which it will ultimately be delivered. Thus, when assessing the effectiveness of a service, researchers may need to gather data on a wider range of variables that allows the researcher to take into account the different perspectives, issues and implications for a range of environments and conditions. Steps could also be taken to establish the preconditions regarding the practice setting and/or personnel requirements for the service to be successful.

Evaluation of health services, generally, involves the measurement of multiple endpoints. Specific clinical objectives may be deemed the most important by practitioners, however, issues such as the feasibility of offering a service in a particular environment or acceptability of a service to potential users may be important determinants of its ultimate success.

Efficiency

Demonstrating that an intervention achieves worthy objectives, may not be sufficient. Researchers may also wish to demonstrate that the programme is a cost-effective method of achieving these objectives, and is thus an appropriate use of limited health care resources. Thus, many researchers will include some assessments of costs and cost implications as part of a service evaluation.

Assessing the costs of a health care programme requires decisions by the researcher regarding which costs to include (e.g. direct and indirect, average or marginal) and who incurs these costs. Costs savings that accrue to a health authority may be offset by consequential costs to service users, or their relatives and friends. Many new programmes will confer advantages and disadvantages that cannot readily be con-

verted into monetary costs. Thus, the comparison of different programmes in terms of costs may be difficult.

A number of methodologies have been developed and employed by
health economists, including cost minimisation analysis, cost-effectiveness analysis, cost-benefit analysis and cost-utility analysis (see
Chapter 23). These techniques have been incorporated into studies in
pharmacy practice and drug use.

Appropriateness, acceptability and accessibility

What to evaluate?

Assessments of efficacy and effectiveness aim to measure the extent to
which specific objectives of a programme are met. In evaluating services,
decisions must be made regarding *'what to evaluate'*. The features on
which an existing or new service is to be evaluated will depend on the
objectives of the service and the objectives of the evaluation. In planning
an evaluation, it is important to remember that different features will be
important to different stakeholders. For instance, from the perspective of
health policy makers, aside from technical standards of care, the costs of
a programme may be of paramount importance. However, service users
(if they do not pay at the point of use) may be more concerned about the
approachability of practitioners, or speed with which a service is delivered. The priorities and concerns of those providing the service will be
different again.

Any new pharmacy intervention will have been devised with
explicit objectives in mind. Endpoints may relate to specific biochemical or clinical measures, improved health status or broader aims
regarding the quality of services. However, the consequences of any
development may be many and impact on other health professionals,
as well as on health care consumers, carers, etc.

In addition to assessing the extent to which specific objectives are
met, an evaluation may also be made of the extent to which a service is
practicable in a pharmacy environment, acceptable to other health professionals and the public, and appropriate to the needs and expectations of the consumers. In considering what to include in an evaluation
all of these issues should be taken into account.

Appropriateness

Appropriateness is a common component in the evaluation of health
care (including pharmacy) interventions. However, in this context,
appropriateness has been variously defined and an interesting debate
exists on how it should be put into practice in health services research.
Common dictionary definitions include *'suitable'* and *'fitting'*, and
researchers are generally aware of the subjectivity involved in decisions regarding the assessment of appropriateness. Policy makers,
pharmacy practitioners and consumers may all differ in what they
believe to be an appropriate service in a particular setting.

Measurements may include aspects of quality of services, or the extent to which they meet a known, but unmet, need of the population. A range of approaches have been applied to measuring appropriateness of pharmacy services. For example, to assess the appropriateness of care, researchers have compared practice against external criteria derived from the literature or an 'expert panel'.

Acceptability

The acceptability of a service, can be assessed from the perspectives of both the health professionals providing it and the users. There may also be implications for other practitioners and, when assessing the acceptability, some attempt should also be made to identify these.

From the perspective of community pharmacists, the acceptability of a service may depend on its practicability in the pharmacy. For example, a programme that requires time of pharmacy staff may be difficult to accommodate at busy times, whilst some pharmacies may not have the space required to offer an extended service. Practitioners may be reluctant to promote a new service that they feel is inappropriate in a pharmacy environment, or when they do not believe that they possess the necessary skills. Factors such as these should be explored when evaluating the acceptability or feasibility of a service.

In evaluating community pharmacy, especially new initiatives, many researchers have included assessments from the perspective of users. Acceptability to consumers, and satisfaction with services, has become an important component of health service evaluation. In the UK, an annual survey of patients' experiences of the National Health Service forms part of the government's strategy of quality assurance in health services.

Satisfaction with services

Donabedian (1980) has stressed the importance of assessing satisfaction with health care, as it provides an indication of the extent to which clients' expectations and wishes are met. Evaluating patient satisfaction presents a number of methodological problems for researchers. Satisfaction will depend on the goals and expectations of the individuals seeking care, and the extent to which they are perceived to have been achieved. Whilst technical standards of care may be the priority of health professionals, service users may feel unable to assess this and/or focus on factors such as the friendliness of staff or the waiting time. Because the sources of dissatisfaction may be many and varied, satisfaction scores can be difficult to interpret. A satisfaction rating by any individual may be a reflection of single (undetermined) aspect of care.

Thus, as a construct, satisfaction comprises many components some of which will be more important to the overall attribute, and particular clients, than others. Further, demonstrating that a series of questions is a reliable and valid measure of an individual's feelings and experiences is problematic, whilst reported satisfaction may be affected by how questions are asked and by whom, and may change over time.

A further issue to be considered is whether or not assessment of satisfaction should be restricted to service users. Clients who use particular community pharmacy services may report that they are satisfied. However, users may be confined to those people who believe their needs and expectations will be met. There may be large numbers of people who do not use a service because they are dissatisfied with its quality, method of provision, or believe it does not meet their needs. Studies confined to service users may consequently miss these sources of dissatisfaction.

Accessibility

Accessibility of pharmacy services, and the availability of the pharmacist, is often identified as a strength of community pharmacy. Whilst accessibility is commonly a component of health service evaluation it is particularly pertinent in the evaluation of community pharmacy services.

Structure-process-outcome

A framework presented by Donabedian (1980) for the evaluation of health care involves the separate consideration of the *structures* of services, *processes* in their delivery and *outcomes*. In employing this framework for evaluating community pharmacy services, structural, process and outcome components may be identified that are important to a service. For example, structural features may include the accessibility of a private area for counselling and the availability of appropriately trained staff. In terms of the processes, the quality of advice with respect to its content and its delivery, appropriate use of protocols, and waiting times may be assessed. Evaluation of outcomes of pharmacy interventions often requires that clients are followed up to establish the extent to which objectives were achieved.

Donabedian does not view structure (appropriate resources and system design) as a measure of quality of care, but he argues that the structural characteristics of the health care setting will influence the process of care and hence its quality. He also views appropriate structures as the most important means of protecting and promoting good quality care. Similarly, if the processes of a service are poor, optimal outcomes (attributable to the intervention) would be unlikely to result.

Once the outcomes of interest have been identified, their measurement, particularly in community pharmacy settings, presents difficulties for researchers. Community pharmacies provide services to regular and casual consumers, unlike secondary care and some other primary care services. Further, records are not kept of many interventions, nor of individuals served. Additionally, services or advice from community pharmacies may be one of a number of considerations influencing an individual's subsequent action. Thus, attributing outcomes to an antecedent intervention can be problematic. Although some of these difficulties can be addressed in evaluation studies, e.g. in randomised controlled trials, these techniques have a number of limitations when applied to health services and pharmacy practice research.

Difficulties in measuring outcomes have led researchers in many instances to evaluate services on the basis of their structures and processes and an anticipated relationship between these components and outcomes. This involves explicit or implicit assumptions regarding the relationship between the structures and processes of care and anticipated health outcomes.

Whilst separate consideration of structures, processes and outcomes provides a useful framework for the evaluation of services, in practice many studies combine structure, process and outcome variables. Aspects of the structure (e.g. availability of a counselling area) and processes of care (e.g. appropriate advice) may be important components in themselves, aside from their relationships with specific health outcomes.

STUDY DESIGN

Randomised controlled trials

In the evaluation of health care, randomised controlled trials (RCTs) are seen as the '*gold standard*'. RCTs are an experimental design whose characteristics are outlined in Box 30.1.

Box 30.1 Characteristics of randomised controlled trials

- Randomisation of participants to achieve equivalence between groups
- Use of control groups for comparison, so differences can be attributed to treatment options
- Blinding of participants and preferably professionals to avoid bias resulting from the 'placebo' effect
- Control of experimental conditions
- Measurement of specific endpoints

The appropriateness of RCTs for the evaluation of health services has been questioned by many researchers. RCTs are generally conducted in a limited range of settings under well-defined conditions. A small number of sites for the study assists the researcher in controlling experimental conditions and procedures which will improve the reliability of the results. However, this may be at the expense of the generalisability of the findings to a wider or more representative range of community pharmacies.

Random allocation of individuals between intervention and control groups may also present practical and ethical problems. For instance, in comparing the impact of counselling areas on the processes of advice giving, the presence or absence of counselling areas in pharmacies is a factor over which a researcher may have no control.

The *'placebo'* effect in health care is well recognised. In clinical trials it is usual practice for subjects not taking the active drug to be given an *'inactive'* placebo, and to be *'blind'* regarding their allocation to either the experimental of control group. In the evaluation of many pharmacy services, blinding of participants will not be possible. Individuals in a pharmacy who are offered an additional intervention, e.g. a home visit, will be aware of this, as will a pharmacist who conducts the visit. Similarly, pharmacists who opt to take part in a training course, will be aware that they have done so in a subsequent evaluation.

Other study designs

A *'quasi-experimental design'* is sometimes employed when randomisation is not possible, e.g. evaluation of a new service offered by a self-selecting group of pharmacists. The researcher may wish to compare outcomes of an intervention group with a control group rather than limit the evaluation to descriptive data on events and views of the study participants. However, when randomisation is not possible, difficulty arises in identifying a control group that is equivalent to the study group in all respects other than the intervention under evaluation.

If systematic differences between the two groups are present (as is likely if the experimental group is self-selecting) it may be these confounding factors to which differences in study-outcomes should be attributed. Every attempt should be made to identify potential confounding factors and to ensure that the control group is similar in these respects to the intervention group. This is referred to as *'matching'*.

'Before and after' studies, are common in the evaluation of pharmacy services. These are more powerful if a control group is also included, they may then also be described as a RCT or a quasi-experimental study, depending on whether allocation to study and control groups is by randomisation or a matching procedure.

Many service developments are evaluated by *'descriptive studies'* in which data may be collected on activities and outcomes regarding the intervention and/or the experiences of participants including pharmacy staff, other health professionals and clients.

Sampling

The sampling procedures and sample size will be determined by the objectives and design of the study. A random sample is defined as one in which every member of the population has an equal chance of being included. A sampling frame (a list of all members of the opulation) is required for the selection of a random sample. In the UK, as in many other countries, sampling of community pharmacies is facilitated by the ready availability of sampling frames. Random or otherwise, representative samples are required for studies in which the researcher wishes to generalise the findings to people or settings beyond the sample. The sample size will depend on the degree of variability in the population and the precision required in the results.

Many evaluation studies are undertaken in one or a few self-selecting locations. For instance, the evaluation of a new service in a community pharmacy environment may, in the first instance, include only one or a small number of pharmacies. Whilst providing a useful indication of the feasibility or problems of a service, caution must be exercised in generalising the findings to other settings.

In studies in which the researcher wishes to compare structures, processes or outcomes among population subgroups, the sample must include sufficient numbers from each of these subgroups. In some studies, researchers have depended on pharmacy staff to identify and recruit participants. The immediate advantage is that a researcher does not have to be present in every pharmacy during the recruitment stages of a study. However, in charging pharmacy staff with this responsibility the researcher may no longer be assured of the extent to which protocols are adhered to, the reliability with which eligible participants are approached, or the comprehensiveness of records of non-responders. Recruitment by pharmacy staff may not be workable. Pharmacy staff may feel unable to put the time aside to discuss participation at busy times; they may feel uncomfortable approaching clients, or may not remember. If random or otherwise representative samples are required researchers must be assured of the reliability of the recruitment procedures.

Response rates in evaluative studies

High response rates greatly improve the value of any study and every effort should be made to achieve the highest rate possible (see also Chapter 25). Unless a sufficiently high rate is achieved, the sample has to be viewed as self-selecting. Increasing the sample size does not compensate for bias introduced by a low response rate. A study protocol should include processes for maximising response rates, as well as collecting data on the number and, if possible, some characteristics of non-responders. In some studies it is possible to gather some data on non-responders retrospectively. In the analysis, differences between responders and non-responders can then be investigated and the implications for the study findings assessed.

Data collection in the community pharmacy setting

Evaluation of services in community pharmacy usually requires the collection of data on the activities and/or views of pharmacy staff and/or their clients. The data collected should be systematic, comprehensive, reliable and valid.

Issues of reliability and validity of data are important considerations in all studies. The reliability of the data refers to the extent to which it is reproducible. For example, had the data been gathered by another researcher on a different occasion, would it be similar? During busy periods, could some information be missed? If data is being recorded retrospectively, might some cases be forgotten?

The validity of data refers to the extent to which it is a true reflection of events, activities or views of individuals. For example, clients questioned about their views on a pharmacy service, may be reluctant to express negative feelings. This may be particularly so if interviews are conducted in the pharmacy and the interviewee believes that the pharmacist may overhear, or be privy to, the information they give. Interviews with clients should be conducted by independent researchers, preferably on neutral territory and with assurances of confidentiality. Questions should be carefully worded to be non-leading and provide equal opportunity for the expression of negative and positive viewpoints.

The presence of a researcher in a pharmacy, and the knowledge that the study is taking place may influence the behaviours of those being observed. This is referred to as the Hawthorne effect, after the Hawthorne experiments which investigated the relationship between factory working conditions and productivity. In these studies, the groups of workers were aware that they were being observed and modified their behaviour to the extent that changes as a result of the working environment were masked. In planning an observation study, researchers should endeavour to keep any effects of their presence to a minimum, e.g. causing minimum hindrance to normal pharmacy activities.

Reliance on pharmacy personnel, rather than on an independent researcher, to collect data can present difficulties in terms of both the reliability and validity of the data acquired. It has the advantage of enabling involvement of a larger number of sites with limited resources, but, in depending on pharmacy staff to collect data, the researcher sacrifices control over the data collection process.

During the course of a working day, it may be difficult for the staff in a pharmacy to collect the comprehensive data required for a research project. The reliability of data gathered by practitioners may be influenced by the workload in the pharmacy, staff holidays etc. If pharmacy personnel are to be involved in data collection, clear protocols and procedures are essential. They should be tested to ensure that they are acceptable and workable in different types of pharmacy and at busy and quieter times. For example, can pharmacy staff be relied upon to systematically approach all eligible participants, irrespective of other activities in the pharmacy? Is the required data collected on all responders and non-responders? Unless protocols and procedures are straightforward and unde- manding, and are workable in a range of pharmacy settings, the resulting compromises to the reliability and validity of the data may be unacceptable, and an independent researcher may be required for the data collection.

Whatever procedures are employed, some attempt should be made by the researchers to establish the extent to which the data obtained are an accurate reflection of the true state of affairs. Comparing data col- lected by a number of different methods (triangulation) is sometimes employed as a means of validation. For example, pharmacists' self- reports may be compared with data collected by an observer. Non- responders should also be followed-up to establish the extent to which they differ from study participants. For example, people who have either positive or negative experiences of a programme may be more likely to agree to participate in an evaluation which would result in bias in the conclusions.

The evaluation of a programme may well include a range of methods to enable the collection of data on different aspects, e.g. obser- vation of events and activities, interviews with pharmacy staff, inter- views or questionnaires to clients. Some validation is often possible by comparing data from one data-set with information in another. This can provide a cross-check on the accuracy of findings and hence the validity of conclusions.

Validity and reliability are also important issues in the choice and development of instruments for an evaluation. The instruments are the questionnaires, interview schedules, data collection forms for observa- tion studies, report forms for data on non-responders etc. Researchers must ensure that their instruments collect data on the relevant aspects of services (e.g. structures, processes and outcomes, pharmacist and client perspectives) according to the objectives of the intervention and the evaluation. They must be workable and reliable, across different settings, environments and conditions, and when used by different personnel.

Many process and outcome variables that researchers may wish to include in an evaluation are difficult to measure. Valid measures may not exist for the assessment of many relevant outcomes. Demons- trating that a series of questions is a valid measure of someone's health status, satisfaction with services, attitudes etc. can be problematic. If suitable measures are not employed, this can threaten the validity of research findings.

CONCLUSION

Given the current emphasis on service development and innovation in community pharmacy services, evaluation is an important activity. Ensuring rigour in the research methods and procedures employed, presents a challenge for researchers. Every evaluation will be unique, presenting its own problems to which researchers have to find solutions.

FURTHER READING

Bowling, A. (1997) *Research Methods in Health,* Open University Press, Buckingham

Smith, F.J. (1999) Health services research methods in pharmacy: evaluating pharmaceutical services: (1) objectives, design, and frameworks. *International Journal of Pharmacy Practice,* **7**, 113–127.

Smith, F.J. (2000) Health services research methods in pharmacy: evaluating pharmaceutical services: (2) methods and measures. *International Journal of Pharmacy Practice,* **8**, 60–76.

St. Leger, A.S., Schneider, H. and Walsworth-Bell, J.P. (1992) *Evaluating Health Services' Effectiveness,* Open University Press, Buckingham

REFERENCES

Donabedian, A. (1980) *Explorations in Quality Assessment and Monitoring Volume 1: The Definition of Quality and Approaches to its Assessment,* Health Administration Press, Michigan.

Hawksworth, G.M. and Chrystyn, H. (1995a) Therapeutic drug and biochemical monitoring in a community pharmacy: Part 1. *International Journal of Pharmacy Practice,* **3**, 133–138.

Hawksworth, G.M. and Chrystyn, H. (1995b) Therapeutic drug and biochemical monitoring in a community pharmacy: Part 2. *International Journal of Pharmacy Practice,* **3**, 139–144.

Shaw, C. (1980) Aspects of audit 1: the background. *British Medical Journal,* **280**, 1256–1258.

Smith, F.J. (1999) Health services research methods in pharmacy: evaluating pharmaceutical services: (1) objectives, design, and frameworks. *International Journal of Pharmacy Practice,* **7**, 113–127.

Smith, F.J. (2000) Health services research methods in pharmacy: evaluating pharmaceutical services: (2) methods and measures. *International Journal of Pharmacy Practice,* **8**, 60–76.

SELF-ASSESSMENT QUESTIONS

Question 1: What are the main study designs that can be employed in the evaluation of pharmacy services? List their main advantages and disadvantages.

Question 2: Why does the assessment of patient satisfaction with health services present problems for researchers? How may some of these be overcome?

Question 3: Provide definitions of reliability and validity. What problems of reliability and validity may arise in the process of data collection?

KEY POINTS FOR ANSWERS

Question 1:

- Randomised controlled trials
- Quasi-experimental designs
- Before and after study with a control group
- Before and after study without a control group
- Descriptive studies

Advantages and disadvantages are based on the extent to which:

- they enable comparison to be made between equivalent groups
- bias from the 'Hawthorne' or 'placebo' effect is minimised
- the study can be conducted in a wide range of settings
- appropriate endpoints can be identified and operationalised

Question 2: Satisfaction comprises many components some of which will be more important to the overall attribute and to particular individuals than others. Assuring that a measure of satisfaction is reliable and valid presents a number of methodological problems.

Question 3:

- *Reliability* – the extent to which measurements are reproducible
- *Validity* – the extent to which a tool or instrument is an accurate reflection of the phenomenon it is designed to measure.

The researcher must ensure that the method of data collection is workable in all settings in which it will be employed, and that the information gathered is a true reflection of events, activities or people's views.

31 Evaluating Hospital Pharmacy Services

Nick Barber and Keith Ridge

INTRODUCTION	524
TYPES OF EVALUATION	524
Evaluation against standards	524
Evaluation by research	525
Clinical services	529
Purchasing and distribution	531
Production and quality control	532
New developments	532
Using the findings	532
The future	533
CONCLUSION	534
FURTHER READING	534
REFERENCES	534
SELF-ASSESSMENT QUESTIONS	535
KEY POINTS FOR ANSWERS	535

INTRODUCTION

Over the past three decades medicines have changed considerably in their range, complexity, cost and availability. Hospital pharmacy has changed in response to these factors. During the 1960s, many medicines used within hospitals were manufactured in hospital pharmacy departments. However the growth of the pharmaceutical industry, together with increased regulation over the manufacture of medicines, meant that the skills of many hospital pharmacy staff could be better utilised elsewhere. It was during this time that ward pharmacy developed. Evidence was emerging that the increased complexity of how medicines were used on wards was leading to an unacceptable level of problems associated with medicines use. Ward pharmacists were able to provide advice on wards to help minimise these problems.

During the 1970s and 1980s, the range of medicines requiring safe manipulation before administration increased (e.g. intravenous cytotoxic treatments, parenteral nutrition), as did the cost of medicines in general. Pharmacists increasingly ensured the clinical and cost-effective use of medicines at both the consumer and policy level. Hospital pharmacists were already beginning to specialise in particular areas, ranging from production to drug information, and in specific clinical areas, such as renal, HIV, paediatrics and oncology.

TYPES OF EVALUATION

In this chapter, two broad types of evaluation will be discussed. The first type of evaluation is evaluation against standards. With this technique, usually applied to long established services, a group of experts decides standards that a particular service should meet. Evaluation then becomes an audit against these standards (see also Chapter 32). This is a quick way of comparing services between hospitals and ensuring a good service. However, such a system can be criticised if the standards are not rooted in evidence.

The second type of evaluation uses research to generate evidence of the effectiveness and efficiency of a service. This area is called health technology assessment. A health technology can be anything from a new drug to a pharmacy service. The principles of evaluation remain the same.

Evaluation against standards

The most basic form of evaluation is testing against standards. An authoritative body decides what is right and converts this into standards of performance. A service will then be evaluated by the number of standards it meets. Hospital pharmacists, like other pharmacists, are expected to abide by a range of legal, ethical and professional principles (see Chapter 13). Prior to the restructuring of the UK's National Health Service (NHS) in the early 1990s, standards for hospital pharmaceutical services were developed by the Regional Pharmaceutical Officers in England (or their equivalents in the rest of the UK). Many of those standards are still applicable today. More recently, other organisations including those from the private sector, have assisted Regions within the NHS to develop a range of standards for hospital pharmaceutical services.

Individual specialities within hospital pharmacy have developed standards applicable to their speciality. For example, the UK Drug Information Pharmacists Group have developed and updated over many years a comprehensive set of standards expected to be delivered by local NHS drug information services.

In response to a fatal incident in 1994 involving contamination of parenteral nutrition prepared in a hospital pharmacy, the Department of Health brought together, in one document, standards expected when delivering aseptic preparation services to NHS patients. Subsequently, the NHS Quality Control Committee and the NHS Production Committee collaborated to further develop standards for the aseptic preparation of medicines in hospital pharmacies. These standards are used during external audit of aseptic dispensing services in hospital pharmacies in the NHS. Other areas have developed standards for the pharmaceutical care of patients in local hospitals.

Evaluation by research

The evaluation of hospital pharmacy services is complex, as a hospital is an enormous network of human and technological systems, and changing one system may adversely affect several others, like ripples flowing out from a stone dropped into a pond. There are several health technology evaluation frameworks. We have suggested a model of such a framework in Box 31.1. This is based on a mixture of technology evaluation models and practice experience.

Box 31.1 A model framework for the evaluation of health technology

- Needs analysis
- Options appraisal
- Development
- Efficacy trials   i)   using outputs
                            ii) using outcomes
- Effectiveness trials

Needs analysis is important as there is a tendency to adopt new technologies or systems without being certain of how well the current system is working, either locally or in general. If the needs analysis shows there is a problem then some form of appraisal of various options should follow. This may involve mathematical modelling. Once the most promising option has been chosen the system needs to be developed, i.e. made to work in practice. The system will continue to be developed in the light of later findings. This stage involves making sure it can work in a sustainable manner. During the development phase, measurements will be made to establish that the system is working.

Efficacy, in this context, refers to how effective the system is under the best conditions. This is usually the case when a system has been developed and is being evaluated. Often people running the system are enthusiasts and extra money has been provided to develop and run the system in its first phases. An efficacy trial is a formal evaluation against a control. Initially, the trials would only measure process measures, such as staff time or some measure of output, such as the number of errors or prescriptions changed. Ideally there would be several measures which may include patient and staff attitudes. If the results of these are satisfactory then health outcome measures would be used – usually in a bigger (more expensive) trial. Finally, if that was satisfactory, effectiveness studies would be conducted. These are to establish the system's effect when in widespread use, e.g. throughout a country. Technically, it aims to generate generalizable findings, rather than those found under ideal conditions, as in efficacy trials. This means that the technology would be used in a wide range of settings, where local conditions and attitudes may make the system more, or (more commonly) less, effective.

The model shown in Box 31.1 is an ideal. Many real evaluations never get beyond an efficacy trial. However, for a pharmacy service to be widely funded and implemented in the future there may need to be more robust evidence than this. Note that this model can be adapted to a continuous cycle of service improvement – the problems found in the trials lead to a new needs analysis, options appraisal and so on. The design of the trial is also important. Ideally, the trial should be randomized and double blind against a control, though this is not always possible. Sometimes early studies use a 'weaker' design, such as employing a historical control, or a 'before and after' study. Then, if the results are promising, a further trial with a more robust design is undertaken. However, for some interventions randomizing and blinding are not possible, and less robust study designs are the only option.

Evaluating hospital pharmacy services in Britain has been difficult and has rarely followed the ideal model outlined. However, the drive for evidence-based health care means future studies will necessarily adopt methodologies similar to the model illustrated. Ideally, an evaluation should focus on health outcomes, which are the ways in which the health of the patient, or their ability to care for themselves, are altered. This often presents difficulties in the evaluation of pharmacy services, as pharmacists tend to facilitate or modulate the basic process of prescribing. This means that large changes in health outcome are rarely going to be apparent, and large (and consequently expensive) trials will be required to show an effect (the smaller the effect, the larger the required trial). Linked to this is another problem – if a service is spread nationwide, such as a ward clinical pharmacy service, then it is almost impossible to create a control group against which it should be compared. In countries in which clinical pharmacy services are not common, it is easier to set up a trial to show the effects of the new service. For example, trials in the USA have shown that pharmacist involvement on wards has had beneficial effects on areas such as the cost and length of stay by patients on the ward.

As health outcome is difficult to measure, hospital pharmacy services tend to be assessed on *'intermediate outputs'* and *'process measures'*. An intermediate output would be some worthwhile end-point that a service was trying to achieve and that could reasonably be expected to benefit patients, such as reducing the number of medication administration errors. Process measures are commonly collected by pharmacy managers and are key markers that show how well the various pharmacy services are running. An example would be the number of drugs that were out of stock when required.

The first part of evaluation is being clear what the services under study should be achieving. To facilitate discussion of issues relating to evaluation, hospital pharmacy may be split into its key services (based on the UK):

- Clinical services, broadly speaking, should have the same aims as those of good prescribing: to achieve the desired clinical effect, to minimise risk of harm, to minimise cost and to respect patient autonomy (Barber 1999)
- Purchasing and distribution services should get the right drug, of the right quality, to the right patient at the right time with a minimum of cost
- Production services should produce a product of the appropriate quality, when it is needed, at a minimal cost

In the following section, we consider how evaluation has been approached in each of these areas.

Clinical services

There are a number of clinical services within hospital pharmacy. Some are policy-based, such as operating a formulary, or evaluating new drugs. Others are closely involved with the act of prescribing, such as participating in consultant ward rounds or being part of a team managing patients' pain. Finally, there are the services that monitor and correct prescriptions.

Evaluation of the policy services is difficult. One may establish whether a formulary or mechanism to consider the acceptance of new drugs is present. However, even if it is present, it does not mean the task is done well. Unfortunately, measures such as the percentage of all drugs that are prescribed from outside the formulary are of little meaning. If it is very small, it could mean either the formulary is poor, as it comprises too many drugs, or that it is good and well enforced.

Studies of pharmacists' involvement in prescribing are currently rare and tend to comprise accounts of the process and the pharmacists' role. However, studies of pharmacists operating warfarin clinics can at least show good intermediate outcomes, such as the proportion of patients who end up with their bleeding times in the required range.

Pharmacists' ward clinical services are the most frequently evaluated. Large studies have been conducted that permit comparisons between hospitals and an understanding of what characteristics are related to success. The pharmacist who monitors a prescription must first ensure there is not a prescribing error, then should look at the quality of prescribing (for instance, might another drug be safer or cheaper?). The prescription should also be examined to ensure it complies with local and national policies and guidelines, and that it is legible and will not confuse the nurse who will administer the drug. The pharmacist will also be giving information about medicines to patients, nurses and doctors. There are several ways of evaluating this sophisticated service.

The largest studies have been of pharmacists' interventions. Not all interventions are designed to change prescribing. For example, they may recommend increasing the monitoring of a patient (such as having the patient's blood concentration of a drug measured), or they may advise a patient regarding their medicines, prior to discharge from a ward. Measuring all interventions gives an idea of the range of actions that a pharmacist makes. Another measure would be the number of prescriptions changed by doctors on the advice of pharmacists. This is generally accepted as a reasonable intermediate outcome. An important role of the pharmacist is encouraging patient adherence to their medication regime after discharge from hospital. A number of discharge schemes have been developed and evaluated by checking patient adherence with their medication at home sometime later.

Mathematical modelling can be used to understand a service. In UK hospitals, there are, on average, 33 prescriptions changed per 100 acute beds per week. There is a considerable degree of variation between sites, and the causes of this variation have been explored using multivariate regression (in other words, lots of variables, such as the type of ward or experience of the pharmacist, were put into a mathematical model to see which ones best predicted the number of interventions made). It was found that the number of interventions was closely related to the mixture of ward beds (for example, Intensive Care Unit beds had many interventions), the grade of the pharmacist (more experienced grades made more interventions) and the time they spent on the ward (Barber *et al.* 1997). This modelling means that it is possible to evaluate differences between hospital services. Comparisons between sites can be made once a correction for the mixture of bed types has been made. The other factors (staff grade, time, etc.) are the responsibility of pharmacy managers, and any differences due to these reflect the services they manage.

An alternative measure of pharmacists' interventions is to use serious prescribing errors as the output. This is of immediate interest to the hospital, and its doctors, as it can be taken as a marker of the value of pharmacists in identifying these problems and preventing them from harming the patient. A pharmacist reports what they consider to be serious prescribing errors and another pharmacist validates them. This is close to a health outcome measure as it is an estimate of health outcome (errors that would cause serious harm). The problem with an estimate is, how good is it? Is it valid and reliable? So far there is no validated, reliable scale for estimating the extent of harm. However, one does exist for estimating the severity of medication administration errors (Dean and Barber 1999).

Other process measures of clinical pharmacy include the number of Adverse Drug Reaction warning cards sent to the Medicines Control Agency by pharmacists, and the quality of the advice provided by a therapeutic drug level monitoring service. Drug information services may be measured by the number of queries per month and the average time to respond to a query, although the relevance of these measures as an evaluation of the service is doubtful.

Purchasing and distribution

These functions are met by systems of work, generally utilising computers. The usual measures are markers of endpoints for the systems, such as the number of drugs out of stock, or markers that the systems are functioning correctly, such as the correlation between the computer's record of stock level and the actual stock level. The focus is on:

- Effectiveness (is the drug where it should be?)
- Efficiency (how much resource was used to get it there?)
- Quality of the drug (is the purchased drug of appropriate quality? Has it been degraded by storage or handling?)

Generally speaking, effective purchasing involves getting the appropriate quality of drug at the lowest price, particularly for drugs used mainly in the hospital. However, cheapness is not the only criteria. The cost implications of drug use continuing in the community must also be considered. It is hard to measure the effectiveness of purchasing pharmacists in negotiating discount, however, they can keep a running total of discounts achieved.

Another measure is the percentage of medicines out of stock when required. This should not be zero however, as this would mean far too wide a range of stock was being held. Pharmacies are usually measured by their 'stock turnover index' – the value of stock purchased in a year divided by the value of stock held in the pharmacy. A high stock turnover index is considered good, as relatively little money is tied up in drugs sitting on shelves. Wasted medicines (destroyed unused) is another measure, and in some countries markers of theft, damage resulting from poor storage, and the existence of poor storage (heat, humidity) are all relevant to evaluating a pharmacy. Computer systems (or, more to the point, the effective use of them by humans) are evaluated by factors such as accuracy of stock records held, 'down time', and their ability to hold, search and report data in various ways.

Dispensaries tend to be evaluated by the waiting time for outpatients to get their prescriptions dispensed. Something routinely measured in most hospitals. There is relatively little work on the dispensing error rate. However, Spencer and Smith (1993) have shown that this is possible in a comparative study which showed that the rate was higher if the dispenser was a pharmacist who was not checked.

The endpoint of the distribution system is generally that wards get the drugs they require when they are needed. Drugs generally reach a ward by one of two mechanisms: stock drugs are commonly sent to the ward in bulk; non-stock drugs are dispensed for a particular patient. A general evaluation of this system would be by the proportion of doses that could not be given because the drug was not on the ward. It would also be by the proportion of doses given from stock versus non-stock (this should be around 80:20), the stockholding of the ward, and the turnover of stock and non-stock drugs (rarely used drugs should not normally be stocked; commonly used ones should normally be stock drugs). Theft from wards (called drug diversion in the USA) is an increasing concern, and recording incidents of theft, particularly involving controlled drugs, is a common measure.

In some countries, unit dose is used as the distribution system. Unit dose was developed in the USA because it produced fewer medication administration errors. In its original form an envelope held all the drugs for a particular patient to take at a given time of day. Nowadays this original system is rarely used because of its cost. Instead each patient has a day's supply of drugs dispensed at a time. More recently several robotic systems have been employed in the USA (a country that has almost totally gone over to unit dose). Studies of robotic and automated systems need to be carefully conducted. Not only must the equipment be carefully studied, but it will result in many different human systems for its input and output. Sometimes these human systems have so many problems that these outweigh the benefits of automation. It is likely that the medication administration error rate of unit dose systems in the USA is similar to that in the UK: medication administration error rate is commonly taken as a measure of the effectiveness of a drug distribution/administration system. When linked to a valid reliable scale that allows people to predict the severity of medication administration errors, this sort of work becomes fairly close to the power of a study involving health outcome.

Studies of medication administration error rate are a good illustration of the problem of using outputs alone without linking them to health outcome. The medication administration rate is generally established by observing nurses on their administration rounds, although the true purpose of the visit is disguised (usually as a *'work study'*). In the UK, around 3–6% of doses are either not given or given incorrectly, around half of these because the drug is not on the wards. In the USA, it is rare for the drug not to be on the wards, although the overall error rate is similar. Many people think a rate of zero percent would be ideal. However, this illustrates the complexity of evaluating pharmacy services, and the weakness of using process measures alone. An error rate of zero could only (if at all) be achieved at enormous cost. Many errors have no effect on the health or care of the patient. The rate alone means little as it needs to be linked to a measure of severity to produce an accurate picture.

Production and quality control

In some circumstances, the clinical needs of patients cannot be met by licensed medicines. For example, a patient may be allergic to a preservative used in a licensed product. In the UK, manufacturing units in hospital pharmacy departments, licensed by the Medicines Control Agency, can produce products, normally as batches, to meet these special needs. Pharmacists can also prepare medicines in response to a prescription.

Across Europe, the size of the manufacturing operation varies from unit to unit and from country to country. For example hospitals in the Netherlands manufacture relatively large quantities of medicines compared to Spain. This variation is due to a range of factors including local economic circumstances and the structure of the national health systems.

In the UK, production units produce a range of products, such as TPN (total parenteral nutrition) fluids and small volume injectables, draw up doses of cytotoxic medicines, run a CIVA (Centralised Intravenous Additives) service, or make non-sterile products, such as creams, ointments and liquid formulations. These services draw on the unique formulation skills of pharmacists and reduce the risk (e.g. from microbial contamination) involved with making medicines on the wards. Some cost savings can also be achieved by centralising the service to reduce wastage. Recent developments in the UK mean that units which are not licensed by the Medicines Control Agency now undergo routine external inspection by NHS Quality Control Pharmacists.

Outside of the formal inspection environment, evaluations tend to be process measures, such as the number of doses wasted, the number of TPN patients treated for less than five days (implying they did not need this expensive treatment in the first place) or the number of occasions a product was available when needed. Quality control services are usually assessed through a range of parameters, which feed into the turnaround time, from receipt of a product sample to release of the batch, e.g. the time for a sterility or chemical test to be completed. Quality control laboratories also usually have in place an external audit arrangement, to make recommendations on practices or equipment.

New developments

Computerisation and robotics are increasingly entering hospital pharmacy services, and their use will undoubtedly continue to grow. In evaluating these systems, it is as well to start with small studies evaluating their claims, then use progressively larger and more rigorous studies. One should be aware that human systems of work exist, and that introducing a computer means that the human systems will change and need to be reassessed. For example, in putting in a system that is expected to make things safer, it is possible that people become less careful in their own practice, thereby nullifying the benefits of the new system. Similarly, long term costs need to be considered – how easy is it to get software or hardware changed? Will the company always keep its rental at that price?

When trials to test equipment or new services cannot be conducted, it may be appropriate to use mathematical modelling. This is relatively rare so far, but has been used to study the most efficient way to dispense, and alternative models of the drug distribution system to reduce medication errors.

Finally, many services are increasingly assessed by checking the perceptions of users. This may be done by interviews (see Chapter 26) or questionnaires (see Chapter 25). This is a very useful technique if used in parallel with others. Ultimately pharmacy services work with, and benefit, others. Therefore, we need to know what they want and think. Patients, doctors and nurses are the groups usually questioned.

Using the findings

Why are we evaluating pharmacy? To improve it, such that patients and society benefit from an efficient, effective system. This means that an evaluation alone is insufficient. Rather, it has to be followed by a process of change, then a re-evaluation to establish whether the changes have been effective. This continues in a quality cycle of continual monitoring, change and re-monitoring (see also Chapter 32). The management of change is difficult and always has been. The main barriers to change should be identified and minimised.

If it seems that the solution to a particular problem has been successfully evaluated elsewhere, consider first the generalisability of the findings, and second (even if the findings are generalisable) consider whether they would work in a particular setting. Sometimes local systems of work, or factors such as ease of recruitment of staff, mean that what is best for others may not be best in the current circumstances.

When the evaluation shows problems that go across disciplines, or even point to a problem with other disciplines, such as doctors or nurses, one has to be diplomatic. Ideally, they should be involved in the evaluation in the first place – and they may highlight aspects of pharmaceutical services that were not previously envisaged as problematic.

THE FUTURE

Hospital pharmacy will have to respond to health service reforms and the development of new technology. Some likely developments are shown in Box 31.2. There will be great competition for money with which to support new services, so more formal evaluation will be required than has hitherto been the case. The high cost of formal evaluation will mean that grant applications have to be written, and only the good ones will be funded. Pharmacists will have to become more skilled in the design and execution of research.

In order to meet these challenges pharmacists will need to continue to develop research tools to measure what they want, and be able to employ qualitative as well as quantitative techniques. A particular area of difficulty will be in representing the patient's perspectives on new services. This area will become increasingly important but is, currently, underdeveloped.

One future development may be that evaluation becomes more theory-based. So far most work has been pragmatic, studying each area afresh. However, common elements and themes are emerging, each with its own academic literature. Pharmacoeconomics is already bringing economic principles into pharmacy. Other areas include information systems (failure of these causes many errors and inefficiencies), psychology (human error, human-computer interface,

New drugs	growth of genomics, hence individualised compounding
Hospitals	will become more intensive high technology centres. Increased use of automation and computer systems
Information	new systems to transfer information within hospitals and to primary care
Patient autonomy	increased recognition, supporting more patient driven choices
Prescribing pharmacists	pharmacists have spent years correcting doctors – Will pharmacists do better?

Box 31.2 Likely future developments in hospital pharmacy

patient beliefs about medicines) sociology (the development of technology in society) and philosophy (values and ethics).

The twin pressures of the increasing need for specialist knowledge of research and of the need for theoretical input is likely to lead to the development of more research pharmacists in hospitals and more integration with university departments.

CONCLUSION

Although we have predicted general trends, we would not wish to generate the impression that all future service developments will have to go through a full service evaluation. A good pharmacy manager, trusted by hospital management and doctors, can often introduce a service quickly by keeping in touch with people who have power, and introducing a service that solves their problems. Because this service has not had a full evaluation does not mean it does not work, it just means that there is little evidence to show if someone wishes to oppose the service. Hospital pharmacy has generally developed as a result of good pharmacists introducing services in this manner. The problem is that, when resources are tight and services reviewed, we have little objective evidence to show sceptical observers. The future of hospital pharmacy depends on development of evaluation skills.

FURTHER READING

Bowling, A. (1997) *Research Methods in Health*, Open University Press, Buckingham.

St. Leger, A.S., Schnieder, H. and Walsworth-Bell, J.P. (1992) *Evaluating Health Services' Effectiveness*, Open University Press Buckingham.

REFERENCES

Barber, N. (1999) A philosophy of clinical pharmacy. In: *Churchill's Clinical Pharmacy Survival Guide*, N. Barber and A. Wilson (Eds.) Churchill Livingstone, Edinburgh, pp 1–4.

Barber, N., Batty, R. and Ridout, D.A. (1997) Predicting the rate of physician-accepted interventions by hospital pharmacists in the United Kingdom. *American Journal of Health-System Pharmacy*, **54** 397–405.

Dean, B. and Barber, N. (1999) A validated, reliable method of scoring the severity of medication errors. *American Journal of Health-System Pharmacy*, **56**, 57–62.

Spencer, M. and Smith, A. (1993) A multicentre study of dispensing errors in British hospitals. *International Journal of Pharmacy Practice*, **2**, 142–146.

SELF-ASSESSMENT QUESTIONS

Question 1: List the stages in an ideal service evaluation.

Question 2: What are the main problems in assessing automated systems?

Question 3: Give five measures suitable for assessing a purchasing and distribution system.

KEY POINTS FOR ANSWERS

Question 1: Needs analysis, options appraisal, development, efficacy trials with outputs, then with outcomes, effectiveness trials.

Question 2: There are several problems but they broadly fall into two groups. First, how well do humans use the system and what are the consequences of this? Second, what are the long-term issues – will it be updated, at what cost, etc.

Question 3: There are several acceptable measures which fall into three areas:

- Are the drugs where they should be?
- What resource was used to get them there?
- Is the drug of sufficient quality?

Examples of measures include: out of stock drugs, stock turnover index, wasted drugs, storage conditions (temperature, humidity, etc.), theft and unavailability of drugs on ward when needed.

Professional Audit and Clinical Governance

Carl Martin

INTRODUCTION	538
HISTORICAL PERSPECTIVE	538
PROFESSIONAL AUDIT: SOME DEFINITIONS	539
THE AUDIT CYCLE	541
Misconceptions hindering successful audit	542
Use of confusing terms and jargon	542
Setting unrealistic standards	542
Inappropriate audit topic	542
Audit is solely about data collection	543
Audit is really about inspection	543
CLINICAL GOVERNANCE	543
Pharmacy's response	545
CONCLUSION	546
FURTHER READING	546
REFERENCES	546
SELF-ASSESSMENT QUESTIONS	547
KEY POINTS FOR ANSWERS	548

Introduction

It can be argued that undertaking professional audit activities is really just part of the *'professional ethic'* or *'duty of care'* principle which is intrinsic to good professional behaviour. The basic concept requires pharmacists to continuously review their work practices with a view to maintaining and improving the quality of patient care. In the UK, the recent undertaking of *'baseline assessments'* of the clinical audit processes, as a first step in the process of *clinical governance*, by both health authorities and primary care groups has underlined the need to reexamine what is meant by the term *'audit'*.

Historical perspective

The White Paper *'Working for Patients'* (Department of Health 1989) was the first to carry a requirement for doctors to participate in medical audit as part of the UK Conservative Government's plans for an internal market within the National Health Service (NHS). This was part of a general shift in making service providers more accountable, through demonstration that they were meeting quality specifications and providing high quality, efficient and cost-effective healthcare. The NHS and Community Care Act (1990) gave further guidance on medical audit and the *'Health of the Nation'* White Paper (Department of Health 1991) set targets for health outcomes in five key areas.

Medical audit was defined in Working for Patients as: *'The systematic, critical analysis of the quality of medical care, including the procedures used for diagnosis and treatment, the use of resources, and the resulting outcome and quality of life for the patient'*. An early dilemma for pharmacy was that the majority of the activities undertaken by a pharmacist, whether in a primary or secondary care setting, could not be described as directly clinical with measurable outcomes. Clearly the supply of the wrong product against a doctor's prescription could be clinically critical. However, whether or not a pharmacist provided *'counselling'* on dispensed medicines could be inferred to be significant, but was not directly measurable.

In November 1991, the Council of the Royal Pharmaceutical Society of Great Britain (RPSGB), established a working group to consider professional audit within community and hospital pharmacy. This group reported in the spring of 1992 (Royal Pharmaceutical Society of Great Britain 1992) and the Council of the RPSGB agreed to promote professional audit in preference to proceeding with proposals for linking assessment of competence to the right to practice. The working group recommended that the Council should seek Department of Health funding to promote audit amongst pharmacists. This was successful and an Audit Development Fellow for England was appointed. The Audit Development Fellow coordinated a range of regional projects linked to the local administrative health authority to promote audit activity within the pharmaceutical profession. As a result a number of pharmacists with community pharmacy experience were appointed as Pharmacy Audit Facilitators, by health authorities, on part-time, two year contracts.

A number of '*get-you-started documents*' were produced. For example, the 'Moving to Audit' distance learning programme, developed in the Centre for Medical Education, University of Dundee (1992), was sent to community pharmacists in England. In Scotland the Pharmacy Practice Division of the NHS in Scotland produced '*Pharmaceutical Audit*', a practical workbook for community pharmacists which included a number of worked examples of audit topics. As a result of the activity of the Audit Development Fellow and his team of audit facilitators, awareness of audit within pharmacy rose by 50% over a twelve month period (1993–1994), with estimates of community pharmacy participation varying from 17% to 35%. Direct funding of audit facilitators has now ceased and the current RPSGB strategy seems to be the development of national audits alongside the publication of guidance documents such as '*Improving Patient Care. A Team Approach*' which encourages community pharmacist participation in multi-professional clinical audit.

A useful document produced as a result of the joint RPSGB/ Department of Health funding was: *Model Standards for Self Audit in Community Pharmacy in England* (Department of Pharmacy and Policy 1994), which covered areas of practice such as:

- The dispensing process
- Information provided with dispensed medicines
- Premises and equipment
- Health promotion
- Services to residential and nursing homes
- Response to symptoms

PROFESSIONAL AUDIT: SOME DEFINITIONS

There are no established definitions of professional audit. Dictionary definitions of audit usually refer to the examination, correction and verification of business accounts. Early experiences of audit facilitators indicated that many community pharmacists expected them to carry out a financial audit and were reluctant to let them visit their premises. Many pharmacists were also confused about the difference between audit and research, with many practitioners expressing a disinterest in research for '*research's sake*' and did not wish to share sensitive business information with '*competitors*'.

The RPSGB working group on Audit in Pharmacy concluded that professional audit is best considered as part of a pharmacist's quality assurance mechanism. Although this reflected the scientific base of pharmacy and quality assurance ensures that the best possible service is delivered to the patient/customer whilst minimising the risk of errors, it unfortunately engendered a *'will I meet national standards?'* fear amongst many pharmacists.

The working group developed a definition of professional audit which was adopted by the RPSGB. This was based upon the model of quality in health care developed by Donabedian (1966):

'Professional audit in pharmacy is the study of some part of the structure, process and outcome of pharmacy practice, carried out by individual pharmacists or groups of practitioners engaged in the activity concerned to measure the level of attainment of agreed objectives, the use of resources and the resulting outcome for patients.'

The much quoted *'structure, process and outcome'* have special meanings, and are discussed in Chapter 30:

- *Structure* – (What do you need?) the physical features, e.g. resources, staff, systems
- *Process* – (How do you do it?) the interaction between practitioner and patient/customer
- *Outcome* – (What do you hope to achieve?) changes in patients' current and future health status as a result of an intervention

One of the difficulties audit facilitators encountered in promoting audit activity to community pharmacists was that not many thought that it had any relevance to their business and was yet another imposition in an already busy day. One of their initial tasks was to develop working definitions and worked audit examples that could be applied to everyday practice by pharmacists. Several attempts were made to produce practical definitions. One such definition, included in the Moving to Audit programme was *'Audit is about taking note of what we do, learning from it and changing if necessary'*.

Another definition which proved useful was: *'Audit is a scientific technique for providing/gathering useful information essential for enabling an informed decision process (in conjunction with colleagues) in both "practice" and "business" issues'*.

A description of audit particularly suited to community pharmacies where there was a heavy dependence on traditional dispensing activities was: *'with reference to a finite part (criteria) of the dispensing/prescribing process, measure the current state of affairs, compare with what you consider a reasonable standard, make a case for changes to the process to improve the standard and implement.'*

Many *'off-the-shelf'* audits, were developed by facilitators. A topic frequently used as a first step was the counting of the number of partially dispensed prescriptions (*'owings'*), assessing which were critical to patient care and evaluating the reasons behind the shortfall in stock. This led to some interesting peer review sessions with a competitive edge. Another popular initial topic was measuring the number of prescriptions returned from the Prescription Pricing Authority unremunerated. The resulting audit discussions led to an increased awareness of the Drug Tariff (a list of authorised medicines and appliances with fees, prescribable by NHS contractors) and resulted in a measurable outcome, i.e. a decrease in the number of returned prescriptions.

THE AUDIT CYCLE

The simple definition used in the Moving to Audit distance learning pack can be converted into the basic audit cycle (Figure 32.1).

Most guides to audit describe implementation in terms of a cycle, although an upward spiral of continuous improvement is more desirable. The *'seven steps cycle'* is most commonly used in pharmacy (Figure 32.2).

Detailed consideration of each step is beyond this chapter and can be found in the document *'Improving Patient Care: A Team Approach'* (Royal Pharmaceutical Society of Great Britain 1997). The key to a successful audit lies in the planning and organisation. Discussions on the What? (audit topic), Why? (objectives), Who? (involvement all staff, definition of roles and responsibilities), How? (of data collection) and the When? (time period) are crucial.

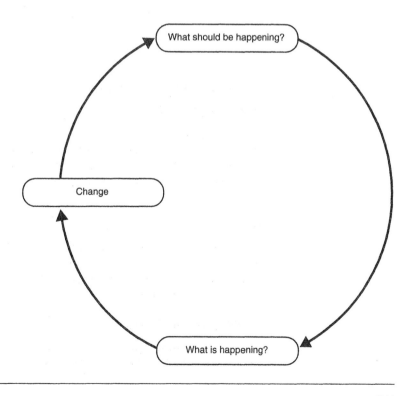

Figure 32.1 The basic audit cycle

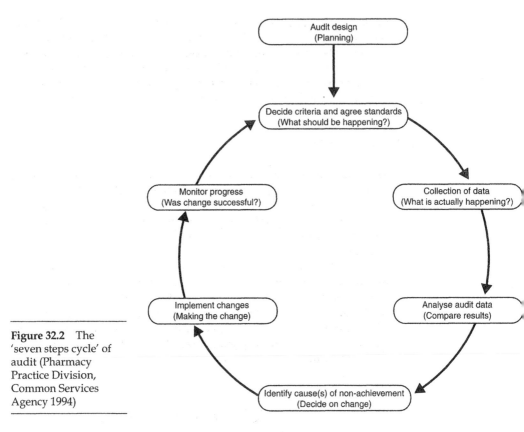

Figure 32.2 The 'seven steps cycle' of audit (Pharmacy Practice Division, Common Services Agency 1994)

Misconceptions hindering successful audit

Use of confusing terms and jargon

Two terms, '*criteria*' and '*standard*', have caused concern. Criteria is an element of care or activity that can be measured (e.g. patients will be counselled on the need to complete a course of antibiotics). Standard is the actual number, count or percentage applied to a criterion (e.g. 90%).

Setting unrealistic standards

Many pharmacists consider that a total (i.e. 100%) outcome is the only standard. Standards should be based on either national standards (if available) or more appropriately what the auditor considers realistically achievable.

Inappropriate audit topic

The choice of audit topic is crucial. Initial choices should not be very wide ranging or difficult, to avoid feelings of failure. Lack of success in audit activity can usually be attributed to a lack of specificity concerning the audit question.

Audit is solely about data collection

Many health care professionals consider that *'doing an audit'* is merely collecting data and then inferring appropriate practice. Consideration of the basic audit cycle highlights a key message, i.e. audit is not just about numbers (or data collection), but is primarily about changing professional practice where it is found necessary to ensure improved patient care.

Audit is really about inspection

A distinction needs to be drawn between the different types of professional audit. The RPSGB Working Group on Audit recognised three types of audit:

- Self audit
- Peer audit
- External audit

Self and peer audit involve an individual or group auditing their own performance against published standards or personal objectives. External audit occurs when visiting professionals (who may be inspectors) audit the practice of an individual or group and do not have their own performance audited. Table 32.1 compares *'audit'* and *'inspection'*.

CLINICAL GOVERNANCE

The White Paper: *The New NHS – Modern, Dependable* (Department of Health 1997) stated that the NHS should have quality at its heart. *Clinical governance,* a concept developed out of corporate governance,

Inspection	Audit
Outside body checks your practice against a minimum standard	You measure your own performance
Standard is set by an outside body	You set the standard you want to aim for
Sanctions can be taken against you for failing to meet minimum requirements	No sanctions
Results of the inspection are the property of the inspector	The results of the audit belong to you

Table 32.1 Audit versus Inspection

was a central plank of the newly elected UK government's health strategy to ensure quality health care. This echos the early days of the NHS, which aimed to ensure that every patient treated received high quality care, wherever they lived and whenever they needed it. The intention of clinical governance is that every part of the NHS, and everyone who works in it, should take responsibility for working to improve quality (Howe 1999).

The quality agenda was further developed in *A First Class Service: Quality in the New NHS* (Department of Health 1998) and clinical governance is defined as: '*A framework through which NHS organisations are accountable for continuously improving the quality of their services and safeguarding high standards of care by creating an environment in which excellence in clinical care will flourish.*'

There is a worry among some health care workers that clinical governance will be used as a '*stick to beat them with*'. Smith (1998) explained that it could be seen positively as a development process, aimed at improving overall quality of care, but highlighted that the context for its introduction was a sequence of serious failures of clinical care, such as failures of NHS cervical cancer screening programmes. Whilst risk management and dealing with poor performance are important features, clinical governance is best seen as part of an overall quality framework, as shown in Figure 32.3.

The National Service Frameworks (NSFs) will produce national standards for the treatment of particular conditions and the National

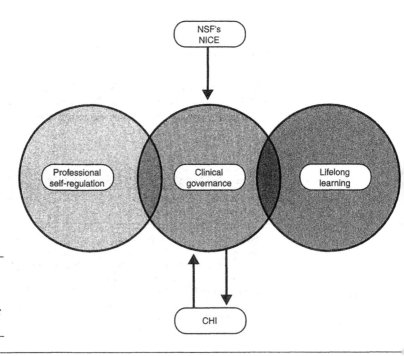

Figure 32.3 Clinical governance as part of an overall quality framework. See text for key to abbreviations.

Institute for Clinical Excellence (NICE) will appraise new and existing treatments for efficacy. These national guidelines will be accepted locally as appropriate. The Commission for Health Improvement (CHI) and patient surveys will monitor how well these standards are being achieved.

All NHS organisations are now appointing a person with specific responsibility for leading the development of clinical governance, who are establishing and implementing local arrangements for continuous quality improvement. These will need to ensure that national standards and guidance are reflected in local services.

Pharmacy's response

As with early discussions on medical or clinical audit in the late 1980s, individual pharmacists were left wondering how does '*clinical*' apply to them and many were waiting for a central lead from the RPSGB. Such a lead came in September 1999, when the Royal Pharmaceutical Society of Great Britain (1999) published *Achieving Excellence in Pharmacy Through Clinical Governance*. It identified four components, which are shown in Box 32.1.

Box 32.1 Four components of clinical governance (Royal Pharmaceutical Society of Great Britain 1999)

- There should be clear lines of responsibility for the overall quality of clinical care
- A comprehensive programme of quality improvement activities including clinical audit, continuous professional development and evidence-based practice
- Risk management policies
- Procedures for identify and remedying poor performance

The RPSGB has also produced a Community Pharmacy Clinical Governance Assessment Questionnaire to help local pharmaceutical committees (LPCs) produce reports on clinical governance in community pharmacy. These assessments cover the pharmacy as a whole, pharmacists' '*continuous professional development*' and additional services (including domiciliary oxygen services, services to care homes, health screening and needle and syringe exchange). The contents of these baseline audits are based upon current professional advice included in the Medicines, Ethics and Practice Guide which is distributed to all pharmacists.

The current RPSGB website contains information about the work of its Clinical Audit Group. Viewing these web pages would suggest that there is a reasonable amount of audit activity incorporated into everyday practice especially in the multiple pharmacy chains. The Clinical Audit Group which has one full time pharmacist, with support brought in for specific projects, provides training, audit design and project management services. The website also provides access to dozens of audit templates and also describes the RPSGB's policy on clinical governance. A current trend is the development of national audits. One was carried out in 1997 on OTC requests for antihistamines licensed for adult sleep disorders, and involved 2,500 pharmacists. Currently, the Clinical Audit Group is developing distance learning audits.

Improving Patient Care A Team Approach (Royal Pharmaceutical Society of Great Britain 1997) reports that awareness of audit amongst community pharmacists is very high (greater than 90%) but that active participation is much lower. Why is this? Is it that there is still considerable misunderstanding about the true nature of *'audit'*?

CONCLUSION

The original concepts behind professional audit need to be re-visited in the light of clinical governance, particularly the professional development/lifelong learning aspect, to enable individual practitioners to become established members of the health care team, as experts in safe and effective medicines management.

It remains to be seen whether the pharmacy profession will accept or reject the challenge of openness and critical review offered by clinical governance. If rejection occurs, this could result in failure to address poor practice, under a cloak of business confidentiality. Conversely, if the challenge is accepted by individual pharmacists and the pharmacy profession, best professional practice (the synergy between professional judgement and the best available evidence) can be achieved and maintained.

FURTHER READING

Irvine, D. and Irvine, S. (Eds.) (1991) *Making Sense of Audit*, Radcliffe Medical Press, Oxford.

Royal Pharmaceutical Society of Great Britain (1997) *Improving Patient Care. A Team Approach*, Royal Pharmaceutical Society of Great Britain, London.

REFERENCES

Centre for Medical Education (1992) *Moving to Audit, What Every Pharmacist Needs to Know About Professional Audit*, University of Dundee, Dundee.

Printed and bound by CPI Group (UK) Ltd, Croydon, CR0 4YY

Department of Health (1989) *Working for Patients*, CM555, HMSO, London.

Department of Health (1991) *The Health of the Nation*, CM1523, HMSO, London.

Department of Health (1997) *The New NHS – Modern, Dependable*, CM3807, HMSO, London.

Department of Health (1998) *A First Class Service: Quality in the New NHS*, CM13175, HMSO, London.

Department of Pharmacy Policy and Practice (1994). *Model Standards for Self Audit in Community Pharmacy in England*, Keele University, Keele.

Donabedian, A. (1966) Evaluating the quality of medical care. *Millbank Memorial Fund Quarterly*, **44**, 166–203.

Howe, J. (1999) Paper to the Hospital Pharmacists Group and Guild of Healthcare Pharmacists joint session on Clinical Governance at the British Pharmaceutical Conference, September 1999.

Pharmacy Practice Division, Common Services Agency, NHS (1994) *Pharmaceutical Audit. A Practical Workbook for Pharmacists*, NHS, Scotland.

Royal Pharmaceutical Society of Great Britain (1992) Audit in Pharmacy. Working Party Report. *Pharmaceutical Journal*, **248**, 505–509.

Royal Pharmaceutical Society of Great Britain (1997) *Improving Patient Care. A Team Approach*, Royal Pharmaceutical Society of Great Britain, London.

Royal Pharmaceutical Society of Great Britain (1999) *Achieving Excellence in Pharmacy Through Clinical Governance. A Discussion Paper*, Royal Pharmaceutical Society of Great Britain, London.

Smith, J. (1998) What clinical governance means. *Pharmacy in Practice*, **8**, 479–482.

SELF-ASSESSMENT QUESTIONS

Question 1: How do you think the definitions of medical audit apply to community pharmacy practice?

Question 2: What are the different types of professional audit?

Question 3: How do audit and quality assurance dovetail together?

Question 4: What are the key questions to ask when designing a pharmacy audit?

Question 5: Consider the pharmacy in which you are now working, or one in which you have previously worked, perhaps in a vacation. Draw up an audit question, using a key question from Question 4.

KEY POINTS FOR ANSWERS

Question 1: Consideration of *'structure, process and outcome'* is a useful starting point. If it is inferred that an aspect of good pharmaceutical practice, e.g. always counselling patients receiving repeat medication for chronic diseases, is beneficial to patient outcomes, the definitions can be applied.

Question 2: The Royal Pharmaceutical Society of Great Britain identified three types of professional audit:

- Self
- Peer
- External

Question 3: Professional audit is one component of a quality assurance system, and complements the other components, which include standard setting, quality procedures and outside external evaluation (which could be inspection).

Question 4: The key questions are:

- What?
- Why?
- How?
- When?

Question 5: A clear uncomplicated audit question is crucial. As a first step choose a topic which has a known national standard, or has an easily measured outcome.

Index

Abstracted empiricism   489
Acheson Report   127–128, 132, 134–135
Achieving Excellence in Pharmacy Through
    Clinical Governance   545
Acquired Immune Deficiency Syndrome (AIDS)
    349, 369
Adherence   165–179, 231, 280, see also
    Compliance, Concordance, Nonadherence
  barriers, see nonadherence
  cost-benefit analysis   176
  drug misuse   360
  mental health   335–336
  perceptions and practicalities approach to
      adherence   178–180
  psychology of   173–177
Adulteration   280
Adverse drug reactions   258, 262, 368–374,
      see also Pharmacovigilance, Side-effects
  classification   373–374
  establishing causality   371–373
  historical examples   368
  reporting systems   370–373
    reasons for under reporting   370–373
    when to report   371
  Type A   373
  Type B   373
  Type C   374
Advertising   74, 145–147, 156
  direct to consumer   74, 145–146
Advice, see also Communication, Drug
    information, Information
  culturally sensitive   275–276
  pharmacist as source   92, 197–198, 204, 220–221,
      238–239, 253, 258, 295–296, 320, 323–324, 359
AIDS   349, 369
Alcohol   355, 357–358
  hepatotoxicity   358
Ali ibn Sina   5
Allopathic medicine   278–279, see also Medicines
Alma-Ata   84
Alternative medicines   64, 67, 107
American Pharmaceutical Association   8
Amphetamine   346, 354, 356–358
Analysis of variance   501–504
Anatomical, Therapeutic, Chemical Classification
    System (ATC)   379–380
Anti-retrovirals   351
ANOVA   501–504
Apoteket   64
Apothecaries   7, 250
Apothecaries Act   8, 24, 250

Apothicaire   7
Asian medicine   278–280
Ask Your Pharmacist campaign   21, 23, 245
Assertiveness   240–241
Assistant pharmacist   63, 66
ATC classification system   379–380
Audio recording   480
Audit   215, 537–546
  audit cycles   541–542
  definitions   538–540
  external   543
  medical   538
  misconceptions   542–543
  peer   543
  professional audit   215, 539–540
  self   543
Audit Development Fellow   538–539
Audit facilitator   539–540
Autonomy   141, 143, 145, 192, 196, 211, 253
Avicenna   5–6
Ayurvedic system of health   277–279

Bamako Initiative   86–87
Beauchamp and Childress   211–212
Before and after studies   517, 526
Behaviour change   157–159
Beneficence   142, 211
Bentham, J.   210
Benzodiazepines   355, 358
Bias   385–387
Birth defects, see teratogenicity
Black Report   125–126, 128
Blood borne viruses (BBV), see also Hepatitis, HIV
    346, 348–349, 358–360
Boot, J.   12, 15–16
Boundary encroachment   197–198, 251
Bradford Hill   371–373
Breastfeeding   304, 306–310
  drug use in   304, 306–310
  pharmacists' role in   308–310
  fasting   282
Budget, drugs/health care   63, 69, 72–73, 142,
    259, 295

Cannabis   356–357
Canon Medicinae   5
Care Programme Approach   332
Carers   315–324, 337–338
  formal carers   317
Caring for People: Community Care in the Next
    Decade and Beyond   332

Case-control study 381–382, 384–385
Causality 435
Chadwick, E. 436
Changing Minds: Every Family in the Land 335
Chemists and Druggists 8, 10, 250
Chemists' Defence Association 16
Chi squared test 501–502
Chinese traditional medicine 93, 278
Children 289–297
    normality 291–291
    recognising illness 290–292, 295
    responding to symptoms 292–295
    self-medication 294–295
Civil liability 206, 208–209
Classification systems
    adverse drug reactions 373–374
    drug use in pregnancy 306–307
    drug use in breastfeeding 307–308
    social class 126
Client groups, see also Patient
    breastfeeding 282, 304, 306, 309–310
        drug use in 304, 306
    carers 315–324
    children 289–297
    disabled 243–244
    drug misusers 256, 345–360
    elderly 313–324
    ethnic minorities 244, 273–284
    mental health problems 337–340
    parents 289–297
    pregnancy 282, 301–310
Clinical governance 537–546
    definition 544
Clinical pharmacy 26, 62, 259, see also Hospital
        pharmacy
    services 67, 527–529
CNS depressants 355
Cocaine 354, 356, 358
Code of ethics 212–213
Cohort Study 381, 383–385
College de Pharmacie 8
College of Mental Health Pharmacists 340
Commercialism 20
Commission for Health Improvement (CHI)
        544–545
Commission for Racial Equality
    Code of Practice in Primary Healthcare
        Services 275
Committee on Safety of Medicines 369
Commodification of medicines 195, 199
Communication 227–245
    advising, see Advice
    assertiveness 240–241
    closing 240
    dialects 275

disability 243–244
    discussing 241–242
    elderly 315
    ethnic minorities 244, 275–276
    explaining 233, 235
    information transfer between pharmacists
        53–54
    inter-professional 254–256
    listening 233, 237
    literacy 275–276
    nonverbal 233, 238
    opening 233, 239
    questioning 233, 235–237
    persuading 242–243
    rapport 233–235
    reassurance 234
    skills 232–244
Community drug agencies, see Injecting drug
        misusers
Community Mental Health Team 337
Community pharmacist, see also Community
        pharmacy, Pharmacist, Pharmacy, Primary
        care pharmacy
    source of income 13
Community pharmacy 32, 52–53, 254,
        see also Pharmacist, Pharmacy, Primary care
        pharmacy, Workforce
    audit 537–546
    evaluation of 509–521
    history 4–22
    in Europe 61–70
    products from 66–67
    services from 67–69
Compliance 165–167, 284, see also Adherence,
        Concordance, Nonadherence
Concordance 165–167, 177–178, 231, 258,
        see also Adherence, Compliance,
        Nonadherence
    initiative 177–178
Confidence intervals 500
Confounding 385–387
Consultations
    medical 171–172
Content analysis 487
Continuous professional development 545, see
        also Lifelong learning
Co-payments 63, 76–77, 86, 133, 169
Corporate governance 543
Cost-benefit analysis 176, 401–402
Cost dumping 51
Cost-effectiveness analysis 402–403
    cost-effectiveness ratio 402
Cost of illness studies 395–396
Cost-utility analysis 403
Counselling, see Advice

Counter prescribing, *see* Over the counter medicines, Self-medication
Counterfeit medicines 95
Crack cocaine 357
Crack lung 357
Criminal liability 206
Cronbach's Alpha 424
Crown Review 62, 140, 257, 260
Cultural Context of Children's Illness Study 290–297
Culture 274
Curriculum, *see* Education

Data, *see also* Reliability, Replicability, Generalisability, Validity
  analysis 467–468, 480, 485–490
  confidentiality 481
  fabrication 441
  generation 440, 463–466
  presentation 441
  processing 441
  recording 466–467
  secondary sources 441–442
Death, premature 355–356
Decision-making 216, *see also* Ethics
Defeat Depression campaign 355
Defined Daily Dose (DDD) 380–381
Dentists 12
Deontological theory 210
Deregulation, *see* Drug deregulation
Descriptive studies 381, 517
De-skilling 197
Deutsche Pharmazeutische Gesellschaft 8
Deutscher Apothekerverein 8
Developing countries 81–97
  pharmacy in 85–87
Diagnostic testing 68, 197–198
Diamorphine, *see* Heroin
Dickson Case 20–21
Diethylstilboestrol 303, 368, 382
Disability
  communication and 243–245
Discharge planning 54
Discorides 5
Disease
  definition 413
  incidence 378–379
  measuring frequency 378–379
  prevalence 378–379
  prevention 110–111
Dispensing 13, 20, 62, 66, 196–197, 204, 208–209, 215, 217–220, 252, 257–258, 540
  extemporaneous 18, 20, 196, 257–258
  doctor dispensing 15, 64, 252
  errors 219–220

pharmacists' monopoly 193–194, 252
Doctor, *see* General practitioner, Inter-professional relationships
Domiciliary visits 314, 316, 321
Donabedian, A. 514–515, 540
Drug, *see also* Medicines, Pharmaceuticals
  abuse, *see* Drug misuse
  addiction, *see* Drug misuse
  adulteration 280
  ATC classification system 379–380
  costs 259, 261, *see also* Budget, Prescribing
  definition 5
  deregulation 140–145, 195, 199, 261–263, 395
    reasons for 144
  discount rate 399–400
    example 400
  distribution system 77–78
  donations 90
  essential, *see* Essential drugs
  information, *see* Drug information
  injectors, *see* Injecting drug misusers
  interactions 258, 279–280, 315
    with traditional remedies 279–280
  misuse, *see* Drug misuse
  orphan 94–95
  over the counter, *see* Over the counter medicines
  policy 88–89, 97, *see also* Health policy
  safety 305
  surveillance, *see* Surveillance
  symbolic transformation to medicines 198–199
  teratogenicity 302–310
  use, *see* Drug use
  utilisation studies 381–382
Drug information 214, *see also* Advice, Information
  to health professionals 69, *see also* Inter-professional relationships
  to public 68–69, 195, 338
Drug misuse, *see also* Alcohol, Amphetamine, Benzodiazepines, Cannabis, Cocaine, Crack Cocaine, Ecstasy, Heroin, Injecting drug misusers, Methadone, Morphine, Naloxone, Opiates, Stimulants
  community pharmacists' role 359–360
  injecting drug misusers, *see* Injecting drug misusers
  morbidity 356–357
  multi-professional communication 256, 346–347
  Routes of administration 349–353
    injecting 349–353
    non-injecting 353
    related health needs 349

Drug Tariff   541
Drug use   374–379
  determinants   375
  information sources   375–377
  irrational   87– 88, 90–92
  measuring   379–387
  outcomes   375
  rational   92
  records   375
Drug Utilisation Review   77
Dual treatment   279
Duncan, W.H.   436

Economic aspects of prevention   403–404
Economics, health   393–406, 513, 533
  characteristics of health care   396–398
    asymmetric information   396–397
    external effects   397–398
    risk and uncertainty   398
  concepts   394
  cost-benefit analysis   401–402
  cost-effectiveness analysis   402–403
  cost-utility analysis   403
  costs, see also Budget, Drug, Prescribing costs
    direct   402
    indirect   403
    intangible   403
    marginal   398–399
    opportunity   398–399, 401
  discount rate   399–400
  efficiency   400–401
  evaluation   398–404
  methods   401–403
  productivity   400–401
  supply and demand   396
  theory   396–398
Ecstasy   358
Education   10–11, 38, 62–63, 66, 95–96
  developing countries   95–96
  European   62–63
  schools of pharmacy   10–11, 38, 95–96
  USA   78
Elderly   313–325
  access to pharmaceutical care   317–318
  carers of   315–324
  drug use in   314–325
  living conditions   315–316
  pharmaceutical services   318–325
  reasons for using pharmacies   317
ENCORE   220–221
Epidemiology, see Pharmacoepidemiology
Essential drugs in developing countries   86–90
  Action Programme on Essential Drugs   89
Essential Drugs List   88–89
Ethics   209–214, 439–441

code of   212–213
  in economic evaluation   401, 404–406
  ethical principles   210–213
  ethical decision-making   213–214, see also
    Decision-making
  ethical dilemmas   213–214, 219
  in research   439–441, 464–465
Ethnic minorities
  adherence   274, 279, 281
  communication   244, 275–276
  morbidity and mortality   274–275
  pharmaceutical services for   273–284
  pharmacists   38–40
Ethnicity   274
Ethnomethodology   487
European Agency for the Evaluation of
    Medical products (EMEA)   62, 305
European Data Protection Act   378
European Union
  medicines regulation   142
Evaluation   509–521, 524–534
  acceptability   514
  accessibility   515
  against standards   424–425
  appropriateness   513–514
  before and after studies   517, 526
  of community pharmacy   509–521
  definition   510
  descriptive studies   517
  development   525
  economic   398–404
  effectiveness   512, 525
  efficacy   511–512, 525–526
  efficiency   512–513
  frameworks   511–516
  future developments   533–534
  generalisability   532–533
  of health services   512
  of hospital pharmacy   524–534
    clinical services   527–529
    drug information services   529
    formulary   527–528
    medication administration error rates
      530–531
    production   527, 531–532
    purchasing and distribution   527, 529–531
    quality control   531–532
    stock turnover index   530
  instruments, see Interviews, Observation,
      Questionnaires, Surveys
  mathematical modelling   528–529, 532
  needs analysis   525–526
  options appraisal   525
  protocols   520
  quasi-experimental design   517

randomised controled trials 516–517, 526
response rates 518–519
sampling 518
structure-process-outcome 515–516, 540
study design 516–520
technology 532
Evidence-based medicine 405
Expert 106, 116–117, 152, 195, 199
Explaining 235
Extemporaneous preparation 18, 20, 62, 196, 258–259
Extended role 22–23, 251, 253–255, 321–324, *see also* individual activities
External effects 397–398

F test 503
Fasting, *see* Ramadan
FIP 9, 67
Floating Sixpence 14
Focus groups 460, 474–481, *see also* Interviews, Qualitative research methods
advantages and disadvantages 460
audio recording 481
co-facilitator 479–480
data analysis 480
ethics 480–481
facilitator 479–480
group number 478
group size 478
group type 476–477
sampling 476–478
venue 479
Folic acid 276–278, 305, 308–309, 359
Follow-up study 383
Food and Drugs Administration (FDA) 74, 305, 369
Formularies 76–77, 259, 262, 527–528
Fraud 441
Friedson, E. 191

Galen 5–6
Gantt chart 444–445
General Household Survey 417
Generalisability 511, 532–533
General practitioner 251–264, 293, *see also* Inter-professional relationships, Prescribing
budget-holding 15, 259
medical information for 69
Good Pharmacy Practice 67, 96
Grocers 7
Gross National Product 395–396
Guild of Public Pharmacists 25

Hakim 277–279
Harm minimisation 347–348

Harm reduction 347–348
Health
definition 109–110, 413
determinants of 83–85
dimensions of 228
indicators 413–414
maintenance 110–111
Health Action Zone (HAZ) 133
Health advice, *see* Advice
Health and illness
measurement 411–427
type of measure 414–419
models 435–436
bio-medical model 435
social model 436
social context 105–119
Health Authorities 133–134
Health care
inequalities 123–136
interface
social context 395–396
systems 63–64, 395
European 63–64
North America 72–79
traditional 276–284
Health centres 256
Health diary 293–294
Health economics, see economics
Health education, see Health promotion
Health Improvement Programme (HimP) 133
Health inequalities 123–136
evidence 126–130
explanations 130–132
history 125
policy response 132–135
Health insurance, see Insurance
Health maintenance 110, 111
Health Maintenance Organisations (HMO) 72, 75
Health measures 414–419, *see also* health status measurement
Health of the Nation 125, 332, 538
Health outcomes
importance of adherence 168
measurement 527, 529
Health policy 50, 134
Health promotion 110, 151–162, *see also* Advice, Drug information, Patient Information Leaflets
drug misuse 347–348, 357–360
goal 152
lifestyle 154–155
models 153–154
myths 154–156

pharmacists' involvement   152–155, 159–162
self-help groups   116
smoking cessation   161
strategies   153
victim blaming   154
Health psychology   173–177
Health-related quality of life   418–419, 421
Health services research   251, 486, 488, 510
Health status measurement   414, 427
   instruments   419–427
      evaluation of   423–427
      interviews   421
      questionnaires   421
      scoring   422–423
   morbidity data   414–416
   mortality data   414–415
   service-use data   414–416
   subjective measures   416–418
Health variation   125, see also Health inequalities
Helicobacter pylori   256, 434
Hepatitis   346, 349, 351–352, see also Blood borne
      viruses
   avoidance   351–352
   harm reduction   352–352
   treatment   353
Heroin   346, 348, 356, 358
Hippocrates   397, 404
HIV   346, 349, 351, 369, see also Blood borne
      viruses
Homelessness   359
Hospital Officers Association   25
Hospital pharmacy   51–52, 254, 319–320,
      524–534, see also Clinical Pharmacy,
      Secondary health care pharmacy, Ward
      Pharmacy
   clinical services   527–529
   evaluation   524–534
   future developments   533–534
   history   23–26
   production   527, 531–532
   purchasing and distribution   527, 529–531
   quality control   531–532
Hot/cold theory   278–279
Human Immuno-deficiency Virus HIV   346,
      349, 351, 369, see also Blood borne viruses
Humours   278–279
Hypothesis testing   494, 496–505, see also
      Statistics

I/T ratio   190–191
Iatrogenic disease   314
Iftar   280–281
Illness
   experience   113–116
   perceptions   174–176

prevention, economic aspects   403–404
   social concept 113–116
Illness behaviour   113–116, 292–295
Improving Patient Care. A Team Approach
      539, 541, 546
Inequalities in health, see Health inequalities
Informal carers, see Carers
Information, see also Advice, Communication,
      Drug information
   asymmetric   146, 396–397
   leaflets   68, 160, 220, 275–276, 302
   oral   315
   recall   315
   transfer between pharmacists   53–54
   written   315
Information Communications Technology   106
Information technology   106, 263
Injecting drug misusers   345–360
   agencies involved in care   347–348, 358
   asthma   357
   compliance   360
   dental health   357
   diabetes   357
   drug interactions   355
   drug-related health needs   354
   epilepsy   357
   harm minimisation   347–348
   harm reduction   347–348, 352–353
   health care   347
   health promotion   347–348, 357–360
   hepatic failure   358
   homelessness   357
   information leaflets   360
   lifestyle   355, 357–358
      related health needs   357–358
   multi-professional working   346–347
   nutrition   357
   overdose   356
   poly-drug use   355
   pregnancy   358–359
   premature death   355–356
   safe sex   349, 351–352, 360
   skin/vein problems   349–350
   stigma   349
   viral infections, see Blood borne viruses,
      Hepatitis, HIV
Injecting equipment   346, 348–349, 351–352, 359,
      see also Syringes
   exchange schemes   348, 359–360
   return to pharmacies   359
   sharing   349, 352
Inspection   543
Insurance, health   72, 74, 85–87, 398
International Conference on Primary Health Care
      84

International Congress of Pharmacy 8
International Pharmaceutical Federation (FIP)
    9, 67
Internet 107–108
Inter-professional relationships 54–55, 69,
    249–263, 346–347
Interviews 421, 457–469
    advantages 460
    bias 421
    colleagues 466
    data analysis 467–468
    disadvantages 460
    ethical issues 464–465
    face to face 445, 451, 459
    groups, see Focus groups
    preparation 461–462
        reflexive bracketing 461–462
    questions 463–466, 480
    recording data 466–467
    recruitment 463
    sampling 445–447, 451–452, 458–459
        combination 459
        deviant case 459
        intensity 459
        maximum variety 459
        snowball 459
        theoretical 459
        typical case 459
    structured 451–452
    telephone 445, 452–453
        response rate 453
    topic guide 462–463, 480
    transcripts 467, 481, 487
Irrational drug use, see Drug use
Inverse Care Law 134

Jenkin Case 15–16
Job satisfaction 42–43
Judgement, see Professional judgement
Justice 211

Kant, E. 210
Knowledge
    indeterminate 190–191
    lay health 108–112
    technical 191

Lactation, see Breastfeeding
Lay carers, see carers
Lay epidemiology 110
Lay health knowledge 108–112
Lay response to illness 289–297
Lay views of medicines 111–113
Learning, see Education
Least developed countries (LDCs) 82, 84

Life expectancy 106, 414
Lifelong learning 214, 217
Linstead Report 24
Listening 233, 237, see also Communication
Local Health Care Co-operative (LHCC)
    260

Mainliners 351, 361
Managed Care 72–75
Managed Care Organisation (MCO) 72–73,
    77
Managed Care Pharmacy 76–77
Mann Whitney Test 502
Manpower, see Workforce
Materia Medica 5
Mathematical modelling 528–529
McMaster Health Index Questionnaire 423
Measuring health, see Health status measurement
Medicaid 72, 75
Medical audit, see Audit
Medicare 72
Medication errors 315
Medication knowledge
    effect on adherence 171
Medication surveillance 67, see also Surveillance
Medicines, see also Drug, Pharmaceuticals,
        Prescribing, Prescriptions
    alternative 64, 67, 107
    Asian 278–280
    charm of 294
    Chinese (traditional) 93, 278
    commodification of 195, 199
    controlling use of 194
    costs, see Budget, Drug, Prescribing costs
    deregulation, see Drug
    dispensing, see Dispensing
    dosage forms 18
    General Sales List 261
    management, see Medicines management
    non-prescription, see Over the counter
        medicines
    over the counter (OTC), see Over the counter
        medicines
    Pharmacy, see Over the counter medicines
    poly-pharmacy, see Poly-pharmacy
    prepackaged 196
    preparation 17, 18
    prescribed 17
    Prescription Only 218, 261
    proprietary, see Over the counter medicines
    safety 279, 302–310
    sale 140, see also Over the counter medicines
    standby 295
    symbolic transformation from drugs
        198–199

teratogenicity 302–310
toxicity 279, 302–310
traditional 93, 277–280
veterinary 64
wastage 258, 332
Western 88, 93, 278
Medicines Control Agency MCA 305, 531
Medicines management 52, 257, 318–319,
 see also Pharmaceutical care
Mental health 329–340
 adherence 335–336
 anxiety disorders 330
 depression 330–332
 eating disorders 330–331
 meeting needs 336–340
 mortality rates 330–331
 pharmacists' role 336–340
 psychotic problems 330–331
 services 330–340
  community care 331–332
  policy guidance on 331–333
 social isolation 334
 stigma 334–335
 suicide 331
 treatment 331
Mercantilism 195
Meta-analysis 499
Methadone 256, 346, 348, 358–360
Mill, J.S. 210
Minor ailments 220–221, see also Over the
 counter medicines, Responding to
 symptoms
Model Standards for Self Audit in Community
 Pharmacy in England 539
Monopoly of practice 65, 140, 193–194, 252
Morality 209
Morbidity
 data 415
 developing countries 82–85
 ethnic minorities 274–275
 mental health 330
 rates 415–416
Morphine 358
Mortality
 data 415–416
 developing countries 82–85
 ethnic minorities 274–275
 mental health 330–331
 infant 83
 rates 415
 regional variations 127
 social class 126–128
 standardised 126–128, 415
Mothers, use of pharmacists 289–297
Moving to Audit 539–540

Multiple pharmacies 11–12, 33, 35, 196, 453
Munchies 358
Muslim, see Ramadan
Myalgic encephalomyelitis (ME) 436

Naloxone 356
National Health Insurance Act 14–15
National Health Service 18–21, 50, 63, 133, 135,
 228, 252, 295, 514, 525, 531, 538
 Act 252
 drugs bill 142, 295
National Health Service Community Care Act
 332
National Institute for Clinical Excellence (NICE)
 544–545
National Insurance Scheme 13–14, 18
National Pharmaceutical Association (NPA) 15,
 21
National Pharmaceutical Union 15
National Service Framework 544
 Mental Health 333
Necessity beliefs 175–177
Needle exchange, see Injecting equipment,
 Syringes
Needles, see Injecting equipment
Needs analysis 525–526
Negligence 206–209, 215
 standard of care 207–208
 Tort of Negligence 207
Neural Tube Defects, see Folic acid
New NHS: Modern, Dependable 543
Nicotine replacement therapy 161
Noel Hall Report 26
Nonadherence 165–179, 231, see also Adherence,
 Compliance, Concordance
 causes 168–176, 231
 consequences 167–168
 mental health 335–336
Non-maleficence 142, 211
Non-prescription medicines, see Over the counter
 medicines
Normal distribution 498, 502
Nuffield
 Committee of Inquiry into Pharmacy 21,
  261
 Foundation 21
 Report 21–22, 250
Nuovo Receptario 6
Nurse practitioner 260
Nurse prescribing 257
Nursing homes 318–319

Observation 460
 advantages 460
 disadvantages 460

Odds Ratio 384–386
Opiates 346, 348, 354, 355, 357–359
    health problems associated with use 354
    overdose 356
Opportunity costs 397–398
Oral contraceptives 385
Original-pack dispensing 196, 258
Orphan drugs 94–95
Osteoporosis 274
OTC, see Over the counter medicines
Over the counter medicines 12, 19, 64–65, 74,
        90–92, 139–147, 220–221, 252, 257, 261–263,
        294–296, 303, 315
    availability in developing countries 90–92
    availability in Europe 64–65
    availability in USA 74
    interactions with prescribed medicines 315
    sales in Europe 143
Overdose 356
    signs of opiate overdose 356

Palermo, Edict of 5
Papyrus Ebers 4
Paradigm 434
Parents, use of pharmacists 289–297
Parsons, T. 113–114
Pathways to Care Study 295–296
Patient, see also Client groups
    beliefs 173–177
    care 52
        pharmacists' role in 50–55, see also
            Pharmaceutical care
    confidentiality 377–378
    satisfaction 171–172, 230–231, 235
Patient information leaflets 68, 160, 220,
        275–276, 302
Patient medication records 52–53
Patient-pack dispensing 196, 258
Patient-practitioner interactions 108, 117–118,
        171–172, 230
Patients' Charter 228, 245
Pen, T'Sao 4
Pepperer 4
Persuading 242–243
Pharmaceutical anthropology 92
Pharmaceutical audit, see Audit
Pharmaceutical Care 52, 67–69, 161, 197–198,
        209, 250–251, 290, 399
    access to 317–318
    barriers to implementation 68
    breastfeeding 306, 309–310
    carers 315–324
    children 289–297
    disability 243–244
    drug misusers 273–284

    elderly 313–324
    ethnic minorities 273–284
    mental health 337–340
        key roles for pharmacists 338
    parents 289–297
    pregnancy 310–310
Pharmaceutical Care: The Future of Community
        Pharmacy 250–251
Pharmaceutical Chemist 10
Pharmaceutical industry 94–95, 143, 167, 261
Pharmaceutical outcomes
    causes of sub-optimal outcome 314–324
Pharmaceuticals, see also Drug, Medicines
    economic evaluation of 398–404
Pharmaceutical Society, see Royal Pharmaceutical
        Society of Great Britain
Pharmaceutical Whitley Council 25
Pharmacien 7, 8
Pharmacist, see also Community Pharmacist,
        Inter-professional relationships, Pharmacy
    alternative to doctors 295–296
    disappearing 19
    extended role, see Extended role
    as first port of call 197, 290, 295
    income 87
    prescribing 62, 260–264
Pharmacoeconomics, see Economics
Pharmacoepidemiology 367–388
    definition 374
    concept 375
    databases 376–377
        strengths 377
        weaknesses 377
    ethics 377
    study design 381–387
        bias 385–387
        case-control studies 381–382, 384–385
        cohort studies 381, 383–385
        confounding 386–387
        descriptive studies 381
        experimental studies 381, 383
Pharmacovigilance 367–388
    aims 369
    information sources 369
    reporting systems 370–373
Pharmacy, see also Community pharmacy,
        Hospital pharmacy, Pharmacist
    Acts 10–12
    care plans 54
    clinical 26, 62, 67, 259
    clinics 323
    community, see Community pharmacy
    degree, see Education
    developing countries 81–97
    education, see Education

ethics   213–214
European   61–70
health centre   256
history   3–30
hospital, *see* Hospital pharmacy
mail services   77–78
monopoly of practice   140, 193–194, 252
North America   71–79
ownership   196
poly-pharmacy   90, 258
primary care   50–55, 254, 260, 296
profession   37, 187–199
  status   192–199
reasons for using   317
regulation, *see* Regulation
remuneration   87, 188
size   65–66
telephone help lines   324
undergraduate curriculum, *see* Education
ward   26, 319–320, 527
workforce, *see* Workforce
Pharmacy and Poisons Act   10, 60
Pharmacy Benefit Management   77
Pharmacy in a New Age (PIANA)   22–23
Pharmacy practice research   251, 436, *see also*
  individual research methods
goals for development   437
Phocomelia   303, 308
Piloting   448–449
Placebo effect   516–517
Poly-drug misuse   355
Poly-pharmacy   90, 258
Poor Law   24
Poor Law Dispensers Association   24
Positivism   434–435
Post-marketing surveillance   370
Pre-eclampsia   305
Pregnancy   276, 278, 301–310
drug use in   278, 280, 302–310, 358, 382
  before pregnancy   304
  drug classification   306–307
  first trimester   304
  late pregnancy   304
  oral contraceptives   309
drug misuse   358
fasting   282
patient information leaflets   302
pharmacists' role in   308–310
Prescribing, *see also* Prescription
budgets   50–51, 259, *see also* Budget, Drug
costs   72, 130, 261, *see also* Budget, Drug
counter, *see* Over the counter medicines
nurses   62
pharmacists' influence on doctors' prescribing
  257–260, 528–529

pharmacists' prescribing   62, 260–264
pregnancy   305–306
primary care   50–51
repeat   321–323
secondary care   50–51
variations   130
Prescription book   17–18
Prescription Pricing Authority   541
Prescriptions, *see also* Prescribing
dispensed   14
earliest   4
errors   215, 218–220
numbers   19–20, 65
private   18
Primary Care Groups   55, 133–134, 260
Primary care pharmacy   50–55, 254, 260, 296,
  see also Community pharmacist, Community
  pharmacy
Primary health care   86, 254, 295
Probability   496–505
Production and quality control, evaluation of
  531–532
Profession   187–199, 253
altruism   195
attributes of   189–190
core features   188–190, 253
definition   188
deprofessionalisation   196
de-skilling   197
monopoly of practice   188, 190
pharmacy, *see* Pharmacy
professionalisation   191, 193, 198
  incomplete   193
  mystification   192, 196
professionalism   20, 215
self-regulation   188, 190, 192
service-orientation   188–191
sociology of   188–199
  functionalist analysis   190–191
status   188, 191–199
technology, implications   196
Trait theory   189–190
  application to pharmacy   193
Professional audit, *see* Audit
Professional judgement   190–191, 195, 205,
  208–209, 213, 216–217
Professional-patient, *see* Patient-practitioner
  interactions
Professional practice   216
Professional Project   188, 192–193, 199
Public Pharmacists and Dispensers Association
  24
Public Pharmacists Association   25
Purchasing and distribution, evaluation   527,
  529–531

Qualitative research methods   436, 443–444, 486,
    see also Focus Groups, Interviews, Research
    methods
  cookbook approach   487–488
  data analysis   485–490
  reliability   468
  sampling strategies   459
    deviant case   459
    intensity   459
    maximum variety   459
    purposive   459
    snowball   459
    theoretical combination   459
    typical case   459
  validity   468, *see also* Validity
Quality Adjusted Life Years (QALYs)   403,
    418
Quality of life   412, 418–419, 421
  enhancing strategies   412
Quantitative research methods   436, 458–469, *see
    also* Questionnaires, Research methods,
    Surveys
  sampling strategies   458–459
Quasi-experimental design   517
Questioning, *see* Communication, Interviews,
    Questionnaires
Questionnaires   421, 443–444, *see also*
    Quantitative research methods, Research
    methods, Surveys
  administration   421, 449–454
  bias   453
  coding   449, 451
  content   440
  covering letter   449
  design   447–448
    of questions   448–449
  length   421
  piloting   448–449
  postal   445
    advantages   450
    disadvantages   450
  processing replies   450–451
  response rate   449, 451, 453–454, 518–519
  self-completion   443
  telephone   445
Qur'an   280

Ramadan   280–294
  compliance   281, 283–284
    pharmacists' role in   284
  fasting   280–284
    breastfeeding and   282
    effect on asthma   281–282
    effect on diabetes   282
    effect on epilepsy   283

effect on gastrointestinal disorders
    281
  exemptions from   280
  pregnancy   282
  information resources   284
Randomised controlled trial (RCT)   160–161, 305,
    383, 387, 435–436, 511–512, 516–517, 526
  characteristics   516
Rapport   234–235, *see also* Communication
Rational drug use, *see* Drug Use
Records, *see* Patient medication records
Receptar   63
Referencing   442
Register of Pharmaceutical Chemists   10–11
Regression   504–505
  multiple   504
Regulation   204–205, *see also* Drug
  ethical   205, 209–214
  legal   205–209
  professional   205, 214–221
Reliability   424, 439, 468, 519–520
Repeat prescribing
  pharmacists' role in   321–323
Replicability   439
Research
  methods, *see* Research methods
  problem-oriented   486–490
  theory-oriented   486–490
  steps in   442
Research methods
  available range   436
  instruments, *see* Evaluation, Focus groups,
      Health status measurement, Interviews,
      Qualitative research methods,
      Quantitative research methods, Surveys
  paradigms   437–438
  triangulation   437, 520
Residential homes, services to   318–219,
    324–325
Responding to symptoms   292–295, 539, *see also*
    Advice
Response rate   449, 451, 453–454, 518–519
Retail Pharmacists Union   15–16
Rhazes   6
Rigour   438
Risk estimates   384–385
  Odds Ratio   384–385
  relative risk   384
Risk management   215–216
Robotic systems   530, 532
Role ambiguity   195
Role strain   195
Royal Pharmaceutical Society of Great
    Britain   7, 9–13, 15, 25, 32, 54, 177, 250, 262,
    545–546

Audit Development Fellow   538–539
Clinical Audit Group   545
coat of arms   6
Council   15, 16, 20, 538
history   9–13
membership   16
Statutory Committee   16

Safe sex   349, 351–352, 360
Sale of medicines   140, *see also* Over the counter
    medicines, Self-medication
    ethical aspects   141–142
    legal aspects   140
Sample size   518, *see also* Sampling
Sampling   445–447, 451–452, 458–459, 518
    business considerations   447
    cluster   446
    combination   459
    convenience   446
    deviant case   459
    focus groups   476–478
    frame   446, 477, 518
    illustrative   446
    intensity   459
    intervals   446
    key concepts   446
    maximum variety   459
    network   446
    purposive   446, 459, 477
    quota   446, 477
    random   446, 518
    snowball   446, 459
    stratified   446
    systematic   446
    theoretical   459
    typical case   459
    units   446
Saving Lives: Our Healthier Nation   128
Schedule for Evaluation of Individual Quality of
    Life (SEIQoL)   420, 423
Schools of pharmacy, *see* Education
Screening   106
Seamless care   51–54
    definition   51
Secondary health care pharmacy   50–55, *see also*
    Hospital pharmacy
Self-help groups   116
Self-medication   90, 92, 97, 145, 294–295, *see also*
    Over the counter medicines
Service-use data   416
Shared care   51
Sick role   113–116
    access to   114
    lay legitimisation of   115–116
Sickness, definition of   413

Side-effects   111, 335, *see also* Adverse drug
    reactions
Smoking cessation   157–158, 161
Social action   487
Social capital   132
Social class   126–127
    classification   126
    health status   126–128
    mortality rates   126–127
    underclass   154
Social closure   193–194
Social distance   192
Social exclusion   154
Social Exclusion Unit   125
Social isolation   333, 340
Social pharmacy   62
Social roles   109
Social surveys, *see* Questionnaires, Surveys
Social theory   487, 489
Spicers   7, 250
Staffing, *see* Workforce
Stages of Change Model of Behaviour Change
    157–159
Standard deviation   498–500
Standard of care   207–208
Statistics   493–505
    analysis of variance   501–504
    chi square test   501–502
    confidence intervals   500
    F test   503
    hypothesis   494, 496–505
    levels of measurement   494–495
    probability   496–505
    regression   504–505
    significance   499–500
    Student's t test   502–503
    t test   502–503
    testing   494–505
        errors   497–499
        hypothesis   494, 496–505
    z test   502
Statutory Committee, *see* Royal Pharmaceutical
    Society of Great Britain
Stigma   334–335, 340, 347, 349, 358
Stimulants   355
    health problems associated with   354, 357
Stock control   530
Structure-process-outcome   215, 515–516,
    540
Student's t test   502
Study design
    case-control   381–382, 384–385
    cohort   381, 383–385
    descriptive   381, 517
    evaluation, *see* Evaluation

follow-up   383
randomised controlled trial, *see* Randomised
    controlled trial
risk estimates   384–385
Subjective health measures   416–417
Substance misuse, *see* Drug misuse
Suhur   280–281
Suicide   356
Supermarket pharmacies, *see* Multiple
    pharmacies
Supply and demand
    economics   396
    workforce   35–43
Surveillance   106
    post-marketing   370
Surveys, *see also* Quantitative research methods
    appraising   438–441
        ethics   439–441
        reliability   439
        replicability   439
        rigour   438
        validity   438–439
        values   439
    design   447–448
    methods   433–454
        historical development in pharmacy   437
    planning   441–445
    sampling   445–447
Symbolic interactionism   487
Symptom iceberg   114
Symptoms   290–295, 539, *see also* Minor
    ailments, Advice
Syringes, exchange schemes   348, 359–360 *see
    also* Injecting equipment

t test   502–503
Tape recording   481
Teratogenicity   302–310
Terrence Higgins Trust   351, 361
Thalidomide   302–303, 308
Traditional Chinese medicine   93, 278
Training, *see* Education
Trait theory   189–190, 193
Transcripts   467, 481, 487
Trans Theoretical Model of Behaviour Change
    157–159
Triangulation   437, 520

Unani system of health   277–279
Underclass   154
UNICEF   86
Unit dose   530
United Kingdom Drug Information Pharmacists
    Group   525

United Kingdom Psychiatric Pharmacy Group
    (UKPPG)   337, 339–340
United Nations   82
United States of America
    health care systems   72–79
Utilitarian theory   210

Validity   425–426, 438–439, 468, 511, 519–520
    concurrent   426
    construct   425
    content   425
    convergent   425
    criterion   425–426
    discriminant   425
    external   438–439
    face   425
    internal   438
    predictive   426
Variance   498
    analysis of   501–504
Veterans Administration   72–73
Veterinary Medicines   64
Victim blaming   154

Ward pharmacy   26, 319–320, 527, *see also*
    Hospital pharmacy
Welfare State   9, *see also* National Health
    Service
Whitley Council   25
Wilcoxon test   502
Women in pharmacy   33–34, 36–37, 40–41
Workforce, pharmacy   31–43
    age   40
    demand factors   34, 35
    dissatisfaction   42–43
    ethnic minorities   38–40
    European   66
    part-time working   36–37, 40–42
    profile   32
    retirement   40
    supply factors   35–43
    surveys   32–33, 41
    USA   78
Working for Patients   538
World Health Organization   81–97, 109, 305,
    369, 379, 413, 510
Western medicine   93, 96, 111, *see also*
    Medicine
World Wide Web   107, 214
WWHAM   220

Yin-yang theory   278

z test   502